Neurosurgery in Transition

The Socioeconomic Transformation of Neurological Surgery

VOLUME 9: CONCEPTS IN NEUROSURGERY

Neurosurgery in Transition

The Socioeconomic Transformation of Neurological Surgery

VOLUME 9: CONCEPTS IN NEUROSURGERY

EDITOR

James R. Bean, M.D.

Neurosurgical Associates
Lexington, Kentucky

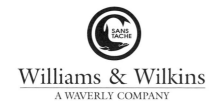

Williams & Wilkins
A WAVERLY COMPANY

BALTIMORE • PHILADELPHIA • LONDON • PARIS • BANGKOK
BUENOS AIRES • HONG KONG • MUNICH • SYDNEY • TOKYO • WROCLAW

Accurate indications, adverse reactions, and dosage schedules for drugs are provided in this book, but it is possible that they may change. The reader is urged to review the package information data of the manufacturers of the medication mentioned.

Printed in the United States of America
(ISBN 0-683-18345-1)

97 98 99
1 2 3 4 5 6 7 8 9 10

Foreword

While revolutions in molecular biology and neurological imaging have transformed the practice of neurosurgery in recent decades, perhaps nothing has changed the daily life of the neurosurgeon in the United States as much as the profound restructuring of the social and economic basis of medical practice. Apparently unlimited potential for scientific and technological advancement has come face-to-face with the recognition of a finite limit on resources and the process of change is taking its toll on hospitals, physicians, insurers, but most importantly on patients and their families. No matter how well trained and experienced, no neurosurgeon can ignore the societal upheaval in the delivery of medical care and expect to continue to serve his or her patients well. Dr. Bean and his colleagues have characterized the place of the neurosurgeon in society at the end of the 20th century, identifying crucial problems that face the profession in the new millennium. Theirs is a guidebook that can help the neurosurgeon direct the forces of change in a positive direction.

Stephen J. Haines, M.D
Charleston, SC

Paul B. Nelson, M.D.
Indianapolis, IN

Preface

"It was the best of times, it was the worst of times, . . ., it was the spring of hope, it was the winter of despair."

—*A Tale of Two Cities,* Charles Dickens

Scanning back over the past decade, one could see it coming. Beginning in the early 1980s, a gathering storm appeared on the horizon. In 1982, Paul Starr published the iconoclastic sociological study of medical practice, *The Social Transformation of American Medicine.* The book was a landmark in understanding the paradoxical entrenchment and vulnerability of American physicians in medical practice. Starr marveled at the historical delay in, and predicted the inevitable conquest by, corporate control of the business of medicine. Compared to other billion dollar, explosive growth industries, medical care was caught in a time warp, stalled in a primitive stage of business maturation and corporate development. The mirage could not last. The huge medical edifice swayed and wobbled on a flimsy, outdated economic foundation: the dispersed not-for-profit hospital system, the "cottage industry" of independent medical practices, and the unrestrained, cost-plus, insurance-financed fee-for-service payment system.

Even Medicare, paradoxically, helped both to feed and to support the customary fee-for-service model, and soon undercut its sustaining roots. Political accommodation in 1965 guaranteed the Medicare program design would mirror the commercial market. Rising Medicare program costs, however, soon spawned successive legislative changes that helped propel corporate takeover of medical business. Three key cost containment policies initiated in the Medicare program in the 1980s invited corporate management, ownership, and profit: hospital prospective payment ("DRGs") in 1983, revised federal HMO payment regulations in 1983, and the Medicare Fee Schedule (RBRVS) in 1989. DRGs converted and accustomed hospitals to risk-based reimbursement and fiscal efficiency; 1983 HMO regulations made Medicare HMOs wildly profitable in traditionally high payment areas (high average adjusted per capita cost, or AAPCC), driving up HMO enrollment; RBRVS began the widespread standardization of fees, shift of reimbursement toward cognitive services and primary care, and reduced market payment rates by adoption of the Medicare conversion factor as a goal in commercial payment.

In 1989, Alain Enthoven and Richard Kronick published back-to-back articles in the *New England Journal of Medicine,* touting the virtues of "managed competition," recommending a complex socioeconomic framework for reform of the health care system in America. Five years later, in 1994, the concept took political root in the proposed Clinton "Health Security Act." The "Act" was resoundingly defeated, and the Democrats later lost their Congressional majority, probably in large measure as a result of the gamble on national health care reform.

But reform didn't go away; it only shifted venue. The political proposal, couched in terms of a rationalized and politically regulated managed care framework, extended its roots as an semiregulated market-driven managed care system. After all, managed care was here to stay, and it was only threatened with political manipulation, not dismemberment.

Traditional medical care as practiced in the United States has been like a Garden of Eden, at least for physicians. Nature was altered to fit an artificial environment, structured according to the vision of the medical profession, and largely to its economic benefit. But the reality of economic consequences intruded, seeding the manicured field of professionally-directed medical care with the entwining and choking vines of marketplace discipline. Physicians have been expelled from the Garden, and must toil in a market-propelled health industry. The sun has set on the "Golden Age" of medicine.

Medicine in general and neurosurgery in particular have arrived at a crossroads. Not only are the financial advantages, social privileges, political influence, and professional stature of physicians threatened with eclipse, but, more profoundly, the self-image and self-understanding of the profession stand on the verge of a metamorphosis. Vying for its allegiance and possession of its soul are two fundamental, powerful, and conflicting forces: the competitive market and altruism. The image of an epic morality struggle is not an exaggeration.

These forces are not mutually exclusive. In fact, their successful compromise and accommodation holds the only promise of successful and satisfying outcome. Alone, business principles corrupt the profession, while undisciplined charitable altruism impoverishes or bankrupts the enterprise. The rising generation of physicians, and the public in general, watches the actions of the profession's members attentively to learn who they have become and who they wish to be. If guided by financial success and self interest, the harsh discipline, guarded distrust, and "every-man-for-himself" exposure of the unprotected market is its fate. If guided by ethical principles, service motive, compassion, and humility, then trust and respect with restrained financial dispensation is its lot. The trick is to preserve the best of the professional character while submitting to the requirements of market controls and incentives, and without surrendering to opportunistic greed, fatalistic despair, or cynical disillusionment.

THE ORIGIN OF THE VOLUME

Concepts in Neurosurgery is a topic-based volume series, published annually for 10 years by the Congress of Neurological Surgeons. Prior volumes have featured purely neuosurgical and scientific topics, such as hydrocephalus, subarachnoid hemorrhage, stereotactic surgery, etc. This volume represents a timely detour from that well-worn path.

Stephen Haines, M.D. and Paul Nelson, M.D., Editors, suggested a volume devoted to the socioeconomic changes occurring in medical and neurosurgical practice. At first envisioned as a general commentary on the conceptual, practical, and ethical alterations in neurosurgical care

and neurosurgeon roles, the idea evolved into a broad survey of the changing, or "transforming," landscape of neurosurgical care. Viewing health care as hovering in the midst of a phase transition, and borrowing from Paul Starr's concept of the transformation of medicine, the title, *Neurosurgery in Transition: the Socioeconomic Transformation of Neurosurgical Practice,* took form.

The purpose of the volume is to dissect the socioeconomic factors controlling or affecting neurosurgical practice into their principal constituent parts. The chapter selection illustrates and organizes current, important aspects of neurosurgical practice, whether academic or private, that can be analyzed as separate subtopics, or clearly outlined branches of the whole tree.

The authorship of this book is no accident. The authors have been selected based on their recognized experience with particular areas of interest. In surveying the field of neurosurgery for its socioeconomic prophets, these authors were chosen as leaders and original thinkers who have expressed their views by persuasive rhetoric or notable action. In contrast with earlier volumes of *Concepts in Neurosurgery,* in which younger authors were particularly favored and a venue created for their academic work, this volume is peopled with a number of seasoned neurosurgical veterans. The subjects of discussion are new to all, young and old, and many of these topics and essays have had no similar prior expression in neurosurgical literature. These authors, therefore, are all "young," in a field with little literary neurosurgical precedent.

THE ORGANIZATION OF THE VOLUME

The general theme of the volume is *change:* change occurring in all aspects of neurosurgical practice related to economic pressures and the resulting growth of managed care. In this context, managed care is more than the annoying micromanagment of medical practice; rather, it is the larger concept of the sprouting and growth of economic principles and business management structures in the conduct of medical practice, teaching, and research.

The aim of the volume is threefold:

1. To explain what changes are occurring and why
2. To predict and describe what form change may or will take

3. To describe Neurosurgery's new roles and how to adjust to them

The problem is approached by reducing neurosurgical practice into its principal component parts and assigning a chapter to each. The common thread running through each chapter is the accommodation to change: the adjustment in thinking and action necessary to survive and thrive in the unsheltered world of business and finance, while identifying (and preserving, if possible) the fundamental historical mission and purpose of neurosurgery. The caveat in this last purpose is the necessity of accommodating or compromising those purely professional goals when they diverge from, or conflict with, public demand or market perspective.

The chapters are divided according to a logical arrangement of the components of practice, training, and research. Perhaps more logical would have been a division according to the traditional business categories of finance, operations, research and development, marketing, and strategic planning. As medicine and neurosurgery complete their transition, that volume may require writing. For the present, the structure of discussion will accommodate commonly understood and practiced medical conventions.

The sequence of topics is:

1. Managed Care
2. Practice Management
3. Office Information Systems
4. Reimbursement
5. Quality
6. Guidelines
7. Manpower
8. Academic Practice
9. Bridging the Academic-Private Practice Divide
10. Residency Training
11. Research
12. Board Certification
13. Professional Organizations
14. Politics
15. Ethical Issues
16. Medical Liability
17. Neurotrauma
18. Lessons from International Neurosurgery

Each chapter is self-contained and can be read independently. However, the sequence is significant. Beginning with an overview of the changing market, the story flows from office practice, payment, and quality maintenance; through training programs, trainee numbers, and oversight; to professional politics, ethics, and liability. Finally, a bird's eye international view completes the survey. The chapters feature the following authors and content:

1. *"Managed Care: The Growth of Cost Containment and the Impact on Neurosurgical Practice,"* is written by John A. Kusske, M.D. Dr. Kusske practices neurosurgey in the vortex of managed care in Orange County, California. He has experienced the full conversion of neurosurgical practice to managed and capitated care and, in the process, has intensively researched and acquired an extensive knowledge of the theory and operation of managed care organizations. Dr. Kusske is chairman of the AANS Managed Care Committee and editor in chief of the Managed Care Handbook for Neurological Surgeons, a publication offered to all AANS and CNS members in 1995. Dr. Kusske conducts the AANS Professional Development Course on Managed Care, given several times annually at various locations throughout the country. He is the southwest Regional Director of the AANS Board of Directors and a member of the AANS/CNS Washington Committee. The chapter is a broad summary of managed care as it relates to neurosurgery, from its historical evolution to working in capitated systems.

2. *"Practice Management,"* is written by Stan Pelofsky, M.D. and Kevin Blaylock. Dr. Pelofsky practices in a private neurosurgical group in Oklahoma City. He is immediate past Chairman of the Joint Council of State Neurosurgical Societies (JCSNS) and is currently Secretary of the Board of Directors of the AANS and member of the AANS/CNS Washington Committee. Dr. Pelofsky analyzes the details of office management from overhead expense control and contracting to marketing and strategic planning for practice under managed care, and increasingly competitive, conditions. The chapter is a primer for the hands-on business management of neurosurgery.

3. *"The Computer Workplace,"* is written by Philip Tally, M.D. Dr. Tally has a private group neurosurgical practice in Tampa, Florida. He is the CNS alternate delegate to the AMA, past Treasurer of the JCSNS, and

former Speaker of the House for the JCSNS delegate assembly. Dr. Tally describes a paperless, fully computerized office information system used in his own practice, with practical details on the advantages of electronic office information systems and how to do it. The chapter complements Dr. Pelofsky's overview of office management and lays the groundwork for tracking quality and outcomes in the chapters to follow.

4. *"Changing Reimbursement for Neurosurgery,"* is written by Richard A. Roski, M.D. Dr. Roski is in private neurosurgical practice in Davenport, Iowa. He is former president of a multispecialty IPA, past President of the Congress of Neurological Surgeons (1994), a member of both the AANS Reimbursement and Managed Care Committees, and he conducts AANS Professional Development Courses on Reimbursement. Dr. Roski has been involved with the AANS's contribution to the development of work values for the Medicare Fee Schedule (RBRVS). He uses his background to describe the structure and rationale for the RBRVS, the avantages and drawbacks of the payment method, and newer payment methods, such as specialty capitation that are now appearing under managed care.

5. *"The Role of Quality in Neurosurgical Practice: The Objective Basis of Clinical Accountability,"* is written by Robert E. Florin, M.D. From Orange County, California, Dr. Florin, with a characteristically probing intellect and compulsive attention to detail, is recognized within organized neurosurgery as the leading authority on Medicare reimbursement and on developing quality and guideline standards. Dr. Florin has directed the guidelines and outcomes development strategy of the AANS and CNS since 1992. He is currently Chairman of the AANS/CNS Committee on Assessment of Quality, the oversight body for four key committees: Guidelines; Outcomes; Drugs, Devices, and Technology; and Practice Assessment. Dr. Florin explores the transition of medical practice to the Age of Accountability and the reasons underlying the demand for explicit and objective demonstration of quality in the evolving world of managed care.

6. *"Guideline Development: The Intersection of Valid Science and the Market,"* is written by Beverly C. Walters, M.D. Dr. Walters specializes in spinal surgery at Brown University in Rhode Island. She is neurosurgery's leading authority, spokesperson, and teacher regarding evidence-based guidelines. Her tireless instruction on critical appraisal of medical literature and unvarying insistence on analysis of evidentiary validity of proposed guidelines has earned her specialty-wide recognition. In this chapter, she reviews the development and use of valid guidelines and the problems with evidence and implementation.

7. *"Neurosurgical Workforce: Public Policy, Professional Constraints, and Market Effect,"* is written by A. John Popp, M.D. Dr. Popp is Chairman of Neurosurgery at Albany Medical Center in New York. He has researched and reported on neurosurgery workforce issues for the JCSNS Manpower Committee. Dr. Popp is Director-at-Large of the AANS Board of Directors. Dr. Popp reviews the evidence of neurosurgical workforce needs and the professional, legal, and market influences affecting increase or reduction of neurosurgical training.

8. *"Health Care Reform and Neurosurgical Training,"* whose principal authors are Julian T. Hoff, M.D., and Michael N. Polinsky, M.D., examines the effects of managed care and reimbursement reductions on academic medical centers and neurosurgical training programs. Dr. Hoff is Chairman of Neurosurgery at the University of Michigan in Ann Arbor. He is a past President of the AANS and has served on the neurosurgery Residency Review Committee of the ACGME. Dr. Hoff uses questionnaire information from 77 neurosurgical program directors to analyze the effects of managed care and reimbursement changes on training program incentives and design.

9. *"Academic Neurosurgical Practice in the Age of Accountability: Bridging the Academic/Private Practice Divide,"* is written by Lyal G. Leibrock, M.D., Chairman of Neurosurgery at the University of Nebraska in Omaha, and Leslie C. Hellbusch, M.D. Dr. Leibrock is Vice Chairman of the JCSNS and chaired the JCSNS Reimbursement Methodologies and Negotiations Committee for 9 years. Dr. Leibrock draws

on his experience in Nebraska to illustrate an academic program's strategy for integrating community and university practices for mutual benefit in the face of mounting cost and competition pressures.

10. *"Assurance of Competency in Residency Training: Neurosurgical Training in the Twenty-first Century,"* is written by Don M. Long, M.D., Chairman of Neurosurgery at Johns Hopkins University. Dr. Long has been outspoken on residency program training requirements and design. In this chapter, he outlines his views on learning theory, residency program redesign for the future, and what steps have been taken in the Johns Hopkins program to adapt to market forces and changing educational and training needs.

11. *"The Reformation of Biomedical Research: Influence of the Market and Society,"* is written by William H. Brooks, M.D. and Thomas L. Roszman, Ph.D. Dr. Brooks is a member of a private group neurosurgery practice in Lexington, Kentucky. For over 20 years, Dr. Brooks and Dr. Roszman have collaborated at the University of Kentucky on NIH-funded basic science research in immunology and applications to human gliomas. This chapter takes a novel approach toward analyzing the political, sociological, and market economic forces affecting basic and clinical research agendas and funding.

12. *"Board Certification: Purposes, Issues, Dilemmas, and the Future in Neurosurgery,"* is written by Sidney Tolchin, M.D. Dr. Tolchin is past President of the AANS (1995–1996) and has served as Secretary of the American Board of Neurological Surgery. Dr. Tolchin paints an overview of the traditional certification process and highlights some of the problems with current Board certification growing out of the changing practice environment.

13. *"'Throw Away the Scabbard': What Neurosurgery Should Do Now,"* is written by Robert E. Draba, Ph.D, M.B.A., Executive Director of the AANS since 1996. Dr. Draba brings a broad perspective of history, politics, the market, and professional organizations to the narrow health care corridor of neurosurgery. The chapter ranges widely over the political and business landscape, generously laced with illustrative anec-

dotes, to bring a well-reasoned view to the role of major neurosurgical organizations and a call to arms for neurosurgeons in today's competitive health care environment.

14. *"Neurosurgery and Politics,"* written by Russell L. Travis, M.D., is the description of a growing role for neurosurgery, that of political lobbyist and activist. As public legislative and regulatory policies grow to control more and more of health care reimbursement and practice conditions, particularly through the direct and indirect effects of Medicare policy, attempts to persuade lawmakers grow in parallel. Dr. Travis brings a lengthy experience in political activity to the discussion, having served as Washington Committee chairman, and as Chairman of the Kentucky Medical Association's Board of Trustees during Kentucky's state legislative health care reform from 1992 to 1994. Dr. Travis is President elect of the AANS.

15. *"Ethical Issues in Neurosurgical Practice,"* is written by John J. Oro, M.D. Dr. Oro is Chairman of Neurosurgery at the University of Missouri, in Columbia. Dr. Oro has long had an interest in ethical issues and the philosophical and social basis of ethical principles. Dr. Oro was featured in the video segment on ethics in practice for the JCSNS socioeconomic educational video series in 1996. The chapter reviews traditional ethical principles, their origins, and application to contemporary dilemmas, such as informed consent, futile care, gene therapy, and the physician-societal relationship in respect to managed care.

16. *"Medical-Legal Aspects of Managed Care,"* is authored by Harold D. Portnoy, M.D. and James M. Pidgeon, Esq. In private neurosurgical practice in Bloomfield, Michigan, Dr. Portnoy has been Chairman of the JCSNS Medicolegal Committee since 1994. The chapter focuses on legal issues unique to managed care, such as physician liability for health plan utilization decisions, vicarious liability of health plans for physician actions, and antitrust restrictions.

17. *"Neurotrauma: Organization, Funding, and Regulation in Neurotrauma Care,"* by John H. McVicker, M.D., is the product of research of a JCSNS ad hoc Committee on Neurotrauma, created in 1996 to research

and report on a series of related resolutions from the JCSNS. Dr. McVicker, in private practice in Colorado, tackles difficult political and socioeconomic issues, including organized neurotrauma systems and funding, EMTALA (Emergency Medical Treatment and Active Labor Act) regulations, managed health plan coverage for out of network trauma care, and reimbursement for emergency call coverage. The issues are controversial, but an intimate part of the changing professional and economic health care environment.

18. *"A View of Neurosurgery Around the World: What It Means to You,"* is a review of international neurosurgery as seen first hand by James I. Ausman, M.D., Chairman of Neurosurgery at the University of Illinois in Chicago and Editor in Chief of *Surgical Neurology*. Dr. Ausman finds historical parallels to American neurosurgery in other nations at various stages of economic development. As a finale, the chapter paints the vision of the future in neurosurgery, reinforcing the need to adapt to changing economic conditions with effective business strategies, including "super-specialization," centralization or regionalization of services, and integration of academic and private neurosurgical practices.

This survey of the socioeconomic field of neurological surgery and the evolving environment in which it lives is intended to challenge thought, create confidence through understanding, and arm the reader to take charge of the future, rather than drift randomly, buffeted about by misconceived events. The focus is in no way meant to detract from the importance of the scientific and technical basis of neurosurgical practice. If anything, it should provide a better framework within which to learn, build, and apply those essential professional skills.

Human history, like nature, is cyclical. Long periods of stability and predictability are interspersed with transitional periods of upheaval, instability, and change, marked by revolution, cataclysm, and species ascent or extinction. Neurosurgery, with medicine generally, is riding the crest of a tidal wave of such change over unfamiliar reefs. Collectively and individually, physicians must pilot their vessel over hazardous water to calmer tides. This book is meant to serve as a guide. If successful, this volume will help the reader reconstruct the role, purpose, character, and future of the medical profession as a whole and neurosurgeons as individual participants in that unstable, confusing, and transforming world.

The volume has been an education to assemble. I, along with the authors, hope it provides useful insight into the future of neurosurgery and practical help in understanding how to adapt to and benefit from changes in the health care marketplace.

James R. Bean, M.D.
Lexington, KY
Volume Editor
Chairman,
Council of State Neurosurgical Societies

Contributors

SERIES EDITORS

Stephen J. Haines, M.D., F.A.C.S.
Professor and Chairman
Department of Neurosurgery
Medical College of South Carolina
Charleston, South Carolina

Paul B. Nelson, M.D.
Professor and Chairman of Neurological Surgery
Indiana University School of Medicine
Indianapolis, Indiana

VOLUME EDITOR

James R. Bean, M.D.
Neurosurgical Associates
Lexington, Kentucky

James I. Ausman, M.D., Ph.D.
Professor and Head
Department of Neurosurgery
University of Illinois at Chicago
Chicago, Illinois

Kevin Blaylock, C.P.A.
Oklahoma Neurological Surgery Clinic, Inc.
Oklahoma City, Oklahoma

James R. Bean, M.D.
Managing Director
Neurosurgical Associates
Lexington, Kentucky

William H. Brooks, M.D.
Neurosurgical Associates
Lexington, Kentucky

Robert E. Draba, Ph.D., MBA
Executive Director
American Association of Neurological Surgeons
Park Ridge, Illinois

Robert E. Florin, M.D.
Chairman
Committee on Assessment of Quality
American Association of Neurological Surgery
Congress of Neurological Surgeons
Park Ridge, Illinois

Leslie C. Hellbusch, M.D.
Neurosurgeon
Methodist-Children's Hospital
Omaha, Nebraska

Julian T. Hoff, M.D.
Section of Neurosurgery
University of Michigan Medical Center
Ann Arbor, Michigan

John A. Kusske, M.D.
Neurological Clinic Medical Group
Laguna Hills, California

Lyal G. Leibrock, M.D., F.A.C.S.
Professor and Section Chief
Neurosurgery
University of Nebraska Medical Center
Omaha, Nebraska

Don M. Long, M.D., Ph.D.
Professor and Director
Department of Neurosurgery
Johns Hopkins University School of Medicine;
Neurosurgeon-in-Chief
Johns Hopkins Hospital
Baltimore, Maryland

John H. McVicker, M.D.
Rocky Mountain Neurosurgical Alliance, PC
Englewood, Colorado

John J. Oro, M.D.
Division of Neurosurgery
University of Missouri
Columbia Health Sciences Center
Columbia, Missouri

Katherine O. Orrico, JD
CLP Associates
Washington, DC

Stan Pelofsky, M.D.
Oklahoma Neurological Surgery Clinic, Inc.
Oklahoma City, Oklahoma

James M. Pidgeon, Esq.
Partner
Portnoy, Pidgeon and Roth, PC
Bloomfield Hills, Michigan

Michael N. Polinsky, M.D.
Section of Neurosurgery
Department of Surgery
University of Michigan Medical Center
Ann Arbor, Michigan

A. John Popp, M.D.
Professor of Surgery and
   Henry and Sally Schaffer
Chair of Surgery
Albany Medical College
Albany, New York

Harold D. Portnoy, M.D.
Chairman, Medical Legal Committee
Joint Council of State Neurological Societies;
Oakland Neurological Clinic, P.C.
Bloomfield Hills, Michigan

Richard A. Roski, M.D., F.A.C.S.
Quad City Neurosurgical Associates, P.C.
Davenport, Iowa

Thomas L. Roszman, Ph.D.
Department of Microbiology and Immunology
University of Kentucky Medical Center
Lexington, Kentucky

Philip W. Tally, M.D.
Neuro-Spinal Associates, P.A.
Bradenton, Florida

Sidney Tolchin, M.D.
San Diego, California

Russell L. Travis, M.D., F.A.C.S.
Neurosurgical Associates
Lexington, Kentucky

**Beverly C. Walters, M.D., M.Sc.,
F.R.C.S.C., F.A.C.S.**
Associate Professor of Clinical Neurosciences
Brown University; Chief of Neurosurgery
The Miriam Hospital
Providence, Rhode Island

Contents

PART III

Other Issues

PART I

Neurosurgical Practice

Managed Care—The Growth of Cost Containment and the Impact on Neurosurgical Practice

JOHN A. KUSSKE, M.D.

"The future ain't what it used to be!"

—Yogi Berra

"He who has a thorough knowledge of his own conditions as well as of the conditions of the enemy is sure to win all battles. He who has a thorough knowledge of his own conditions but not the conditions of the enemy has an even chance of winning and losing a battle. He who has neither a thorough knowledge of his own conditions nor of the enemy's is sure to lose every battle."

—Sun Tzu, The Art of War

INTRODUCTION

First, one might ask, what is managed care? Broadly speaking, managed care describes a health care delivery system in which a party other than the physician or the patient influences the type, nature, and extent of medical care delivered. The characteristics most common to managed care include: arrangements with selected providers, who furnish a package of services to enrollees; explicit criteria for selection of providers; quality assurance, utilization review, and outcome measures; financial or program coverage incentives or penalties to enrollees who do not use selected providers; provider risk-sharing arrangements; management by providers to assure that enrollees or members receive appropriate care from the most cost-efficient mix of providers (1).

A conceptual definition of managed care has been proposed: ''Managed care is the process of the application of standard business practices to the delivery of health care in the traditions of the American free enterprise system'' (2). As the author of this proposed definition, E. F. Hughes points out, managed care is a process. He states that it is change itself—a process that is inexorable. There is, and will be, no rollback to a preexisting status quo. As this chapter will illustrate, this is because of deep-seated forces in the American business and consumer communities. Managed care is an American invention, and, like other American inventions, it will ultimately grow to dominate the world. This is so because there really is no alternative to managed care to rationalize the cost and quality of care (2). According to Hughes, the disciplining of the health care sector by the invisible hand of Adam Smith entails squeezing out of it excess supply and excess profits, so that they may be used for more productive social purposes. This is what markets do in general and why many feel markets are our best social rationing system.

D. M. Eddy points out that, in comparing fee-for-service health care with managed care, it is germane to consider how trade-offs between quality and cost are made in each system (3). According to Eddy, the fee-for-service tradeoffs include the following: there is no defined population for which the insurance company is responsible; contacts with the system are initiated by patients; the main focus is on treating sick patients; the responsibility of the insurance company is to pay the bills; physicians are left alone to decide what care their patients should receive;

where there is uncertainty about the appropriate level of care, physicians have a financial incentive to overuse care; the insurance company has no managerial control over the providers, and there is no capacity for centralized decision making; the locus of the conflict between quality and cost is split between physicians, who have income incentives to maximize the services they deliver to patients, and administrators, who have market incentives to keep premiums low.

On the other hand, characteristics of managed care that affect the cost/quality tradeoff include the following: the managed care organization (MCO) has responsibility for the health of a defined population, i.e., all of the people who have paid premiums; for this defined population, the MCO is responsible for the entire spectrum of care; physicians are not left alone to practice as they see fit; the MCO has a variety of clinical management systems for modifying the actions of physicians; the MCO has the capacity for centralized decision making; while the tension between quality and cost is felt differently in different parts of the organization, the conflict comes together at the level of the medical director.

Managed care is rapidly dominating the health care financing and delivery system in the United States. Neurosurgeons have little choice regarding participation in managed care plans. Nearly three-quarters of U.S. workers with health insurance now receive their coverage through a health maintenance organization (HMO), a preferred provider organization (PPO), or a point-of-service plan (POS). Managed care plans are now commonplace in small firms as well as large ones (4). The government is increasingly relying on managed care options to bring down costs (and to improve quality) for both the Medicare and Medicaid programs. About 4.6 million (or 12%) of Medicare beneficiaries have enrolled in HMOs with Medicare risk contracts, and, every 30 seconds, one senior citizen joins an HMO (5). Similarly about 8.5 million (24%) of the Medicaid population has enrolled in managed care programs (3). Even traditional plans are adopting principles of managed care: for example, hospital precertification and large case management, which were daring innovations as recently as a decade ago, have become common in indemnity insurance (6).

Managed care has also become big business. Some 36.7 million HMO enrollees are in multistate firms, including nonprofit organizations such as Kaiser and the HMOs which are owned by the various Blue Cross and Blue Shield plans (7). The HMOs are also an industry in the throes of massive consolidation. In California only 6 HMOs now account for 85% of the state's 13 million enrollees (8). Many of the large managed care companies are traded on the New York Stock Exchange and other stock exchanges, and the general business press reports their profits along with the compensation of their chief executive officers, compensation which can amount to millions of dollars annually.

When thinking of managed care, a distinction should be made between the techniques of managed care and the organization that performs the various functions. A wide body of techniques are embodied in managed care, including a mix of financial incentives for providers, promotion of wellness, early identification of disease, patient education, self care, and all aspects of utilization management. Many organizations can implement managed care techniques. The HMO has the potential to align financing and delivery most closely because, with few exceptions, enrollees are required to use network providers. However, managed care methods can also be used by employers, insurers, union-management (as with the Taft-Hartley law) trust funds, and the Medicare and Medicaid programs. PPOs use them also. A variety of hybrid arrangements have evolved, with one example being the POS program, which operates as a PPO—except that to receive the highest level of benefits, the enrollee must obtain a referral from a primary care physician who is part of the contracted network. The arrangements, increasingly, are difficult to characterize, let alone to profile statistically in a meaningful manner (6).

The same forces that have encouraged the expansion of managed care have also brought about change in HMOs. These changes have included: the growth of for-profit plans and the relative decline of nonprofits; the shift from vertically integrated group/staff models to virtually integrated individual practice associations/network models; industry consolidation through mergers and acquisitions; increased cost sharing; the shift to capitation payment for primary care and some specialty physicians (9).

HEALTH CARE REFORM

As the health care reform debate continues throughout the remainder of this century and possibly into the next, managed care will be a central component. At the heart of this debate is the struggle to accept the concept that a managed system has greater benefit than one that relies on solo practitioners and fee-for-service. Cost containment and incremental reforms are the prevailing themes at the heart of the present debate over national health care reform. At the federal level, the emphasis has shifted from universal access to cost containment, because of the issues the Congress is dealing with, including: reducing the federal deficit, balancing the federal budget, addressing the insolvency of the Medicare Trust Fund, and decreasing the size of government.

The health care system has multidimensional effects on federal, state, and private sector spending, as well as on business innovation and competitiveness. The drivers of federal health policy include: the United States budget deficit; the public debt, which is $5 trillion and growing; the Medicare Trust Fund, approaching insolvency by 2002; state budget shortfalls, strapped by an average 12% Medicaid growth rate; public perception of change and reluctance to accept larger roles for government; an aging population and changing demographics, represented by a 23% increase in the over-85 population (10, 11).

In recent years, neither the federal government nor most state governments have had major roles in shaping the forces that drive health system change. Nevertheless, their future actions may be particularly influential. The implications of Medicare's shift toward managed care will be felt throughout the health care system. Medicare's health plan standards, market rules, quality assurance, grievance procedures, and consumer information, as well as its national consumer choice system for 37 million enrollees, may provide models for national reforms (11).

Legislators, at the state level, are becoming increasingly concerned that competitive pressure and risk-sharing contractual agreements are skewing health plans incentives toward withholding care. As a result, they have developed regulations that are collectively referred to as health plan accountability laws. These laws cover a variety of issues, all truly relevant to managed care. They include: grievance procedures, health information, confidentiality standards, credentialing, utilization review, quality assurance, and provider contracting.

At the federal level, the debate ranges from the government's running a fee-driven health program to standardizing a private health plan market that is held accountable for cost and quality of service. In the meantime, health care is likely to continue on the path of incremental changes that will moderately support the continued development of managed care plans in each marketplace (10).

It has been suggested (10, 12) that to enable the continuation of these incremental changes, Congress will need to address a number of areas, each sector having an independent and collective impact on the development of managed care organizations. These areas include: defining a health benefits package that would be standardized to all markets; deciding the level of responsibility and risk to be assumed by health care consumers; legitimizing Integrated Delivery Systems (IDSs) or provider-sponsored health plans as a model of managed care; establishing administrative reporting requirements to support fiscal integrity and development of practice guidelines; determining the role of supplemental insurance; initiating changes in tax laws to limit the amount of employer-deductible health coverage expenses; implementing changes in tax laws so that money accumulated in employees medical savings accounts (MSAs) is tax exempt; refining the definition of an insurance company to clarify the requirements of tax exempt organizations; and affirming the role of academic medical centers.

The reader should be aware of incremental health care and entitlement reform legislation enacted in the remainder of this century, since that will point the way for the future direction of the private market and the public sector. The daunting task of defining new roles and responsibilities among state and federal governments, patients, businesses, insurers, and health-care providers cannot be completed with the enactment of a single piece of legislation. As the defeat of the Clinton Health Care proposals demonstrated, a comprehensive enactment of a single health plan for everyone would be too revolutionary for Americans.

THE EVOLUTION OF MANAGED CARE

Managed care had humble origins and fought to survive in the early years. It was strictly an outgrowth of the private sector, dating back some 80 years. Sometimes cited as the first example of an HMO (or prepaid group practice as it was known) is the Western Clinic in Tacoma, Washington (13). Started in 1910, the Clinic offered, through its own providers, a broad range of medical services for a premium of $0.50 per member per month. The clinic was later expanded to 20 sites in Oregon and Washington.

A rural farmers' cooperative health plan was established in 1929 by Michael Shadid, M.D. in Elk City, Oklahoma. Participating farmers purchased shares for $50 each to raise capital for a new hospital and in return they received medical care at a discount (14). That same year, two physicians in Los Angeles, Donald Ross, M.D. and H. Clifford Loos, M.D. entered into a prepaid contract to provide comprehensive health services to about 2000 water company employees (14). These plans were harbingers of managed care.

Health insurance itself is of relatively recent origin. In 1929, Baylor Hospital in Texas agreed to provide prepaid care to 1500 teachers at its hospital, an arrangement that represented the origins of Blue Cross. Starting in 1939, state medical societies in California and elsewhere created, generally statewide, Blue Shield plans, which reimbursed for physician services. At the time, commercial health insurance was not a factor (15). The formation of the various Blue Cross and Blue Shield plans in the midst of the great depression, as well as that of many HMOs, reflected not consumers demanding coverage or nonphysician entrepreneurs seeking to establish a business, but rather providers wanting to protect and enhance patient revenues (6). The American Medical Association (AMA), in 1932, adopted a strong position opposing prepaid group practices, favoring instead indemnity insurance. The AMA's stance at a national level set the tone for continued state and local opposition to prepaid group practice.

World War II saw the formation of HMOs that are among the leaders today. They encountered varying degrees of opposition from local medical societies. A diversity of origins was seen coming from employers, providers seeking patient revenues, and consumers seeking access to improved and affordable health care. The following are examples of early HMOs:

1. The Kaiser Foundation Health Plans were started in 1937 by Dr. Sidney Garfield at the behest of the Kaiser construction company building the Colorado River Aqueduct in California and the Grand Coulee Dam in Washington. A similar plan was established in 1942 at Kaiser shipbuilding plants in the San Francisco Bay area.
2. The Group Health Association (GHA) was started in 1937 in Washington, D.C., at the direction of the Home Owner's Loan Corporation, to reduce the number of mortgage foreclosures resulting from large medical expenses.
3. The Health Insurance Plan (HIP) of Greater New York was established in 1944 at the behest of New York City seeking coverage for its employees.
4. Group Health Cooperative of Puget Sound was organized in 1947 by consumers in Seattle.

Only in later years did nonprovider entrepreneurs form for-profit HMOs in significant numbers.

A variant of the prepaid group practice plan appeared in 1954, when a prototype independent practice association (IPA) was established by the San Joaquin County Foundation for Medical Care in Stockton, California. The San Joaquin Medical Society, fearing competition from Kaiser-Permanente, set up a prepaid foundation for medical care, later to be called an IPA. A relative value fee schedule for guaranteeing payment was adopted; all grievances were heard by a voluntary board of physicians, and an attempt was made to monitor the quality of care. It became licensed by the state to accept capitation payment, making it the first IPA model HMO (16).

HMOs played only a modest role in the financing and delivery of health care through the 1960s and into the early 1970s. The total number of HMOs numbered between 30 and 40 in 1970, the exact number depending on the definition applied (13). The years since the early 1970s represent a period of accelerating developments, which are still unfolding.

In 1973, the federal HMO act was passed. That act authorized start-up funding and, more importantly, ensured access to the employer-based insurance market. It evolved from discussions that Paul Ellwood, M.D. had in 1970 with the leadership of the United States Department of Health, Education, and Welfare, which later became the Department of Health and Human Services (17). Ellwood, sometimes referred to as the father of the modern HMO movement, was asked in the early years of the Nixon administration to devise ways of constraining the rise in the Medicare budget. Out of these discussions evolved both a proposal to capitate HMOs for Medicare beneficiaries, which was not enacted until 1982, and the development of the outline for the HMO Act of 1973 (P.L. 73-222).

The Act provided start-up funding, required many employers to offer an HMO option, and removed state regulations blocking HMO development. The start-up funding provided for federally qualified HMOs, that is, those meeting federal requirements for fiscal responsibility and quality of care. The act removed state legislative prohibitions on the corporate practice of medicine that restricted HMO development in many states. It identified three HMO types: group, staff, and independent practice association; in 1976, the act was amended to make it more ''user friendly'' for HMOs. Among other things, the 1976 amendments spurred the development of the IPA model (18, 19).

Other managed care developments also occurred during the 1970s and early 1980s. Of note was the evolution of PPOs. These organizations are generally regarded as differing from HMOs in two respects. First, they do not accept capitation risk; rather, risk remains with the insurance company. Second, enrollees may access providers that are not in the contracted network, but they are burdened with higher out-of-pocket costs for doing this. PPOs are generally regarded as originating in Denver in the early 1970s (20).

From 1985 until the present, managed care has come of age. The era has been characterized by innovation and maturation.

Three areas of innovation are important. First, in many communities, hospitals and physicians have collaborated to form physician-hospital organizations (PHOs). These are primarily vehicles for contracting with MCOs. Most PHOs, historically, have sought to enter fee-for-service arrangements with HMOs and PPOs, although an increasing number are accepting capitation. The role of PHOs is frequently debated, and the question as to whether they are an important development or little more than a temporary transition model still has not been settled. The unsettled questions revolve around domination of PHOs by hospital administrators and physician specialists and about the (customary) practice of allowing participation in the PHO of all physicians with admitting privileges at a particular

PHO hospital rather than selecting the more efficient ones. Some PHOs also are weakened by organizational segmentation, poor information systems, inexperienced management, and lack of capital (6).

A second innovation has been the development of carve-outs. These are organizations made up of specialized provider networks and are paid on a capitation or other basis for a specific service, such as neurosurgery. The carve-out companies market their services principally to HMOs and large self-insured employers. Similar in concept are groups of specialists, such as ophthalmologists and radiologists, that accept capitation risk for their services, sometimes referred to as subcapitation, through contracts with health plans and employer groups.

Advances in computer technology have made a third set of innovations possible. Computer programs marketed by private firms or developed by MCOs have become available that generate statistical profiles of the use of services rendered by neurosurgeons and other physicians. These profiles assess efficiency and quality, and they may also serve to adjust payment levels to providers paid under capitation or risk-sharing arrangements so as to reflect the severity of patient conditions (21, 22). Computer technology has also changed the ways of processing medical and drug claims, which is increasingly being performed by being downloaded electronically rather than by paper submission and manual entry. These electronic claims have resulted in significantly lower administrative costs and superior information. Management information systems can be expected to improve further in the next few years as providers, almost universally, will submit claims electronically. Providers are also likely to be assigned unique identification numbers, enabling profiling systems to cross multiple payers. Technology-enabled systems are now viewed as an investment in the future of each provider's enterprise, rather than an expense (23).

Problems remain, however, with the development of health information networks. As Starr recently described it, computer networks should help raise the quality of health care, reduce its cost, and enable consumers and providers to make smarter decisions (24). But, because government and the private sector have failed to resolve such problems as the protection of medical privacy and production of reliable comparative data on plans and providers, the development of systems is lagging. He points out that an information revolution in health care is in the making, but the hope that it will allow consumers and providers to make smarter choices is still far from being realized.

The maturation of managed care can be seen from several vantage points. The first relates to HMO and PPO growth. Between 1992 and 1994, HMO enrollment rose 23%, reaching 51 million, and PPO enrollment, which is more difficult to estimate, has reached similar levels (7, 25). Medicare and Medicaid have also increasingly relied on managed care. While fully capitated Medicare HMOs have been available since 1985, the risk-contract program has only recently exploded in terms of beneficiary enrollment, HMO participation, and new areas of penetration throughout the United States (26). In 1996, for the first time, Medicare enrollment in risk-contract HMOs exceeded 10% of all beneficiaries, and between 1994 and 1996 risk-contract enrollment increased at an average annual rate of more than 40% (26). The enrollment in Medicare risk-contract HMOs is expected to increase to more than one-third of all beneficiaries in the next 10 years (27). Many HMOs regard Medicare risk-contracting, that is, capitation programs that HMOs enter into with the Medicare program, as an essential part of their business strategy.

Another phenomenon is the maturation of external quality oversight activities. Starting in 1991, the National Committee for Quality Assurance (NCQA) began to accredit HMOs (28). The interests of employers and the HMO plans themselves have catapulted the NCQA, a private, not-for-profit organization, virtually unknown until recently, into an important new role as the leading accreditor of managed care plans (29). The NCQA accredits managed care plans that voluntarily request a review of their operations. It develops performance measures for plans through the Health Plan Employer Data and Information Set (HEDIS), the most prominent of recent private efforts to develop, collect, standardize, and report measures of plan performance (30). Many employers are demanding or strongly encouraging NCQA accreditation of HMOs with which they contract, and accreditation is coming to replace federal qualification as the "Good Housekeeping Seal of Approval." Of about 575 managed care plans currently oper-

ating, the NCQA has reviewed 230. Of those reviewed, 90 have been granted full accreditation for 3 years; 88 , accreditation for 1 year; and 23, provisional accreditation. Accreditation was denied to 26 plans and several others are under review (29).

NCQA has also developed a variety of products directly aimed at consumers. These include the Accreditation Status List (ASL), which is a register of all health plans on which NCQA has granted decisions, showing only their overall accreditation status. In July 1996, NCQA released the first of its Accreditation Summary Reports (ASRs), which provide more detail on individual health plan accreditation decisions. An ASR is a two-page synopsis of a health plan's in-depth technical NCQA accreditation report. These reports are available on NCQA's World Wide Web Site. Also in July 1996, NCQA launched "Quality Compass," a national database of comparative information about the quality of the nation's managed care plans. Finally, in September 1996, NCQA established the Practicing Physicians Advisory Committee (PPAC), which is an advisory committee organized to address concerns raised about having regular insight into the impact that many NCQA activities have on practicing physicians (31).

As the number of plans offering managed care grows, the business of accrediting them has become highly competitive. The NCQA's competitors are the Joint Commission on Accreditation of Health Care Organizations, the Accreditation Association for Ambulatory Health Care, the Foundation for Accountability, the Medical Quality Commission, and the Utilization Review Accreditation Commission (URAC) (32). The leading accreditation agency for utilization review (UR) is URAC. It was established as the result of provider frustration with the diversity of UR procedures and the growing impact of UR on physicians and hospitals. The URAC accreditation process was developed in large part as a response and alternative to legislative initiatives that sought to limit UR (28). URAC's stated goal is to improve continually the quality and efficiency of the interaction between the UR industry and the providers, payers, and purchasers of health care.

In addition, performance measurement systems, or report cards as they are known, are evolving, although they are at an early stage. The most prominent is HEDIS, which was developed by the NCQA at the urging of several large employers and health plans (31, 33). The July, 1996 release of HEDIS, version 3.0, was major news in health quality circles. The most significant change was a new emphasis on patient health status and medical outcomes, whereas the measurements have been previously almost exclusively measurements of processes and standard operating procedures (33). One of the reasons for establishing the PPAC was to promote cooperation with physicians on the use and misuse of report cards. It appears that the combined weight of employer groups and the managed care industry is helping to make HEDIS a powerful tool in the eye of the public. Providers will have little choice but to learn how they too can earn an "A" in health care reporting. Unfortunately, as many physicians are aware, there are multiple problems with measuring the quality of care (34).

THE FIVE STAGES OF MANAGED CARE

Russell Coile describes five stages of managed care, based on the extent of HMO market penetration, with limited primary care capitation beginning in stage 2 and professional capitation at stage 4 (35).

In stage 1, less than 5% of the population are enrolled in HMOs. PPOs are the most common type of managed care plans. Employers are just beginning to offer HMO options, but few are available in their service area. At this stage, employers may not be enthusiastic about HMO options because they fear favorable selection to the managed care plan, leaving the fee-for-service plan with higher risk members. Individual and small physician groups may join open panel IPAs to maintain their patient base and to position themselves, if HMO penetration grows. Hospitals are attempting to go it alone and frequently organize open panel physician organizations for receiving patients from health insurers. Based on 1995 data, Coile lists Boise, Idaho; El Paso, Texas; Fargo, North Dakota; Ft. Meyers, Florida; Knoxville, Tennessee; Muncie, Indiana; and Wilmington, North Carolina at stage 1. He reports that even in these areas, physician management companies are purchasing primary care physician practices and hospitals are being acquired by Columbia/HCA and other large systems.

At stage 2, HMO penetration ranges from 5 to 15%, and HMOs begin to contract with primary care groups for primary care capitation. Insurance companies, attempting to compete with their PPOs, demand deeper discounts and tougher controls. Urban HMOs may attempt to establish themselves, adding choice for employers concerned about rising health-care costs. Employers may also form coalitions to share data on utilization and costs. Small medical groups may merge into "groups without walls" to reduce overhead costs and to compete for capitation and reduced fee contracts. Hospitals may be absorbed into systems and use system capital to purchase medical office buildings to align physicians more closely. Coile lists Charlotte, North Carolina; Indianapolis, Indiana; New Orleans, Louisiana; Omaha, Nebraska; San Antonio, Texas; and Topeka, Kansas at stage 2. He states that employer coalitions may act to select hospitals based on price and quality. Data on quality and cost become useful for selection and price negotiations.

At stage 3, HMO penetration is at 15 to 25%, allowing HMOs to use their market power aggressively. Fees become sharply discounted and hospital per-diem rates may drop below costs. Primary care capitation becomes widespread, as indemnity plans fall below 15% of total population. Specialists feel the impact of managed care with declining utilization, from fewer primary care physician referrals, and begin to form local networks. Hospitals initiate the formation of PHOs to compete for HMO contracts, and they also attempt direct employer contracting. However, many physicians do not want to be dependent on a single hospital and so they form their own groups for HMO contracting. In some cases, IPAs evolve into integrated medical groups. More often, multispecialty groups and hospitals are buying primary care groups or adding primary care physicians. Coile lists Chicago, Baltimore, Kansas City, and Hawaii at stage 3.

At stage 4, HMO penetration is 25 to 40%. Employers are demanding lower costs from HMOs, usually by a coalition requiring all HMO bids to adhere to a standard benefit package. The bids may be negotiated lower in subsequent years. HMOs, such as those in California, seek to export more of their risk through professional capitation contracts with IPAs and medical groups, as well as through hospital capitation. Capitation rates may fall with the result that

IPAs and medical groups are forced to merge or, at least, to consolidate their administrative functions to reduce costs. Specialist capitation becomes more common, although not at an individual physician level. Rather, the specialty is given a budget with affected specialists having the responsibility for monitoring and controlling utilization to meet budgetary targets. IPAs may also help the specialists develop systems for monitoring utilization and developing clinical pathways. Coile lists Boston, Los Angeles, San Francisco, Tallahassee, Milwaukee, Salt Lake City and San Diego at stage 4.

At stage 5, HMO penetration exceeds 40%, the 1996 estimate for the Los Angeles and San Francisco metropolitan areas. As Medicare and Medicaid HMO enrollment soars, mergers of IPAs and medical groups increase. The reasons for the mergers are greater influence with HMOs, the possibility of direct contracting for Medicare, Medicaid, and with employers, and greater administrative efficiencies. HMOs may purchase provider entities and selected hospitals, forming more integrated delivery systems, or providers may obtain an HMO license. More integration results regardless of which trend predominates, as employer coalitions work to drive down HMO premiums. Hospitals facing high levels of uninsured populations will be forced to consolidate or close, as subsidies from employers, Medicare and Medicaid evaporate. Under Coile's scenario, increased pressure is put on federal and state governments to determine how employers' demands for cost containment and government cutbacks can allow for the financing of safety-net hospitals serving the uninsured. Whatever solutions are adopted, reimbursement for physicians will continue to fall for specialists and level off for primary care physicians. Early data for 1997 reveals that health insurance premiums are again beginning to rise, suggesting that there will be greater pressure exerted on providers to reduce costs (36).

Further cost reductions will require integration of financing and delivery with health plans and providers, reducing mutual administrative costs, such as utilization management, quality assurance, credentialing and network management. This administrative streamlining could result from further delegation of HMO administration to integrated delivery networks, HMO acquisition of the networks, or networks becoming HMOs. Also, increasing mergers between

HMOs could reduce their per-member administrative costs and make networks more likely to integrate with a single HMO. It has been predicted that in 5 years, there will be three to five dominant networks in most market regions (35). It is also believed that capitation to the network will be the dominant form of payment, which has far-reaching implications for health care delivery and for neurosurgeons.

TYPES OF MANAGED CARE ORGANIZATIONS

The various types of managed care organizations were reasonably distinct as recently as 1988. Originally, HMOs, PPOs, and traditional forms of indemnity insurance were discrete, mutually exclusive products and mechanisms for providing health care coverage. Today, an observer may be hard pressed to uncover the differences among products that bill themselves as HMOs, PPOs, or managed care overlays to health insurance. As a result of recent changes, descriptions of the different types of managed care systems that follow provide only a guideline for determining the form of a particular managed care organization. In many instances, or in most cases in some markets, the managed health care organization will be a hybrid of several specific types (37, 38).

Some controversy exists about whether the term "managed care," alluded to at the outset, with its six essential elements, accurately describes the new generation of health care delivery and financing mechanisms. Those who object raise the question about what is being managed by a managed care organization. The question boils down to this: is the individual patient's medical care being managed, or is the organization simply managing the composition and reimbursement of the provider delivery system? Those who favor the term "managed care" believe that managing the provider-delivery system can be equivalent in outcome to managing the medical care delivered to the patient. In contrast to the historical methods of financing health care delivery in the United States, the current generation of financing mechanisms includes far more active management of both the delivery system through which care is provided and the medical care that is actually delivered to individual patients (37).

HMOs are organized health care systems that

are responsible for both the financing and the delivery of a broad range of health services to an enrolled population. The original definition of an HMO also included the aspect of financing health care for a prepaid fixed fee (thus, the term, prepaid health plans), and, although that portion of the definition is no longer absolute, it is still a common one. An HMO can be viewed as a combination health insurer and health care delivery system. HMOs are responsible for providing health care services to members through affiliated providers who are reimbursed under various methods, which will be discussed subsequently. In addition, HMOs generally are responsible for ensuring the quality and appropriateness of the health services they provide to their members. The five common models of HMOs are staff, group practice network, network, IPA, and direct contract. The primary differences among these models are based on how the HMO relates to its participating physicians. These models are discussed at some length in other publications (37, 38).

So far as neurosurgeons are concerned there is a great deal of significance in how an HMO is structured. In a staff model HMO, the physicians who serve the HMO's beneficiaries are employed by the HMO. These physicians are typically paid on a salary basis and may also receive bonus or incentive payments based on their performance and productivity. Staff model HMOs must employ physicians in all the common specialties to provide health care. These HMOs often contract with selected specialists in the community, such as neurosurgeons, for infrequently needed health services. A well-known example of staff model HMOs is Group Health Cooperative of Puget Sound in Seattle, Washington. Many staff model HMOs are incorporating other types of physician relationships into their delivery systems.

In pure group model HMOs, the HMO contracts with a multispecialty physician group practice to provide all physician services to the HMOs members. The physicians in the group practice are employed by the group practice and not by the HMO. There are two broad categories of group models.

In a captive group model, the physician group practice exists solely to provide services to the HMO's beneficiaries. The most prominent example of this type of HMO is the Kaiser Foundation Medical Plan, where the Permanente Medi-

cal Groups provide all physician services for Kaiser's members. The Permanente Medical Group often hires neurosurgeons to provide care for its members. The Kaiser Foundation Health Plan, as the licensed HMO, is responsible for marketing the benefit plans, enrolling members, collecting premium payments, and performing other HMO functions. The Permanente Medical Groups are responsible for rendering physician services to Kaiser's members under an exclusive contractual relationship with Kaiser. Kaiser is sometimes mistakenly thought to be a staff model HMO because of the close relationship between itself and the Permanente Medical Group.

In the independent group model HMO, the HMO contracts with an existing, independent, multispecialty physician group to provide physician services to its members. An example of the independent group model HMO is Geisinger Health Plan of Danville, Pennsylvania. The Geisinger Clinic, which is a large, multispecialty physician group practice, is the independent group associated with the Geisinger Health Plan. Typically, the physician group in an independent group model HMO continues to provide services to non-HMO patients, while it participates in the HMO. Of additional interest here is the recent announcement that Pennsylvania State's Milton S. Hershey Medical Center and the Geisinger Health System will merge (39). Both the Geisinger Clinic and the Hershey Medical Center hire neurosurgeons.

In network model HMOs, the HMO contracts with more than one group practice to provide physician services to the HMO's members. These group practices may be broad-based multispecialty groups, in which case, the HMO resembles the group practice model. An example of this type of HMO is Health Insurance Plan of Greater New York, which contracts with many multispecialty physician group practices in the New York area. Alternatively, the HMO may contract with several small groups of primary care physicians, in which case, the HMO can be classified as a primary care network model. Typically, the HMO compensates these groups on an all-inclusive physician capitation basis. The group is responsible for providing all physician services to the HMO's members assigned to the group and it may make referrals to other physicians as necessary. The group is responsible for reimbursing other physicians for any referrals it makes. An example is the Bristol Park Medical Group of Southern California.

The network model HMO addresses many of the disadvantages associated with staff and group model HMOs. The broader physician participation identified with the network model HMO helps overcome the marketing disadvantage associated with the closed panel staff and group model plans. Nevertheless, network model HMOs usually have more limited physician participation than either IPA models or direct contract models.

IPA model HMOs contract with an association of physicians to provide services to their members. The physicians are members of the IPA, which is a separate legal entity, but they remain individual practitioners and retain their separate offices and identities. IPA physicians continue to see their non-HMO patients and maintain their own offices, medical records, and support staff. IPA model HMOs are open panel plans because they open participation to all community physicians who meet the HMO's and IPA's selection criteria. IPA's generally try to recruit physicians from all specialties to participate in their plans. This allows the IPA to provide all necessary physician services through participating physicians and minimizes the need by IPA physicians to refer HMO members to nonparticipating physicians. In addition, the broad participation of physicians can help make the IPA model HMO more attractive to potential HMO members.

HMOs may contract with IPAs that have been independently established by community physicians. There may be a large number of plans that contract with such an IPA on a nonexclusive basis. The HMO, alternatively, may assist community physicians in establishing an HMO and recruit physicians to participate in it. In this instance, the contract is usually on an exclusive basis, because of the HMO's lead in forming the IPA. The formation of the IPA can be on a community-wide basis, where physicians participate without regard to the hospital with which they have privileges. Or, IPAs may be hospital-based and formed so that only physicians from one to three hospitals are eligible to participate in the IPA. Hospital-based IPAs are sometimes preferred by HMOs over larger, community-based IPAs for at least two reasons. First, hospital-based IPAs can restrict the panel of physicians to those who are familiar with each other's

practice patterns. This may make utilization management easier. Second, by using several hospital-based IPAs, an HMO can limit the impact of termination of one its IPA agreements to a smaller group of physician (39).

IPAs are compensated by HMOs on an all-inclusive physician capitation basis to provide services to HMO members. That is to say, the HMO establishes a budget for physician services based on actuarially determined projected expenses. Typically, HMO allocations for neurosurgeons amount to 1 to 2% of the physician budget (40). The IPA then compensates its participating physicians on either a fee-for-service basis or a combination of fee-for-service and primary care capitation. In the fee-for-service variation, IPAs pay all their participating physicians on the basis of a fee schedule and may withhold a portion of each payment for incentive and risk sharing purposes. Typically, this withhold is within the range of 10 to 15%. Under one capitation approach, the primary care physicians are paid on a capitation basis and the specialists on a fee-for-service approach using a negotiated fee schedule with similar withholds.

From an HMO's perspective, there are two major disadvantages of an IPA. The first is that the IPA creates an organized forum for physicians to negotiate as a group with an HMO. This can help the physician members achieve some of the negotiating leverage of belonging to a group practice. Unlike a group practice, however, the individual physicians retain their ability to negotiate and contract directly with managed care plans. Because IPAs accept capitated risk payments, they are generally immune from antitrust restrictions on group activities by physicians, as long as they do not prevent their member physicians from participating directly with an HMO. The second disadvantage seen by some for IPAs relates to the perceived difficulty of utilization management, because physicians remain individual practitioners. Notwithstanding this historical disadvantage, recent studies have demonstrated that some IPA model HMOs have overcome the challenge and have succeeded in managing utilization as well as, or better than, their closed panel counterparts (41).

Direct contract model HMOs contract directly with individual physicians to provide physician services to their members. With the exception of their direct contracting relationship with participating physicians, direct contract model

HMOs are similar to IPA model plans. A well known example of a direct contract model is US Healthcare and its subsidiary HMOs. Direct contract model HMOs attempt to recruit broad panels of community physicians to provide services as participating providers. These HMOs usually recruit both primary care and specialist physicians, and typically use a primary care management approach, sometimes referred to as a gatekeeper arrangement.

Modes of compensation are similar to those described earlier for IPA model plans. Unlike IPA model plans, however, direct contract models retain most of the financial risk for providing physician services, while IPA model plans transfer the risk to their IPAs. Although this model may have many of the advantages of the IPA model, they eliminate the physicians bargaining potential to a great extent. The direct contract model HMOs may have several disadvantages—including added expense because of overutilization by the primary care physicians. In addition, it is difficult for nonphysician administrators to recruit physicians into the plans. There may also be little incentive for physicians to participate in utilization management programs.

In recent years, the oversupply of specialists in some markets, along with the increasing penetration of MCOs, like those described above, has led specialty physicians (SPs) in those marketplaces to actively pursue contracts with MCOs. Concomitant with that shift in attitude, many HMOs and other forms of MCOs, such as PPOs and even some integrated delivery systems, have closed their panels to new SPs and have even deselected some SPs with existing contracts (42). By reducing the number of specialists, IPAs are able to increase the primary-to-specialist ratio needed for capitation, thereby gaining leverage to reduce fees and to increase volume for the remaining physicians and retaining physicians with the most proven cost effectiveness or ability to draw members (18).

In reaction to this, physicians are strongly pushing any willing-provider laws at the state level in order to limit this practice of deselection. As of 1995, approximately 20 states had adopted such laws (43). The relevance of these laws to both managed care and integrated delivery systems is clear. As has been stated (44), "Although 'anti-managed care' legislation can take several forms, it can be reduced to one essential result: it removes the right of health care plans to selectively and competitively negotiate contracts with the highest qualified and most cost effective providers." It is essential to understand the effect of these laws, because they become a major impediment to the effective development and operation of MCOs (45).

By contrast, in other markets, SPs remain in strong financial positions or may not be in excess supply, or managed care may not yet be in a strong market position. In those areas, nevertheless, MCOs may set a high priority on contracting for specialty services for a number of reasons. Contractual arrangements aid in getting and holding a specialist's attention, and they help in the administration of the system, allowing the plan to forecast and budget medical expenses more accurately. They also make the MCO more attractive to the potential enrollees. The MCO may be able to save money through a capitation system or by having a financially advantageous contract, such as a discounted fee schedule.

Specialists in such markets will be interested in the total volume of referrals. If there is evidence that the plan expects to restrict the size of the provider panel and if the plan has a good-sized membership base, then the specialist can easily determine the expected number of referrals. In some instances, it makes good sense for the SP to contract with a plan before someone else gets there first. The contract may provide a reliable revenue source and may enhance fee-for-service referrals by bolstering relations with primary care physicians.

The number of SPs of each type that an IPA, or other type of MCO, may require is not easy to determine. In one widely read study, the number of SPs required was estimated to be between 80 and 110 per 100,000 population depending on the type of MCO (46). Other authors used a study of group model HMOs to project the number of covered lives needed for each of a variety of specialists in nonrural areas. In that report, it was suggested that there was a need for one neurosurgeon for every 150,000 covered lives (47). More recently, a study of two staff model HMOs revealed a staffing ratio of 180 physicians per 100,000 enrollees, a number which is near the national average and far above the figures alluded to above (48). Other commentators have stated that this latter number is too high and does not represent the declining appeal of the staff model HMO and does not reflect the staffing requirements for the rapidly growing IPA model (49). In the marketplace, the MCO must balance between the lowest possible number of SPs required for the purposes of medical management and a somewhat higher number of SPs required for the purposes of access and marketing. The projections by Weiner and by Kronick et al. given above, therefore reflect the maximum efficient use of SPs and are not based on other real-world considerations. The MCO must provide good access to services by members and PCPs, thus improving satisfaction and retention of members and PCPs, and thus requires more SPs.

INTEGRATED HEALTH CARE DELIVERY SYSTEMS

Managed care has placed increasing pressures on health care providers both to reduce costs and to improve quality, as well as to find ways to protect their market share. The prospect of impending reform of the health care system, whether through regulatory reform or market-driven reform, provides even greater impetus for change. This has led to a still-evolving desire on the part of health care providers to become aligned. Such alignment provides, at least on a theoretical basis, greater economies of scale, the ability to deploy clinical resources most cost effectively, a greater ability to influence provider behavior, and greater negotiating strength (50). This is an area of continual evolution, as is managed care in general, so it is to be expected that some of the terms and definitions will change while the concepts will remain valid.

IDSs can be classified into three broad categories: systems in which physicians only are integrated, systems in which the physicians are integrated with facilities such as hospitals, and systems that include the insurance function as well as the other two functions (50). For a more complete discussion of this topic, a number of reviews have been listed (51–55) that will be of interest. IDSs also fall along a continuum, and as one proceeds from one end of the spectrum to the other, the degree of integration increases as does the capability of the organization to operate effectively in a managed care environment. It should be noted that the complexity of formation and operation, required capital investment, and political difficulties all increase from one end of

the continuum to the other as well. The primary political difficulty, at least in the systems that are tightly managed, is that all providers cannot participate. It can be assumed that the regulatory environment at the state and federal level will continue to evolve, which may alter the form and methods used in alignment, but not the need for IDSs (56–59).

At the low end of the spectrum, the IPA and its member physicians are at risk for at least some portion of medical costs in that, if the capitation payment is lower than the required reimbursement to the physicians, the member physicians must accept less income. It is this risk sharing that sets the IPA apart from a negotiating vehicle that does not bear risk.

The usual form of an IPA is that of an umbrella organization for participation in managed care by physicians in all specialties. Recently, however, IPAs that only represent a single specialty have emerged. These IPAs are not common, but the recent increase in vertical integration activities such as physician-hospital organizations has led to an increase in specialty capitation. The specialty IPA, operating like a standard IPA, accepts capitation from the HMO, but usually pays a modified fee-for-service schedule to the participating physicians. Capitation of individual SPs within the specialty IPA is possible, but is rarely seen, because specialty IPAs are often created to preserve the opportunity for multiple, unrelated SPs to participate with HMOs. Recently, in California, such an organization for neurosurgeons was formed and is now in full operation. A second IPA, which is made up of a wider variety of neuroscience providers including neurologists and neuroradiologists, has also recently been established and has begun receiving capitation payments from HMOs.

The early history of IPAs was varied, with a number going out of business. Recently, IPAs have enjoyed considerable success, particularly in the western United States. Hospitals usually have no role in IPAs, although some hospitals have begun sponsoring IPA development as an alternative to a PHO. The newly successful IPAs are those that allow more convenient geographic access, have succeeded in bearing risk, and have limited specialist membership. Also, in nonurban areas, they may be the only model available. They require much less capital to start and operate, and they may motivate their physicians more successfully than models that depend on salary. Later in this chapter, we will discuss the role of the IPA in the growing "virtual" integration of health-care systems.

It has been stated that the IPA is inherently unwieldy, because it is usually made up of a large number of independent physicians whose only commonality is the contracting vehicle of the IPA. Since an IPA may be initiated to preserve private practice, it also may have an inability to leverage resources, achieve economies of scale, or change behavior to the greatest degree possible. Also, many IPAs may contain a surplus of specialists, resulting in upward pressure on resource consumption.

The "expert" argument across the last several years was that the IPA was at a terminally competitive disadvantage against the more completely integrated group practices and staff models. However, this view has been shown to be incorrect. IPAs are proving the equal of other physician models in managing costs and attracting covered lives. Sudden market discipline has been displayed by some IPAs and their member physicians. These IPAs have instituted strong central government by fiat, reduced hospital utilization rates by 40%, decreased specialist utilization by 60%, and trebled their enrolled covered lives. The IPA, well managed, can be competitive and remain so across time (49).

Physician practice management (PPM) organizations are recent arrivals on the integration scene (60). Some have considered PPMs to be variants of management service organizations (MSOs), but unlike MSOs, which are usually a part of the vertical integration scheme between hospitals and physicians, PPMs are physician-only enterprises. The CEO of MedPartners/Mullikin, a large national PPM, has stated, "We built and designed a company specifically for the purpose of consolidating this industry (60)." In a melding of Wall Street and the physician's office, entrepreneurs have capitalized for-profit PPMs operating independently of hospitals. These most often have purchased physician practices, beginning with primary care groups, but including large specialty groups as well, and have signed multi-year contracts with those physicians (50). The physicians may be given varying degrees of equity participation in the PPM and a voice in governance. In some cases, the PPM may not offer equity to physicians, or it may offer equity only to those physicians who

are early participants. In other instances, equity is offered in exchange for the value of the acquired practice, but, in other cases, there is no equity offer, if cash is paid for the practice.

In general, the PPM provides management for all support functions (e.g., billing and collections, purchasing, negotiating contracts), but it remains relatively uninvolved with the clinical aspects of the practice. In many cases, the physician remains an independent practitioner, although the PPM owns all the tangible assets of the practice. The PPM usually takes a percentage of the practice revenue, often at a rate equal to or slightly below what the physician was already experiencing for overhead expense. The physician agrees to a long-term commitment, as well as noncompetition covenants. It is too early to enunciate clear advantages and disadvantages for PPMs. All practice acquisitions make the physician an employee, or employee-like, for many years; however, this brings with it all the attendant motivational concerns. It may be that the early success of PPMs is related to the virtue of an integrated delivery system that is physician-driven as opposed to hospital-driven or insurer-driven. This value derives in part from the fact that physicians control or direct between 75 and 90% of health resources consumed.

From its inception in 1988, PhyCor has appeared to be deliberate and discriminating in its growth strategy (60). It has looked for larger, stable group practices in nonmanaged care markets. PhyCor appears to be working diligently to prepare all their groups for managed care. One of their top priorities has been to install an information system to support management of capitation, adjudication and payment of claims, practice guidelines and protocols, physician profiling and outcomes management. In 1995, they started a pilot automated patient record system. They also initiated the PhyCor Institute for Healthcare Management, which provides an environment for affiliated physician group presidents, medical directors, managed care directors, and clinic directors to convene periodically for education, training, and practical exercises in medical management and associated information systems. They offer training in capitation, business management, clinical protocols, epidemiology, outcomes management, and leadership skills (60).

A variation on the comprehensive PPM is the specialty PPM, which has taken most of the comprehensive PPM features into consideration for a single specialty's market share preservation or expansion. The most common specialties involved are oncology and cardiology, and multistate networks are now in place. Other specialties, such as ophthalmology, orthopedics, radiology, anesthesiology and occupational medicine are also involved in this process. The future of the specialty PPM depends upon whether two conditions are met, however: first is the ability to bear financial risk, and second is the willingness on the part of the PPM's customers to deal with yet another carve-out vendor. The potential ability of a PPM to be successful may relate to the existence of the PPM network in a region before the HMO provider relations manager begins recruiting specialists. Thus, the in-place network could become the dedicated specialty network for the HMO. An HMO may also choose to use such a specialty PPM if it allows the HMO to improve quality and lower cost compared with using a less organized network of private specialists.

The primary advantage of a PPM is that its sole purpose is to manage physicians practices. This means that it will have, or will acquire, expertise that is not available from a hospital or a payer. Also the PPM has the ability to obtain substantial purchasing power through combining the needs of many physicians. The PPM can also provide a greater sense of ownership to the participating physicians in an equity model, thereby aligning incentives and goals.

The primary disadvantage is that the PPM may not achieve sufficient mass in the market to influence the course of events or negotiate favorable contracts. Also, physicians may chafe under the long terms required and may not change their practice habits sufficiently to be truly effective in managed care. This last issue is critical if the PPM is seen as a vehicle to negotiate fees rather than a system to lower costs and improve quality. It must be kept in mind that investor-owned PPMs are businesses that are expected to return a profit. If that profit does not materialize, it may be expected that investors will begin to demand action, some of which may not be palatable to participating physicians.

Group practice without walls (GPWW), sometimes known as the clinic without walls, is a significant step toward integration of physician services. The GPWW does not require the participation of a hospital. In some instances, GPWWs have been formed to leverage negotiating strength not only with MCOs, but with hospitals as well. The basic strategy is for private practice physicians to aggregate their practices into a single legal entity, with the physicians continuing to practice in their independent locations. Thus, from the point of view of the patient, the physician appears to be independent; however, from the vantage point of the contracting entity (usually an MCO), they are a single group. The GPWW is owned solely by the member physicians and not by any outside investors. The GPWW is a legal entity, merging all assets of the physicians' practices, rather than the acquisition of only the tangible assets. The governance of the GPWW is also by the physicians. It should be noted that, to be considered a medical group, the physicians must have their personal income affected by the performance of the group as a whole. The Sacramento-Sierra Medical Group in Sacramento, California was probably the first of these groups to be organized (61). The GPWW is not generally applicable to neurosurgery practices, except in large urban areas where several practices exist.

An advantage of the GPWW is that it has the legal ability to negotiate and commit to binding contract on behalf of all members of the group. Perhaps the key advantage is that income is affected by the performance of the group as a whole. Therefore, the GPWW has some ability to influence practice behavior. A member physician who practices in such a manner as to have an adverse affect on the group as a whole can be influenced by considerable peer pressure. The group can even expel a physician, if the problems are serious and remain uncorrected. The primary disadvantage of the GPWW is that the physicians essentially remain in independent practice. The ability of the group to manage practice behavior is therefore significantly limited. Thus, optimal efficiencies are not achieved. The GPWW may also face significant difficulties in obtaining new sources of capital for further growth and development. There are other controversies related to GPWW, which should be reviewed before entering into such an arrangement (62).

The term "consolidated medical group" or medical group practice, refers to a traditional structure in which physicians have combined their resources to be a true medical group practice. This entity has a strong appeal for neurosurgical practices or neuroscience providers.

Unlike the GPWW, the true medical group is located in a few sites and functions in a group setting. This means a great deal of interaction among members of the group and common goals and objectives for group success. The group is usually a partnership or professional corporation, although other forms are possible. The group can employ other physicians as well.

Medical groups have the ability to achieve substantial economies of scale, have strong negotiating leverage, and have the ability to influence physician behavior. Many times, groups are attractive to MCOs because they can deliver a large block of physicians with one contract and they also have the ability to manage their own resources. On the whole, medical groups are in a superior position to benefit from managed care, compared with many other models, certainly in comparison with independent private physicians. The disadvantages of medical groups are centered on management issues and the cultural mindset of the group. Such problems as uncontrolled overhead or poor utilization patterns can affect performance (50).

The PHO is an entity that, at a minimum, allows a hospital and its physicians to negotiate with third-party payers. PHOs may do little more than this, or they may actively manage the relationship between the providers and MCOs. They may provide other services, at which point they may look more like MSOs. At the lowest level, the PHO is considered a messenger model (63). This means that the PHO analyzes the terms and conditions offered by an MCO and transmits its analysis and the contract to each physician, who then individually decides whether to participate. PHOs are thought to be the first step on the evolutionary ladder to vertical integration for physicians and hospitals. Many times they are organized as a reaction to market forces from managed care. Some have stated that PHOs are an easy step in vertical integration, and, while providing some integration, they preserve the independence and autonomy of physicians. Many times, the formation of the PHO occurs at the hospital's behest; often as a defensive mechanism to deal with increased managed care contracting efforts in the community (50). There are two categories of PHOs, open and closed.

The open PHO is available to virtually any member of the hospital medical staff. Specialists usually dominate open PHOs. Many times, the specialists create the PHO, because they are worried that selective contracting by MCOs will reduce the business that, as a group, the specialists are doing. The political reality of an open PHO is that it is often difficult to bring sufficient discipline to bear on the medical staff members who wield significant influence. Also, the inability of the PHO to attend to the needs of the medical staff may lead to serious problems for hospital administrators charged with managing such organizations. Most commonly, physicians remain independent and contract as individuals with the PHOs, although they could be organized in IPAs or GPWWs.

The closed PHO proactively restricts physician membership. From a political vantage point, this is more difficult than an open model, but it carries more chance of success. Two general approaches have been used to limit membership to the PHO; membership is based either on specialty type or practice profiling. The limitation on the number of specialists is most often accomplished by projecting the covered lives that the PHO is expected to cover over a specified period, usually several years, and then by recruiting specialists according to predetermined ratios of numbers of specialists to enrollment size. The second type of limitation, based on practice profiling, is much more difficult to carry out for technical reasons. Some objective form of practice data is needed, and most organizations have no access to information adequate to perform this analysis. However, if the PHO has the ability to capture and analyze practice behavior and clinical quality data, then that data may be used to manage the physician membership and finally terminate those physicians who depart from the PHOs practice guidelines.

The singular advantage of a PHO is its ability to negotiate for a large group of physicians. The PHO may be an expeditious way to develop a delivery system. MCOs may find closed PHOs more to their liking than open PHOs. Many physicians may view the PHO as a facilitator to arrange for direct contracts with self-insured employers and with the Health Care Finance Administration (HCFA) for Medicare risk contracts. Theoretically, the PHO should be able to track and utilize data from the standpoint of UR (utilization review) and QA (quality assessment). More likely, this advantage will be found in a closed PHO, since it has greater control over a smaller number of physicians. Finally, the PHO may be the first step to greater integration between a hospital and its medical staff.

The primary disadvantage of the PHO is that it often fails to develop any improvement in contracting ability. MCOs may view these organizations as little more than a vehicle to keep their reimbursements high. PHOs may be at a disadvantage if the MCO does not want all the physicians in the PHO to be participating with the plan. Even closed PHOs may suffer from this problem if the MCOs wish to avoid contracting with certain physicians who are members of the PHO. Also, the PHO may be seen as a barrier to efficient communication with the physicians by the MCO. The PHO must have a strong story to tell about its ability to manage utilization, otherwise the MCO may believe it can do a better job itself. Because physicians who are members of a PHO remain, for the most part, completely independent, the PHO's effect on provider behavior is limited. This can have a direct bearing on UM and also impede changes the organization may need to make to prosper in the managed care environment (50).

Management service organizations (MSOs) represent the evolution of the PHO into an entity that provides additional services for the physicians. An MSO provides a means of negotiating with MCOs and also has support services for physician practices. The physician continues to be independent, however. MSOs are usually based upon a hospital or hospital system. The rationale for the formation of the MSO is similar to that for the PHO. In its simplest form, the MSO operates as a service bureau providing billing and collection, administrative support, electronic data interchange, such as electronic billing, and other services.

The MSO must receive compensation from the physician at fair market value to avoid legal problems for both the physician and the hospital (64). The MSO may, in addition to providing all services described above, purchase many of the assets of the physician's practice, including the office space or office equipment at fair market value. The MSO can serve as employer of the physician's office support staff as well. MSOs can also incorporate functions such as UM, provider relations, member services, and claims processing. The MSO does not usually have direct contracts with MCOs for two reasons. Many MCOs insist on the provider being the contracting agent, and some states do not allow MCOs to have contracts with an entity that does not have the legal authority to bind the provider (64).

The primary advantage of an MSO over a PHO is the ability of the MSO to build a closer relationship between the provider and the hospital. The MSO can bring economies of scale and management to the physician's office services, thus potentially lowering overhead costs. If the MSO provides more advanced functions, such as UM and claims processing, it has the potential ability to capture data regarding practice behavior that can be used to enable physicians to practice more cost effectively.

The disadvantages of an MSO are similar to those of a PHO. The physician remains an independent practitioner with the ability to change allegiance with relative ease. Also, if the MSO does not employ the physician, it has a limited handle to effect change or redeploy resources because of changing market priorities. Special problems may arise when an MSO purchases a physician's practice. These are the problems of the transaction being thought of as not-for-profit assets inuring to the benefit of the physician in an illegal fashion, and of fraud and abuse for federally funded patients (64).

A foundation model IDS is one in which a hospital creates a nonprofit foundation, which actually purchases physician practices, including tangible and intangible assets, such as good will. This model usually is seen when the hospital cannot employ the physicians directly or cannot use hospital funds to purchase practices (50, 65). A second form of foundation model is one in which the foundation is an entity that exists on its own and contracts with a medical group and a hospital. The foundation is governed by a board that is not dominated by either the hospital or the physicians. The intricacies of the foundation model are many and will not be discussed here, but the reader is referred to reference articles for further insights (65–68).

A major issue for all IDSs is the management of utilization of referral physicians and consultants. This is an area of importance to all types of MCOs, and the most successful physician organizations will be those that learn to manage utilization well. In most managed care health plans, the costs associated with nonprimary care professional services will be substantially greater than the cost of primary care services, often between 1.5 and 2.0 times as high (69). This is due to the increased fees associated with consultant services and to the hospital-intensive and procedure-oriented nature of those services.

In other words, more than half the costs of consultant services may be associated with hospital or procedural cases. Often overlooked are the associated utilization costs generated by consultants. It is not only the fees of the consultants themselves that add to the cost of care but also the cost of services ordered by consultants. One study, in a nonmanaged care environment, found that each referral from a PCP generated nearly $3,000 in combined hospital charges and professional fees within a 6-month period after the referral (70). It can easily be assumed that those costs are much higher now.

The consensus of opinion, until recently, held that regional health care markets will be dominated by large integrated delivery systems that offer a closed panel of providers. However, there is not universal consensus on that issue. Goldsmith has argued that many of the structurally rigid vertical integration models are not going to work (71). He has argued that success will be more likely with models of virtual integration, in which parties otherwise independent come together for the purpose of behaving like an IDS under managed care, but retain their own identities and missions. Goldsmith points out that the idea for ''integration'' in health care came from firms like General Motors, DuPont, and Standard Oil, who followed a common pattern— acquiring competing firms and integrating suppliers and distributors into their organizations, incorporating the middlemen and their profits into the larger organization. By coordinating the production and marketing of their goods, the large integrated firms created a crushing cost and service advantage over their less-integrated competitors, enabling those large firms to dominate their respective industries (71). He states that it is difficult to find hard evidence of economic advantage or market share accruing from similar system development in health care.

In virtual integration, each major segment of the health care enterprise acts in concert for a common cause, but none is an employee or subdivision of another. This allows each party to manage its own affairs and meet its own financial goals without being managed by another segment of the industry. In this model, there is greater horizontal integration, as, for example, between hospitals or between physicians, with each of these horizontally integrated systems forming relationships with other parts of the healthcare system.

In its classic form, virtual organizations are developed by integrating core competencies and resources around market opportunities (72). Typically, virtual organizations are held together by a system of agreements and protocols between the parties that outline responsibilities and contributions and align incentives that govern how each party will profit from their effort. Its main assets are information, people resources, and the capability to combine capital and knowledge assets quickly and inexpensively.

Goldsmith and others have concluded that a virtual organization may be a more appropriate vehicle on the road to successful integration (73, 74). As the result of a 4-year study of 11 large health systems, it was found that the upfront costs associated with creating a virtual organization were substantially less than alternative models (74).

Integrated health care systems combine health care delivery and financing under one-umbrella organization. The larger organization owns, or sometimes contracts, for all elements of the health care system, including physicians, hospitals, nursing homes, ambulatory surgery centers, and other components of the system. A vertically integrated system is one that coordinates all the components of service that it needs to deliver health care under one ''organizational roof.'' Virtually integrated organizations, however, distinguish themselves from traditional capital-intensive structural organizations by creating a network of partners with different or complementary services and competencies. These virtual organizations attempt to act in a central and coordinated manner, but tend to stay away from the outright purchase or merger of their partners. ''The virtual organization emphasizes coordination through patient-management agreements, provider incentives and information systems, rather than investing in ownership and building all elements from scratch or through merger (72).'' Examples of applications of virtual health care systems are seen throughout the United States today (72).

More recently, it has been stated that: ''The reality is that employers and consumers are asking the health care system for something very different, a seemingly incongruous mixture of broad choice and economic discipline (47).'' The authors add that closed panels offer consumers and providers no real benefits.

The recent experience and actions taken by

historically integrated health systems suggest they understand the potential advantages of a virtually integrated system. Kaiser-Permanente, for example, has demonstrated that it can improve its cost structure, enhance quality through consolidation of volume, and improve access by developing strategic partnerships with community hospitals and hospital systems, in lieu of building new proprietary hospitals in its key markets. Kaiser has also introduced external physician networks in selected markets in order to support expansion and higher-choice products such as POS. Family Health Plan (FHP) divested its hospitals and staff physician organization, but through its successor, PacifiCare, continues to maintain a contractual relationship with its former provider entities. Harvard/Pilgrim is reassessing the role and relationships it wants to maintain with its staff model health centers. Several other integrated health systems are also reevaluating the relationship between the physician group and the health plan (75).

CONTRACTING AND REIMBURSEMENT

Contracting is the starting point for physician participation in managed care. Participation is not automatic; physicians must apply for and be accepted into the managed care family. Initial stages of contracting can be a surprising and unpleasant experience for physicians unused to discussing long and seemingly overcomplicated personal service documents. These documents may go into the smallest details and contain clauses that physicians may consider inappropriate, insulting, oppressive, prying, and downright absurd (38). The most important thing to remember, and the most difficult hurdle for a physician to clear, in entering into a managed care agreement, is that he or she will lose a certain amount of freedom of independent action, as will the patients in managed care. There is a subtle, but critical, difference between the supervised control that is managed care and the total control that is traditional medicine.

Keep in mind that managed-care physicians are always playing by someone else's rules and on the "other guy's" home field. The manner in which physicians receive and refer patients will be drastically changed. The practice may be subject to the inquiring eyes of the health care plan, IPA medical directors, utilization/quality assurance review boards, state and federal regu-

latory agencies, and even health care plan committees made up of enrollees and consumer affairs staff—and physicians will be contractually bound by the findings of those committees.

Virtually everything good or bad in managed care is a direct result of how well physicians negotiate agreements that they did not have to worry about in the "good old days." Thus, a necessary, but difficult, consequence of the rapidly changing face of health care is that physicians are having to learn to deal with new issues: contract analysis and negotiation. Particularly in the managed care arena, these acts have such an influence on success or failure that physicians can no longer pay only passing attention to contractual terms and payment methodologies.

In the past it was common for a physician to review a contract by turning to the end, looking at the discounted fee-for-service reimbursement schedule and making a decision to sign or not based on how closely the proposed fees approached usual and customary figures. The very nature of the document—long, convoluted, and full of terminology that even the physician's personal attorney might not understand—should have encouraged careful review, but did not. Now times have changed and so have the rules of the game. With fixed prepayments and risk-shifting more the rule than the exception, physicians must conduct a careful review of every page, every paragraph, every term of any proposed managed care agreement. Entering into any agreement without careful personal review and review by qualified legal counsel is an open invitation to disaster.

Keep in mind there is no such thing as a "standard" managed care agreement. Although contract language will be state-specific and health-care-plan-specific, managed care agreements generally follow one of two formats: one designed for a modified fee-for-service arrangement and one covering capitation. In any contract analysis, it is important to know which conditions or terms are negotiable and which are not, including certain language specific to federal or state regulation that cannot be modified. One must attempt to modify or delete sections including terminology indicating that the physician holds the health care plan "harmless." Such a stipulation may actually negate some or all of the physician's malpractice coverage. In any contract discussion involving multiple independent practices, care should be taken to avoid any issues that might be considered to be inappropriate—for example, group agreement on individual fees or the group holding out for a particular fee (76). For a full discussion of contracts and contracting issues, the reader may refer to a list of references (38, 77–84) dealing with these issues.

Of particular concern are professional liability issues in managed care. Clearly, increased accountability will be required from managed care plans through reporting on quality assurance systems, patient satisfaction, and patient care outcomes. A recent review details the techniques now in use for holding managed care organizations accountable for quality, ranging from those grounded in the law to more market-based approaches (85). These trends will increase the emphasis on the ways physicians are selected, retained, and monitored, as well as the manner in which utilization review systems are designed and implemented. Moreover, the effect of provider payment systems on the quality of care in managed care environments is likely to receive more attention (86).

A health plan can be held vicariously liable for the negligent acts of an independent contracting provider, if the provider is reasonably perceived by the plan member as the plan's apparent or ostensible agent (87). HMOs that use limited panels of contracting providers who are licensed to provide or arrange care and that use capitation payment systems may be more vulnerable to ostensible agency claims than more open-panel, fee-for-service PPO programs. Negligence might also be alleged against a health plan if it did not properly credential its physicians, since physician credentialing is the HMO's corporate responsibility (87).

Health plans may be held liable for the alleged malpractice of contracting physicians on the theory that the physician-incentive payment system used by the plan contributed to the malpractice. Even though many courts recognize physician risk sharing and incentive payments as valid and central components of managed care, the use of excessive financial incentives could possibly be a basis for both physician and plan liability, when negligent treatment occurs (86).

The plan's conduct of its utilization review program may also be the basis for liability. Similarly, a physician who fails to provide needed care because of the plan's contrary utilization review decision may also face liability. Two key cases in California underscore how important it is for a physician to actively protest any of the payer's medical necessity determinations with which the physician disagrees (88, 89). Physician responsibilities vis-a-vis patient care cannot be limited by any health plan protocols. Ultimately, if required care is withheld, the physician may be responsible for the outcome, despite the protocols imposed by the health plan. In addition, the payer can be held liable when utilization review processes and criteria are negligently designed or implemented. In any event, physicians contracting with managed care plans should understand and exercise any appeal rights available under the health plan's utilization review program (86).

Utilization management (UM) and quality assurance (QA) should, therefore, be of concern to every physician during the contract review process. Since there will probably be prospective, concurrent, and retrospective review of the care rendered, it is vital that physicians know exactly who will conduct such a review and how it will be accomplished. There must be reasonable and efficient mechanisms for appeal. The contract should specifically state how the results of UM/QA are communicated to the patient. In many circumstances, the specifics of UM/QA are detailed in a document "incorporated by reference" into the contract. Obtain a copy and review it carefully before signing (38). Anything incorporated by reference is an integral part of the agreement and is, therefore, the physician's responsibility to know about. Such reference documents may contain very specific and important obligations that could cause much distress if they come as a future surprise.

Another issue of extreme concern to physicians are contract clauses that may require the physician to hold the MCO harmless and indemnify the MCO for claims or liabilities made against the MCO for the failures of the physician, such as malpractice or other types of negligence (79). Do not sign any agreement with a clause requiring you to indemnify anyone without checking with your malpractice carrier first. Some malpractice insurance carriers will protect a physician for malpractice in the context of services provided to an MCO. Others will not provide coverage for this type of "contracted" liability. It is essential to determine whether your malpractice carrier will cover you for this agreement (79). Also, if you perform any administrative functions for the MCO, such as utilization review, including denial notices or function as medical director, be sure that the MCO has insurance protecting you for those administrative functions and check with your own insurer to determine whether your insurance will protect you if you indemnify for these functions.

The other aspect of "hold harmless" clauses in MCO contracts that physicians cannot abrogate are those that state that the physicians will not charge the MCO member anything for covered services other than applicable copayments and deductibles. In other words, the physician "holds harmless" and indemnifies the member for any and all charges if the health plan ultimately fails to pay the bill. In most MCO contracts, one cannot negotiate on this provision (38).

Defining the scope of services provided is an important issue for specialists, such as neurosurgeons, when negotiating managed care contracts. Unless specifically stated otherwise in the agreement, usually as a limitation or exclusion, assume that everything is covered and that you are obligated to perform the services or to arrange for another physician to perform them. Two questions should immediately come to mind: "Will I be obligated to deliver services I am not prepared to deliver or have not subcontracted? If I do deliver the services will I bankrupt my practice?" (38).

One section of most contracts identifies the term of the contract and the term of any subsequent contract renewals. Many contracts have automatic renewal provisions if no party exercises its right to terminate. Providers should give careful thought to the length of the contract and the renewal periods. The automatic renewal of a contract is often referred to as an "evergreen clause." This provision can be beneficial if things are going well, as physicians have a lock-in for continued participation. If things are not progressing well, one could be forced to endure an unacceptable situation for another year or more. Physicians should seek to have automatic renewal included in any agreement, but with provisions for renegotiation before the renewal date as well as some acceptable termination-without-cause language (38).

Termination provisions fall into two categories: termination without cause, and termination with cause (77, 90). Termination refers to contractual provisions that permit parties to end the

relationship at an earlier date, during the term of the contract. Many managed care contracts provide that either party can terminate the arrangement "without cause" or "without cause or penalty." Typically, this can be done at any time after giving an advance written notice to the nonterminating party or at regular intervals by written notice before the contract anniversary or renewal date. The provider as well as the MCO should have this right in any contract, with a 90-day notice period being fairly common. As the term implies, "termination without cause" means that the party invoking termination cannot, in normal circumstances, be made to state any reason for ending the relationship. It is not even necessary for the party to have a reason. The value to the managed care plan of this type of clause is that the MCO need not defend a challenge by the provider on the substantive issue of whether the grounds were met. The value to the physician is that an unsatisfactory arrangement can be concluded earlier than the contract term. Many states, either by statute or by judicial interpretation, will not permit a party to exercise a right to terminate a contract without cause, if it can be shown that the terminating party in effect had a prohibited motive for the termination, as in the form of retaliation or prohibited discrimination (90).

Physicians who advocate for medically appropriate health care for their patients are now protected from retaliation by MCOs. Some states may have statutes that give a physician a right to recover damages if a health organization terminates employment or a contract or otherwise penalizes a physician in retaliation against the physician's efforts to challenge decisions, policies, or practices that impair the physician's ability to provide medically appropriate health care to his or her patients (90). For example, California statutes hold that penalizing for advocating for medically appropriate health care violates public policy. Although the MCO is not prohibited from deciding not to pay for a particular medical treatment, nor for conducting necessary peer or utilization review, these laws provide an important protection for physicians who face retaliatory activities by MCOs (91).

In general, "termination for cause" consists of a failure of some required condition of the contractual relationship, such as the licensure of the HMO or the physician, or the occurrence of some other event that qualifies as a "material breach'' of the contract. A material breach is generally a failure of one party to comply with a contractual requirement that is not merely technical, but rather goes to the basic noncompliance of the party with the requirements of the agreement (90). The grounds specified for termination for cause fall into two general categories. The first, such as loss of a license, is not subject to remedy. The second category, a more general description of a material breach, can be remedied within a stated period of time during which the party receiving the notice can still maintain the contract in force.

An essential part of each managed care agreement is the mode of compensation for the physician. The payment structure of the agreement often represents the most important provision for the provider and the managed health care plan. The payment terms are frequently set forth in an exhibit appended to the contract and are cross-referenced in the body of the agreement. From the provider's perspective there needs to be a clear understanding of what is necessary for a service to be authorized. If the provider submits a claim to the MCO, the contract should set out the manner in which the claim is to be made and the type of information to be included with the claim. The agreement should also obligate the provider to submit claims within a specified period and obligate the MCO to pay claims within a certain number of days (38).

The most complex aspects of provider contracts are often risk-sharing arrangements. Risk can be shared with providers in varying degrees depending on the initial amount of risk transferred, the services for which the provider is at risk, and whether the MCO offers stop-loss protection. Risk pools with complicated formulas determining distributions are often used both where services are capitated and when payments are based on a fee schedule. The primary objective of these arrangements is to create incentives to discourage unnecessary utilization (77, 92).

The reimbursement of specialist physicians can be thought of in the context of the relationship between the MCO and the provider. It is possible that a contracting entity, such as an IPA, an MSO, or a PHO may accept reimbursement from a plan but compensate individual physicians in a separate manner; for example, the IPA receives a capitated payment, or a percentage of premium, but pays the specialist on a modified fee for service agreed to in the provider's contract (93). Approximately 20 to 30% of HMO specialists were paid through capitation as the predominant form of reimbursement in 1994 (94, 95). That percentage had not changed significantly two years later (96). The majority of specialists are paid through fee-for-service, the rest by other mechanisms, such as salary, retainer, hourly, and so forth (94).

The simplest arrangement to understand, although not a highly satisfactory one for an MCO, is straight fee for service (FFS) The specialist sends a claim and the plan pays it. Then why should the MCO bother to contract at all if it is simply paying like an insurance plan? The answer is to get the specialist physician to agree to the National Association of Insurance Commissioners (NAIC) sole source of payment clause (97). Although not a preferred arrangement from the point of view of the MCO, it is, occasionally, all the managed care plan can get, particularly in high cost specialties, or when there are no good alternatives, or in small start-up plans without significant enrollment (98).

Another simple arrangement is discounted FFS. Two variations are commonly seen: a straight discount on charges, such as 20%, and a discount based on volume or a sliding scale. In the latter arrangement, the degree of discount is based on an agreed set of figures. For example, for a neurosurgeon who performs 0 to 5 neurosurgical procedures per year there is a 10% discount, for 6 to 10 per year there is a 15% discount, and so forth. Some plans combine a discount scheme with a fee maximum. The fee maximum is a fee allowance schedule; the plan pays the lesser of the specialist's discounted charges or the maximum allowance.

The most common form of FFS is the relative value scale, such as the resource-based relative value scale (RBRVS), or a fee allowance schedule. The RBRVS fee schedule, originally adopted by the HCFA, is now employed by many private payers and by physician groups (99). The difference between a relative value scale and a fee allowance schedule is that, in the former, each procedure is assigned a relative value, usually on the basis of current procedural terminology revision 4 (CPT-4) (100). The value is multiplied by another figure, the conversion factor (specified in dollars), to arrive at a payment. The contract should specify the amount of the conversion factor and the version of the CPT-4 that is being used. Rather than negotiate separate fees, one negotiates the conversion factor. In a fee allowance schedule, the fees for procedures, again on the basis of the CPT-4, are explicitly defined in the contract. The specialist agrees to accept those fees as full payment unless the discounted charges are less than the fee schedule, in which case, the plan pays the lesser of the two. The majority of MCOs that use FFS use the RBRVS, and the majority of those set the conversion factor somewhat higher than those used by Medicare (94). However, in competitive managed care markets, conversion factors are used that are somewhat less than Medicare. The advantage for the MCO, of RBRVS or a fee allowance schedule, is the avoidance of fee hikes, but they do not put the provider at risk.

One common risk adjustment is the withhold. A withhold is simply a percentage, typically 5 to 20%, of the fee which is withheld every month and used to pay for cost overruns in utilization (101). The withhold amount is held by the plan and used at year end for reconciliation of cost overruns. The agreement must specify how, when, and under what conditions any such reserves are distributed. Physicians should be concerned that the agreement specifies if the withholds are the limit of each physician's risk or if the physician can be held financially responsible for losses in excess of his or her withhold. If the latter is the case, there must be limits, and those limits can be covered with special insurance. If utilization does not exceed projections, and if the plan costs are within budget, some or all of the withhold is returned to the physician. Physicians must take special measures to account for withholds so that they actually know the amount of withhold funds owed to them at the end of each contract year (38).

A variation on FFS is the global rate, flat rate, or case rate. These all represent single fees that are paid for a procedure, and the fee is the same regardless of how much or how little time and effort are expended. The most common example of this is in obstetrics, where plans use the same flat rate for either a vaginal delivery or a cesarean section, thereby eliminating any financial incentive to perform one or the other (102). Related to the flat rate is the global fee. A global fee is a flat rate that encompasses more than a single type of service. For example, a global fee for surgery may include all preoperative and postoperative care as well as follow-up office visits. Global fees must be carefully defined in the provider contract, as to what they include and what may be billed outside them.

Bundled case rates refer to a reimbursement that combines both the institutional and the professional charges into a single payment. For example, a plan may negotiate a bundled case rate of $15,000 for lumbar disk surgery. That fee covers the charges from the hospital, the surgeon, the anesthesiologist, as well as preoperative and postoperative care, including any preoperative imaging that may be required. Bundled case rates sometimes have outlier provisions for cases that become catastrophic and grossly exceed expected utilization. Bundled payment arrangements for neurosurgical services have been established in some mature managed care markets (Lanman, T., personal communication, 1997.).

Although only 20 to 30% of HMOs use capitation as the predominant form of reimbursement to specialists, a much higher percentage of plans do use capitation to reimburse individual specialties. The majority of HMOs have stated that they plan to increase the use of specialty capitation (94). Capitation refers to a fixed payment per-member per-month (PMPM) for services. This is the monthly fee physicians will be paid prospectively for each eligible enrollee assigned to the practice. Payments are made each month whether the enrollee presents for services or not, but the amount physicians are paid is all they get, and physicians must provide or arrange for the provision of all covered services regardless of cost, duration or frequency. The capitation payment may be adjusted for age, sex, and type of service. The expected volume of services must be calculated along with the average cost of providing those services. The providers ability to control utilization must be factored in, and the negotiating strength of the provider(s) also plays a major role in arriving at adequate capitation fees. The provider may have past data from the practice to guide these calculations, or may need to rely on an actuary, or a best guess, to derive the correct capitation amount.

The numbers involved in specialty capitation are often much smaller for any given specialty than those for primary care. For example, PCP capitation may average $14.00 PMPM, while the capitation rate for neurosurgery may range from $.07 to $1.20 PMPM. Thus, adjustments based on demographic variables become very small and may not be worth considering. Because the capitation fees are smaller, a specialist, such as a neurosurgeon, requires a much larger number of members for capitation to have any meaning. Where a PCP may achieve stability in capitation at a membership level of 1000 to 1500 a neurosurgeon may require 50,000 or more enrollees to avoid the problem of random chance having more effect than medical management on utilization.

The easiest form of specialty capitation is through organized medical groups, in which case it is assumed that any member assigned to a PCP in that group will likewise be assigned to the specialists in the group. Specialty-specific IPAs are not common, but interest in them is growing. The specialty IPA, as noted previously, operates like a standard IPA and accepts capitation from the MCO but usually pays discounted FFS to the participating specialists. The specialty IPA can also offer bundled services to add value to their managed care contracts. Capitation of individual specialists within the specialty IPA is certainly possible, but it is not often seen because the specialty IPA is established to enhance the opportunity for multiple, unrelated specialists to participate with aggressive HMOs.

Carve-outs are another issue to consider when negotiating a capitated contract. A carve-out is a particular service that the specialist does not include in the capitation rate. For example, neurosurgeons may capitate for all services except trauma care, for which they might negotiate a specified discount on fee-for-service charges. One might seek to carve-out a service since it may be difficult to estimate the actual incidence of service or the population involved. A variation on the carve-out issue arises when the provider cannot handle all services. The provider must negotiate the terms of the contract so that services that are referred out because he/she can truly not perform them are not deducted from the pool of capitation funds.

Often the capitation of specialists individually is impractical. It is difficult to "parcel out" enrolled covered lives to individual specialists in advance of need for specialty care. Receiving capitation for a small number of covered lives creates excessive actuarial risk for the majority of specialists. At the same time, a common dilemma faced by most MCOs is that the specialists control the majority of health system expenditures, yet have no incentive to decrease cost

under FFS, and gatekeepers and utilization review go only so far in reducing costs without specialist cooperation. An inadequate, but all too common, solution is to capitate a specialty department. The funds are then divided among individuals based upon proportion of claims submitted (41). This is an incentive to maximize fees in order to capture a greater share of the dollars. This often leads to higher costs because of overutilization of inpatient and ancillary services. At the same time, incentive for the individual specialist to "churn," that is, do more procedures and schedule more repeat visits, leads to greater and greater discount for all specialists in the department. Although division of specialty department capitation by production may motivate "gaming" to maximize share of income, the effects of this can be greatly diminished in tightly-knit specialty groups where department capitation may be an adequate solution.

With this in mind, a handful of IPAs are giving individual specialists incentive to eliminate unnecessary costs through *contact capitation*; that is, a capitated specialty budget is divided among physicians by the number of referrals that each receives. The payment covers all professional care within that specialty for a set period of time (41). The strength of contact capitation is the ability to bring cost containment incentives to the individual level without the difficulties inherent in true capitation; incentive to conduct unnecessary procedures is eliminated as well as the bulk of downstream costs.

There are two key elements to contact capitation. First, the IPA capitates the specialty department and awards the individual specialist one point for each referral; that is to say, physicians share in the specialty capitation budget in proportion to points earned. Second, the specialist provides all care within the specialty for a set period. That period is determined by the likely length of the episode of care for the average condition within that specialty. The author's experience has been that one year is the typical period used for neurosurgery. Contact capitation has been recommended as an effective partner to primary care cost reduction incentives and, according to some, is the best way to reduce utilization costs that the PCPs are not qualified to eliminate (41). There is compelling evidence of immediate and large cost reductions with the introduction of contact capitation. It is clear that contact capitation is the superior means of specialist compensation for IPAs, but it is also good for groups as well. High productivity is motivated in the group setting while breaking the proceduralist culture common to groups under FFS. Contact capitation is said to be particularly effective in high-cost specialties, such as orthopedics, where physicians have significant discretion over care costs. However, in specialties with low discretion and in specialties that generate few costs, contact capitation will likely do little for cost savings and may put specialists at unnecessary risk (41).

SPECIALTY NETWORKS

As managed care grows more dominant in today's markets, purchasers of health care services are increasingly concerned about the value they are receiving for their dollars. Astute purchasers have begun to examine and question variations in cost, treatment, and outcome among providers, and there is now explicit data to assist them in the process (103). The frustration common to both purchasers and providers is the difficulty of demonstrating the relationship of quality and value with the provision of health services. Pressures for accountability are mounting on providers. As a result, specialists are struggling with the challenge of providing services for less money in a system that once rewarded them based primarily on production; that is, volume and the number of procedures.

The demands of managed care organizations, insurers, and other purchasers on providers to improve health care services without raising prices are changing the roles of specialists and primary care physicians. The PCP assumes the role of risk manager, in many instances, when the patient first approaches the provider group. Specialists, like PCPs, are being asked to assume at least a portion of the economic responsibility of caring for a certain population by furnishing services on a discounted fee-for-service basis or in a capitated arrangement with a MCO. This has led, in some instances, to deselection of specialists, particularly if panels are large (41). Those most likely not to be asked back are specialists with consistent patterns of overutilization, low volume, or no observable commitment to managed care objectives (104).

In those areas where managed care is limited, neurosurgeons continue to be sanguine about their practices. But time is fleet-footed. Neurosurgeons, everywhere, need to assess their market conditions. Every area is different in terms of demographics, psychographics, health care demand and supply, and degrees of managed care competition and penetration. Even so, the number of markets is growing where managed care penetration has precipitously increased or is expected to increase. For example, recent data from the St. Louis area demonstrates that HMO membership has increased 30%, and has achieved a relatively high penetration of 28 to 33%, in just 6 months (105). Similar numbers are seen in Pittsburgh and Tampa (105).

Specialists in general, and perhaps neurosurgeons in particular, have not been generally proactive in changing their practices to fit the times. Neurosurgeons must get organized, develop single specialty networks, develop capitated programs that include risk assessment, demand management, disease management, treatment protocols, outcomes measurement, and both cost and clinical results reporting. Even where managed care has made inroads, physicians don't have to abandon their single specialty practices (106). They need, however, to conduct a situation assessment that will enable them to identify the competition and evaluate their strengths and weaknesses; they need to understand the concern of insurers, managed care organizations, and employers, to determine the level of commitment and interest of network physicians, to understand the needs of PCPs, and to identify other specialty providers offering similar services (107). A market assessment should follow to determine the attitude of payers toward specialty providers and the volume of specialty services utilized. Consideration must also be given to the extent of current competition and the likelihood of increased competition as other physicians form group practices.

To satisfy payers, specialty networks must be focused on becoming effective in terms of quality and outcomes. Single specialty groups also may have lower overhead than multispecialty groups and as a result may be able to deliver lower costs. Whether HMOs and primary care groups will continue to be attracted to single specialty groups in the future is hard to tell. But specialty carve-outs and subcapitation appears to be a growing trend (107). Certainly, groups are better at managing the risk under these arrangements than are solo practitioners. An alternative is simply to absorb the specialists and develop multispecialty groups that can go at risk under global capitation arrangements. But many specialists, it seems, are developing or joining larger networks of their peers. Some of these networks are only designed to enter into risk contracts, while others are more fully integrated and are managed by emerging publicly owned practice management companies. In a few short years, an entire industry has developed. Local networks are also forming in heavy managed care areas with the goal of obtaining carve-out arrangements for entire regions. Some of these networks involve setting up physician-owned MSOs. Others involve IPAs.

Are single specialty neurosurgery groups the answer? They're vastly superior to private solo practice in their ability to deal with managed care. Their success, however, will depend on how they relate to managed care organizations. In the short term, those groups with the lowest prices will probably get the contracts. Over the long term, single specialty groups will need disease management programs with full information systems support. They will need to consolidate their administrative costs and streamline clinical practice costs. Single specialty groups won't succeed as unions or cartels, only as the best solution to the medical cost, quality, and access equation.

CONCLUSION

There is a strong sense of optimism in some quarters about the private sector's ability to continue to ratchet down health care spending. But this optimism must be tempered by a realization of social and cultural problems that have not been addressed. While managed care has been the primary force behind price stabilization, in order for these levels to continue, the future for health care in this country is likely to mean closed provider panels, capitated contracts, sole-source contracting and large integrated systems. Yet the public wants more choice and no restriction on service utilization. There is intense pressure to open physician panels and introduce point-of-service plans that allow patients to go outside prescribed physician networks.

The managed care market remains unstable, with premiums dropping and costs rising and investment capital fleeing to more profitable sectors. And the problem of the uninsured continues to worsen. Some have predicted a return to a single payer system as the problem of uninsurance again creeps up "high into the middle class." Consumers in this market-based system are going to be given more control over the purchasing of their health care plans with the advent of medical savings accounts, Medicare HMO options, and even voucher systems. But the information needed to make such informed decisions is often limited, not standardized, or objective, and generally incomprehensible to the lay public. The result is that for most purchasers, whether employers or individuals, price continues to be the primary factor in plan choice. According to recent surveys, growing numbers of seniors are unwilling to join managed care plans and, in the near term, the Medicare Hospital Insurance Trust Fund may not be able to support mandated pay-out levels as early as mid-2000 (108). The mixed message is that for the strong, the current changes in the health-care marketplace offer opportunity and growth; for the weak, it can end the "safety net." The trip is not over.

REFERENCES

1. Dasco ST, Dasco CC. Introduction to managed care. In: Dasco ST, Dasco CC. Managed Care Answer Book. New York: Panel Publishers, 1997:1–25.
2. Hughes EFX. The ascendancy of management: National health care reform, managed competition and its implications for physician executives. In: New Leadership in Healthcare Management. The Physician Executive. Tampa, FL: American College of Physician Executives, 1994.
3. Eddy DM. Balancing cost and quality in fee-for-service versus managed care. Health Aff 1997;16:162–173.
4. Jensen CA, Morrisey MA, Gaffney S, Liston DK. The new dominance of managed care. Insurance trends in the 1990s. Health Aff 1997;16:125–136.
5. Health care megatrends, 1997. In: Cochrane JE, ed. Integrated Healthcare Report. Lake Arrowhead, CA: December 1996/January 1997.
6. Fox CD. An overview of managed care. In: Kongstvedt PR, ed. The managed health are handbook. 3rd ed. Gaithersburg, MD: Aspen, 1996;3–15.
7. Hamer R. HMO Industry Report. Interstudy Competitive Edge. 1995:5(1)1–105.
8. Health care megatrends, 1997. In: Cochrane JE, ed. Integrated Healthcare Report. Lake Arrowhead, CA: December 1996/January 1997.
9. Gabel J. Ten ways HMOs have changed during the 1990s. Health Aff. 1997;16:134–145.
10. Abbey FB. Managed care and health care reform. Evolution or revolution? In: Kongstvedt PR, ed. The managed health care handbook. 3rd ed. Gaithersburg, MD: Aspen, 1996:16–32.
11. Etheredge L, Jones SB, Lewin L. What is driving health system change? Health Aff 1996;15:93–104.

12. Helms RB, ed. American health policy. Competition and controls. Washington DC: American Enterprise Institute Press, 1993.

13. Mayer TR, Mayer GG. HMOs: Origin and development. N Engl J Med 1985;312:590–594.

14. MacLeod GK. An overview of managed care. In: Kongstvedt PR, ed. The managed health care handbook, 2nd ed. Gaithersburg, MD: Aspen, 1993:3–11.

15. Starr P. The social transformation of American medicine. New York: HarperCollins, 1982.

16. MacColl WA. Group practice and prepayment of medical care. Washington DC: Public Affairs Press, 1966.

17. Stumpf GB. Historical evolution and political process. In: Mackie DL, Decker DK, eds. Group and IPA HMOs. Gaithersburg, MD: Aspen, 1981, 17–36.

18. Penner MJ. Capitation in California. A study of physician organizations managing risk. Chicago IL: Health Administration Press, 1997.

19. Soper MR, Stallmeyer JM, Bopp KD, Wood MB. Balancing the triad: Cost containment, quality of service and quality of care. Kansas City: National Center for Managed Health Care Administration, 1995.

20. Spies JJ. Alternative health care delivery systems: HMOs and PPOs. In: Fox, PD, ed. Health care cost management: Private sector initiatives. Ann Arbor MI: Health Administration Press, 1984, 43–68.

21. Kongstvedt PR. Using data in medical management in managed care. In Kongstvedt, PR, ed. The managed health care handbook. 3rd ed. Gaithersburg, MD: Aspen, 1996, 440–452.

22. Hughes RG, Lee, DE. Using data describing physician inpatient practice patterns. Issues and opportunities. Health Care Manage Rev J 1991;16:33–40.

23. Reese R. Information systems: Operations and organization structures. In: Kongstvedt, PR, ed. The managed health care handbook, 3rd ed. Gaithersburg, MD: Aspen, 1996: 455–468.

24. Starr P. Smart technology. Stunted policy. Developing health information networks. Health Aff 1997;16: 91–105.

25. Patterns in HMO enrollment. Washington DC: Group Health Association of America, 1995.

26. Lamphere JA, Neuman P, Langwell K, Sherman D. The surge in Medicare managed care: An update. Health Aff 1997;16:127–133.

27. Congressional Budget Office. Jan 1, 1997.

28. O'Kane M. External accreditation of managed care plans. In Kongstvedt PR, ed. The managed health care handbook. 3rd ed. Gaithersburg, MD: Aspen, 1996:593–607.

29. Iglehart JK. The national committee for quality assurance. N Engl J Med 1996;335:995–999.

30. Epstein D. Performance reports on quality, prototypes, problems and prospects. N Engl J Med 1995;333: 57–61.

31. Inglehart JD. The national committee for quality assurance. N Engl J Med 1996; 335:995–999.

32. Guide to accreditation. Washington DC: American Association of Health Plans, 1996.

33. Kenkel P. The new HEDIS: Boon or burden? Health Sys Rev. 1996;29:17–19.

34. Kassirer JR. The quality of care and the quality of measuring it. N Engl J Med 1993;329:263–265.

35. Coile RC. The five stages of managed care. Strategies for providers, HMOs and suppliers. Chicago IL: Health Administration Press, 1997.

36. Rosenblatt RA. Cost of health care for state's big firms falls 2.5% in 1996. The honeymoon for premium rate cuts may be coming to an end, however. Los Angeles Times. January 21, 1997.D:1.

37. Wagner ER. Types of managed care organizations. In: Kongstvedt PR, ed. The managed health care handbook. 3rd ed. Gaithersburg, MD: Aspen, 1996: 33–45.

38. Kusske JA, ed. Managed care handbook for neurological surgeons. Park Ridge IL: American Association of Neurological Surgeons, 1994.

39. Health care megatrends 1997 In: Cochrane JE, ed. Integrated healthcare report. Lake Arrowhead, CA: December 1996/January 1997.

40. Wilmes AL. Preparing neurosurgeons for capitation: Managed care survival for neurosurgeons. Professional development program. Boston: American Association of Neurological Surgeons. Nov. 11, 1995.

41. To the greater good. Recovering the American physician enterprise . Washington DC: The Advisory Board Company, 1995:83–100.

42. Specialist survival strategies. In: Cochrane JE, ed. Integrated Healthcare Report. Lake Arrowhead, CA: November 1996.

43. Francesconi GA. ERISA preemption of "any willing provider" laws. An essential step toward national health care reform. Washington Univ Law Q 1995; 73.

44. Any willing provider. In: Cochrane JE, ed. Integrated Healthcare Report. Lake Arrowhead, CA: April 1995.

45. Kopit WG, Bouton AB. Antitrust implications of provider exclusion. In: Kongstvedt, PR, ed. The managed health care handbook. 3rd ed. Gaithersburg MD. Aspen: 1996:906–929.

46. Weiner JD. Forecasting the effects of health reform on U.S. physician workforce. Evidence from HMO staffing patterns. J Am Med Ass 1994;272:222–230.

47. Kronick R, Goodman DC, Wennberg J. Wagner E. The marketplace in healthcare reform. The demographic limitations of managed competition. N Engll J Med 1993;328:148–151.

48. Hart LG et al. Physician staffing ratios in staff model HMOs. A cautionary tale. Health Aff 1997;16: 55–70.

49. Mullan F. Iconoclasm and physician workforce research. Health Aff 1997;16:87–90.

50. Kongstvedt PR, Plocher DW. Integrated healthcare delivery systems. In: Kongstvedt PR, ed. The handbook of managed health care. 3rd ed. Gaithersburg, MD: Aspen, 1996:46–65.

51. Beckham JD. Redefining work in the integrated delivery system. Healthcare Forum J 1995;May/June: 76–82.

52. Burns IR, Thorpe DP. Trends and models in physician-hospital organizations. Health Care Manage Rev J 1993;18:7–20.

53. Conrad D, Hoare G, eds. Strategic alignment in managing integrated health systems. Ann Arbor MI: Health Administration Press, 1994.

54. Fine A, ed. Integrated health care delivery systems: A guide to successful strategies for hospital and physi-

cian collaboration. New York: Thompson Publishing Group, 1995.

55. Traska E. Managed care strategies: 1996. New York: Faulkner and Gray, 1996.
56. Blumenthal D. Health care reform: Past and future. N Engl J Med 1995;332:465–468.
57. Helms RB, ed. American health policy: Competition and controls. Washington DC: American Enterprise Institute Press, 1993.
58. Carneal G, Marsan D. State oversight of HMO sponsored point of service products. Medical Interface 1993 (August)105–108.
59. Iglehart JK. Health care reform. The labyrinth of congress. 1993;329:1593–1595.
60. The future of practice management companies. In: Cochrane JE, ed. Integrated Health Care Report. Lake Arrowhead, CA: June 1996.
61. Clinic without walls: A futuristic model In: Cochrane JE, ed. Integrated Health Care Report. Los Angeles, CA: September 1992.
62. The clinic without walls controversy. In: Cochrane JE, ed. Integrated Health Care Report. Lake Arrowhead, CA: August 1993.
63. Back K. Antitrust's expanding universe. Health Systems Rev 1996:November/December:11–14.
64. Peters GR. Health care integration. A legal manual for constructing integrated organizations. Washington DC: National Health Care Lawyers Association, 1995.
65. A new era of foundations, MSOs and clinics without walls. In: Cochrane JE, ed. Integrated Healthcare Report. Los Angeles: July 1992.
66. A designer world for integrated systems. In: Cochrane JE, ed. Integrated Healthcare Report. Los Angeles: October 1992.
67. IRS breakthroughs for foundations. In: Cochrane JE, ed. Integrated Healthcare Report. Los Angeles: February 1993.
68. The Palo Alto medical foundation. In: Cochrane JE, ed. Integrated Healthcare Report. Lake Arrowhead, CA: October 1994.
69. Kongstvedt PR: Managing basic medical and surgical utilization. In: Kongstvedt PR, ed. The handbook of managed healthcare, 3rd ed. Gaithersburg MD: Aspen, 1996:249–273.
70. Glenn JK: Physician referrals in a competitive environment: An estimate of the economic impact of a referral. J Am Med Assn 1987;257:1920–1923.
71. Goldsmith JC. The illusive logic of integration. Healthcare Forum J 1994;37:26–31.
72. How virtuous is vertical integration? In: Cochrane JE, ed. Integrated Healthcare Report. Lake Arrowhead, CA: June 1996.
73. Shortell SM, Gillies RR, Anderson DA, Erickson EM, Mitchell JB. Remaking healthcare in America. Building organized delivery systems. San Francisco: Jossey-Bass, 1996.
74. Goldsmith JC, Gorun MJ. Managed care mythology. Supply-side dreams die hard. Healthcare Forum J 1996;39:42–47.
75. Health Care Megatrends 1997. In: Cochrane JE, ed. Integrated Healthcare Report. Lake Arrowhead, CA. December 1996/January 1997.
76. Wieland BJ, Berenson RA. Physicians survival guide: Legal pitfalls and solutions. Washington DC: National Health Lawyers Association, 1994.
77. Joffe MS. Legal issues in provider contracting. In: Kongstvedt PR, ed. The handbook of managed healthcare. 3rd ed. Gaithersburg, MD: Aspen, 1996: 849–886.
78. Peters GR. Healthcare integration. A legal manual for constructing integrated organizations. Washington DC: National Health Lawyers Association, 1995.
79. Gosfield AG. A physicians guide to managed care contracting. Chicago IL: American Medical Association, 1993.
80. Ile ML, Lerner AN. Antitrust and managed care. Chicago IL: American Medical Association, 1993.
81. Korenchuk KM. Physician-hospital organizations. Series on integration document design and analysis. Englewood, CO: Medical Group Management Association, 1994.
82. Korenchuk KM. Management services organizations. Series on integration document design and analysis. Englewood, CO: Medical Group Management Association, 1994.
83. Korenchuk KM. Physician equity model. Series on integration document design and analysis. Englewood, CO: Medical Group Management Association, 1996.
84. Dechene JC. Establishing a physician organization. Chicago IL: American Medical Association, 1993.
85. Gosfield AG. Who is holding whom accountable for quality? Health Aff 1997;16:26–40.
86. Michaels JL. The regulation of managed care organizations. A legal perspective. Chicago IL: American Medical Association, 1994.
87. Boyd vs. Albert Einstein Medical Center. 547 A2d 1229 (Pa Super 1988).
88. Wickline vs. California. 192 Cal App 3d (1986), rev dismissed 741 P2d 613 (Cal 1987).
89. Wilson vs. Blue Cross of So. California. 222 Cal App 3d 680 (1990), rev denied 1990 Cal Lexis 4574 (Cal Oct. 11 1990).
90. Wieland JB, Quan KP, Meghrigian A, Askansas AV. Physician rights when a managed care contract is denied or terminated. Chicago IL: American Medical Association, 1994.
91. California Business and Professions Code §2056 (effective January 1, 1994).
92. Pauly MV, Eisenberg JM, Radany MA. Paying physicians. Options for controlling cost, volume and intensity of services. Ann Arbor MI: Health Administration Press, 1992.
93. Robinson JC, Casalino LP. The growth of medical groups through capitation in California. N Engl J Med 1995;333:1681–1687.
94. Gold M. Arrangements between managed care plans and physicians. Results from a 1994 survey of managed care plans. Washington DC: Physician Payment Review Commission, 1995.
95. Hamer R. HMO Industry Report, Part II. Interstudy Competitive Edge. 1994;4:1–121.
96. Medical Economics. October 1996.
97. HMO examination handbook. Kansas City, MO: National Association of Insurance Commissioners 1990.
98. Kongstvedt PR. Contracting and reimbursement of

specialty physicians. In: Kongstvedt PR, ed. The handbook of managed health care. Gaithersburg MD. Aspen, 1996:176–190.

99. Clements B. RBRVS. Its not just for Medicare anymore. AM News 1997:Jan 13, 1.

100. Current Procedural Terminology, 4th ed. Chicago IL: American Medical Association, 1997.

101. Hillman AC. HMO managers views on financial incentives and quality. Health Aff 1991;10:207–219.

102. Keeler EB, Brodie M. Economic incentives in the choice between vaginal delivery and caesarian section. Milbank Q 1993;71:365–404.

103. Wennberg JE, ed. Dartmouth atlas of healthcare in the United States. Chicago IL: American Hospital Publishing, 1996.

104. Rowe CS. The impact of managed care on specialty practices. Medical Group Management Association. 1994;41:36–41.

105. Singing the St. Louis Blues. In: Cochrane JE, ed. Integrated Healthcare Report. Lake Arrowhead, CA. February 1997.

106. Specialist survival strategies. In: Cochrane JE, ed. Integrated Healthcare Report. Lake Arrowhead, CA. November 1996.

107. Fine A. Specialty networks from the specialists view. In: Kongstvedt PR, ed. The handbook of managed health care. Gaithersburg, MD. Aspen: 1996: 191–201.

108. Fabini S. The mixed message of today's health care market. Healthcare Trends Rep 1996;10(6):1–2.

CHAPTER 2

Practice Management

STANLEY PELOFSKY, M.D., KEVIN BLAYLOCK, CPA

INTRODUCTION

Achieving success in neurosurgical practice has become a complicated matter. To survive, neurosurgeons must be well-trained, talented, and highly professional; in today's health care environment, however, survival also requires personality and business sense. Neurosurgeons without these characteristics, who are abrasive toward others or who are foolhardy in business, will find themselves enmeshed in malpractice cases with patients, damaged by workers who lack loyalty, and limited in productivity and income. The days are gone when neurosurgeons could rely on the high regard in which both society and the medical community held them, insuring built-in respect and high compensation—in this new health care environment, the pyramid has been reversed and neurosurgeons, once the prima donnas of medicine, are now referred to by the managed care industry as "cost generating centers." Amazingly enough, this rearrangement of the medical hierarchy has occurred at daunting speed, bringing with it confusion, resentment, insecurity, and distrust at many points on the medical continuum, from patient to doctor to hospital to insurance company. These changes have caught many neurosurgeons off guard, or perhaps in a state of denial, about where they fit into the new structure, how to maintain high professional standards, how to protect traditional incomes, and how to manage day-to-day practices. Within this context of change, this chapter attempts to offer sound advice to neurosurgeons on managing their practices with savvy in a world where the only certainty is that change is inevitable.

Nowhere have the changes in health care affected us more dramatically than in day-to-day practice. As little as 5 years ago, most neurosurgeons' offices were usually run by a "business manager" with a high school education and some prior business experience, who handled appointments, sent bills, worked the ledger, and answered phones. Some offices, especially those of solo practitioners, were managed by either the neurosurgeon himself or his wife. Times have most certainly changed, because for practices to survive and flourish in the marketplace today, it is essential to have professional business managers skilled in economics, finance, marketing, accounting, demographics, statistics, and management information systems.

MANAGEMENT FUNCTIONS

Managing a busy neurosurgical office seems intimidating and complicated, but, in the simplest terms, it can be divided into two major management functions: *strategic* and *administrative*.

Strategic Management Functions

Strategic management functions are the macro aspects of management, such as organizational structure and form; number of physicians and their respective specialties; planning; and marketing/strategic relationships. Ultimately, of course, responsibility for the most important strategic functions must fall at the feet of the physician-owner or committee of physician-owners, although other strategic functions may be delegated to one managing physician, a team of managing physicians, or to a (nonphysician) administrator. As neurosurgeons merge into partnerships and group practices, many will become managing partners and work alongside the in-house administrator to steer the practice.

Organizational Structure and Form

Since any neurosurgeon's time is too valuable to be consumed by mundane management functions, managing neurosurgeons must in turn delegate much of the responsibility for these matters to subordinates. Depending on the size of the practice, there may be a need for one, or more than one, nonphysician manager. Figure 2.1 illustrates two possible configurations for practice management, with strategic functions appearing at the top of the structure, and administrative functions appearing nearer the bottom.

Number of Physicians and Their Respective Specialties

Once an appropriate organizational structure has been agreed on, the most fundamental strategic issue is to determine the optimal number of physicians in the practice and the specific specialty of each. Solo practitioners of the future will no doubt find themselves with some independence, but with little or no power; therefore, the only reason neurosurgeons should be in solo practice is if they are the only act in town. The more physicians a practice can profitably integrate into the group, the greater the concentration of capital, and the greater the market power of the practice. In fact, the present and future marketplace will most certainly require that neurosurgeons join together to form a sufficient power-base to contend with managed care, contracting, and competition. Additionally, statistics indicate that more profitable single-specialty neurosurgical practices have at least three physicians, and the most profitable have five or more. Perhaps even more important to most neurosurgeons than profitability, capital, or power-base, though, is the greater quality of life obtained via additional physicians, allowing for the sharing of call duties.

Neurosurgeons must also consider whether or not to include nonneurosurgical physicians in the group. Certainly a multi-specialty group poses many complexities, not the least of which is the problem of allocating practice earnings among different specialties. Since neurosurgery constitutes a small portion of total medical costs, incorporating neurosurgery into a large full-service multi-specialty group is not efficient and is generally not favorable to the neurosurgeon. Combining neurosurgeons with a limited number of related specialists, however, can be an effective organization and could include medical and surgical specialties, such as neurology, physical medicine, orthopedics, and even limited license practices, such as physical therapy

and chiropractic. In deciding the optimal size and composition of physicians in a practice, however, one must keep in mind that there are antitrust statutes and regulations that may bear on the decision. The details of these laws are beyond the scope of this chapter, but suffice it to say that failure to consider these laws could be disastrous.

After determining the appropriate number and specialty of your physicians, recruiting the best candidates becomes critical. This may actually be the most important strategic assignment to be implemented, as recruiting the wrong physician could be worse than recruiting none at all. The managing physician, assisted by the practice administrator and other physicians where needed, should be responsible for physician recruitment. Of course, maintaining physician numbers involves not only recruiting new physicians, but also addressing the needs of senior members. In order to avoid difficult situations of succession, retirement considerations must be planned well in advance.

Planning

Recruitment and retirement issues are not the only matters that must be thought out and planned for; many other problems and questions arise as we endeavor to make our practices successful. Consequently, all physicians and administrators should eventually participate in formal strategic planning sessions (conducted by trained strategic planning professionals), which are intended to assist groups of physicians to learn from the past, deal with the present, and plan for the future. If done properly, these are usually annual sessions lasting 2 to 3 days and are well worth the time spent out of the operating room; some are even held as weekend ''retreats,'' reducing the amount of work-time lost and allowing for fewer distractions on the part of the participants. At the end of the strategic planning session, your professional planner should provide you with a formal document outlining all of the crucial themes your group discussed, a time-line for the completion of certain tasks, and a chart indicating who is accountable for following through on specific areas of concern. If it is to be effective, great pains should be taken to ensure that this document does not become static—rather, it should be dynamic and fluid, providing a long-range business plan while at the same time allowing for appropriate

ORGANIZATIONAL CHART # 1 : ONE NON–PHYSICIAN MANAGER

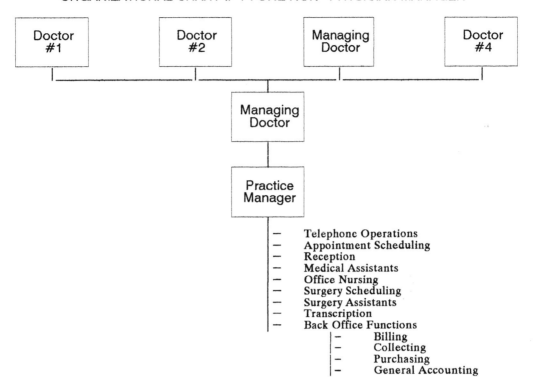

ORGANIZATIONAL CHART # 2 : MULTIPLE NON–PHYSICIAN MANAGERS

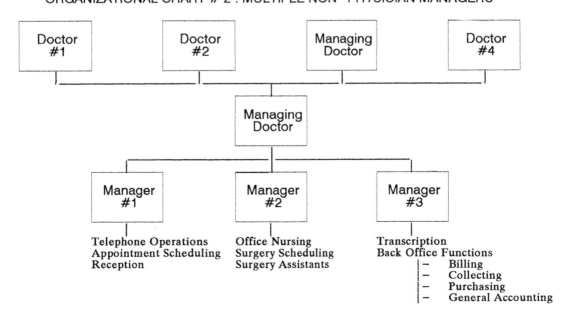

Figure 2.1. Two examples of practice organizational charts

responses to rapid changes in business conditions. This sort of rapid-fire response is best handled via weekly meetings (attended by the physicians who have strategic interests invested in the practice) instead of at the annual strategic planning session, so it is imperative that scheduling such meetings is a part of the overall strategic plan.

Marketing and Strategic Relationships

Strategic planning is especially pressing as it relates to marketing neurosurgical services. Despite the fact that physicians have rarely been trained in marketing or basic business principles, "the business of medicine" marches on, leaving behind it anyone who remains naive or unsophisticated in marketing and business related concepts. It is incumbent on those who wish to remain financially viable to learn such business skills, just as in the past we have learned our surgical skills.

The principle marketing questions that neurosurgeons must always keep in mind are, "What am I selling?" and "Who are my customers?" Although some physicians might find these questions crass in a medical context, they are, nevertheless, the reality of doing business in the current marketplace. For neurosurgeons to prosper in the future, they must not only determine a way to sell the skill it takes to perform current neurosurgical procedures, but they must also consider how to sell the skills necessary to reclaim former neurosurgical arenas, such as carotid artery disease, pain management, peripheral nerve surgery, and trauma, markets recently penetrated by vascular surgeons, cardiologists, physiatrists, plastic surgeons, anesthesiologists, orthopaedists, and general surgeons. In addition, neurosurgeons and their administrators must determine who their customers are by analyzing and understanding the demographics of their geographical area and by evaluating their competition, especially the effect the competition has on their population base. In order to have access to a large enough population base, it may be necessary to develop relationships with several hospitals in the practice area, or to maintain offices in proximity to more than one hospital. In particularly difficult markets, neurosurgeons may be forced to establish satellite offices or clinics in relatively remote areas. While this may seem extreme, it cannot be overlooked as a way to develop or protect a market population of ade-

quate size and composition to ensure that your practice is economically successful.

There is no set number of potential patients required to support a successful neurosurgical practice. If the United States population of 260,000,000 is divided by 4000 (the approximate number of neurosurgeons in practice in the country), the quotient is an average of 65,000 people per neurosurgeon. These numbers are often misleading, however, since it is not uncommon for a neurosurgical practice to thrive in an isolated town of 40,000, or for a practice to flounder in a city of millions. The most obvious factor bearing on the adequacy of the population base is the competition serving the same population. While this competition might come from neurosurgeons or other specialists, it is clear that the demographics of the population will influence the ability to prosper in its service. And increasingly more important, the extent to which the population served is covered by various forms of managed care insurance will determine the ability to practice successfully in that market location.

Geography and demographics aside, marketing actually begins with neurosurgeons themselves, as there is no better marketing strategy than presenting to the public and the medical world a group of talented, caring physicians with pleasant personalities. It is certainly no secret that many neurosurgeons have reputations for displaying arrogance, abrasiveness, and insensitivity toward other medical personnel and even toward patients. Keep in mind that neurosurgery is practiced in a litigious society that has produced a certain mind set among many patients; these patients are quick to sue, especially when they feel that their physician doesn't care about them. Within this context, taking the time to develop positive relationships with your patients becomes especially meaningful. As an extension of the physician, office staff can also make a substantial difference, since staff members often spend more time with patients than does the physician. Efficient, engaging office personnel also encourage referrals; they should, therefore, be trained in communication skills and required to attend courses that help them address the needs of patients. Staff members should also be trained to seek out and find solutions for potential barriers preventing patients from easily accessing the practice.

One relatively simple solution for addressing

office accessibility, as well as enhancing the marketability of the practice, is to evaluate the adequacy of the telephone system. Nothing infuriates patients and referring doctors more than busy phone lines, automated phone messages, and voice mail; it is essential, therefore, to invest in a telephone system with a sufficient number of lines, and one that retains the personal touch. Such a system is an excellent marketing tool, and any money invested in it will be returned to the practice many times over.

Marketing continues via written communication after the patient has been seen in the office. A dictated letter sent to the referring doctor (or third party carrier) as quickly as possible, documenting the evaluation, clinical impression, and recommended treatment plan, becomes a superb marketing tool and one of the most effective means of ensuring future referrals. This prompt documentation of the patient's evaluation also improves efficiency in the implementation of the patient's treatment plan and billing process, and prevents potential medical-legal problems. Pamphlets explaining patients' injuries, diseases, and recommended therapies and brochures detailing the services that are rendered in neurosurgical practices are also useful as written communication techniques. These brochures, especially when combined with favorable outcome studies and profiles of physician credentials, make for excellent third party payer communications. Other successful written communications have taken the form of medical newsletters, doctor referral guides, and satisfaction surveys. Surveying patients to obtain their opinions concerning their care, as well their thoughts on the effectiveness of the office staff, is extremely useful. These surveys can be compiled and used to market the practice to third party carriers, other physicians, workers' compensation companies, and individual employers. Compilations of patient and referring physician satisfaction surveys can be the basis for the best written communication to third party payers.

It is also reasonable for practicing neurosurgeons to expect the hospitals with which they are affiliated to contribute financially to mutually beneficial marketing efforts. These shared marketing strategies might be in the form of advertising, or perhaps in the creation of what has come to be known as "centers of excellence," i.e., cooperative relationships among neurosurgeons, a particular hospital, various therapists,

diagnosticians, and related physician specialists, which take on strategic importance. These centers are often good marketing ventures, as well as efficient vehicles for providing care to patients. If the professionals with whom a practice is affiliated prove uncooperative or inefficient in providing appropriate care to patients, consider other alternatives. For example, related specialists, therapists, and diagnosticians might be incorporated into the practice, in order to enhance the quality of care and perhaps even to contribute to overall practice profitability. A practice might also consider acquiring its own outpatient diagnostic and surgical facilities, in order to gain control over quality and to develop additional profit potential.

Not all marketing consists of mammoth efforts to obtain outside facilities or centers of excellence, nor is it always packaged and slick; much of it, in fact, is the natural outgrowth of such "extracurricular activities" as producing clinical articles for publication locally, statewide, or nationally; delivering lectures to fellow physicians, hospital staff, and medical school students; and giving civic lectures and participating in civic projects. All such endeavors improve the relationships of neurosurgeons within their communities and add to their prestige and patient flow.

In the future, neurosurgeons will be assisted in their marketing efforts by their national organizations. The American Association of Neurological Surgeons (AANS) and the Congress of Neurological Surgeons (CNS) are producing marketing programs that focus on specific skills and treatment plans for diseases, such as lumbar stenosis, herniated cervical and lumbar disc disease, carpal tunnel syndrome, and carotid artery disease, among others. These marketing programs, developed and designed for membership, should be invaluable to neurosurgeons wishing to become more competitive in the future marketplace. Professional development programs will also be conducted to help teach marketing and communications techniques to neurosurgeons attending the national meetings.

Administrative Management Functions

In contrast to strategic functions, *administrative management functions* deal with the more tactical, micro aspects of practice, such as nonphysician staffing patterns and personnel management, productivity matters, cost management (see Cost Management/Data Management below) and profitability issues. The following are just some of the administrative functions present in all practices:

- telephone operations;
- office appointment scheduling;
- incoming pre-certification;
- office reception;
- patient interviewing;
- patient flow management and medical assistance;
- out-going pre-certification and authorization;
- surgery scheduling and coordination;
- nonphysician surgery assistance and inpatient care;
- office nursing;
- transcription;
- medical records administration;
- service coding;
- third party payer claims filing;
- payment processing and auditing;
- patient billing;
- collections;
- purchasing;
- general accounting;
- managed care contracting.

These administrative management functions should be delegated to the managing physician, the administrator or the middle level managers, or to teams comprised of combinations of these people. It is vital, too, that management functions designated as administrative be respected by the nonmanaging physicians in the practice, since interference with administrative management functions will undoubtedly lead to great frustration on everyone's part.

An alternative for neurosurgeons not wishing to manage their own practices is the relatively new option in practice management called a Management Service Organization (MSO). MSOs provide practice management services, as well as managed care contract administrative services, to individual physicians or groups of physicians, and can be owned by private investors, hospitals, or physicians, or by combinations of all three. Some MSOs buy the physician's "hard assets," (so the physician and the office staff actually become paid employees), then provide contract management services to the physician, which could include evaluation, analysis, and negotiations with managed care companies. Because the MSO may also be responsible for

scheduling, billing and collections, and supervision of the physician's staff, some physicians may find that utilizing MSO services is a more efficient and economical way of managing the demands of the practice than hiring an in-house professional administrator. The point that should not be missed, however, is that it takes *professional business managers*, not just physicians themselves, to lead a neurosurgical practice to financial success.

Nonphysician Staffing Patterns and Personnel Management

The goal of personnel management is straightforward: to have the right employees assigned to the right jobs and to have these people motivated to be efficient, effective, and committed to profitability and patient care. In fact, it is not an exaggeration to say that the quality of the employees of a practice is second only to the quality of the neurosurgeons as predictors of financial success. While most aspects of personnel management are best left to administrators, certain aspects of this critical administrative function demand involvement by the managing neurosurgeon. This is especially true when it comes to employee motivation. Because the practice may not be able to pay its employees as much as they would like, it is particularly important that the managing neurosurgeon personally articulate the goals and philosophies of the practice to them, as this can serve to inspire employees to work hard and to take satisfaction from participating in a good and profitable business. Never forget that words of encouragement from "the boss" are a great (and inexpensive) motivating force.

Other important aspects of personnel management that merit attention include decisions regarding hiring and firing, as well as decisions related to employee compensation and benefits. In order to contribute usefully to these decisions, the physician manager should have a fair understanding of the key functions for which the employees are responsible within the office. While it is not necessary for managing physicians to know every detail of these functions, periodic discussions with practice administrators and staff are necessary to provide general guidance and useful input into the most significant aspects of practice management.

Productivity

The average neurosurgeon's week breaks down as follows: 16 hours seeing patients in the office, 20 hours performing surgery, 9 hours making hospital rounds, 6 hours on other patient care activities, and 5 hours on administration. Of course, because the amount of the neurosurgeon's available time is finite, careful management of that time is the most important contributor to a successful practice. Interestingly enough, a recent survey (1) indicates that while only 9% of neurosurgeons would like to see more patients in the office, almost 32 % have time for more surgical volume. And, as the number of surgeries performed tends to be a function of the number of patients seen in the office, the preferences revealed in the survey seem to present a dilemma. One solution is to attempt to increase the number of patients that can be seen in the office without increasing the amount of surgeon's time devoted to that activity; this may be accomplished most effectively by using physician extenders, such as physician assistants or clinical nurse specialists.

Profitability

While careful management of practice costs can enhance the neurosurgeon's productivity and contribute greatly to the practice's profitability, careful management of the types of patients, and the patients' sources of payment, can be equally determinative of profitability. The trend away from commercial indemnity insurance and traditional fee-for-service payments, toward managed care and all its permutations, is mentioned elsewhere in this chapter; three other sources of payment, however, which figure prominently in the economics and profitability of neurosurgery and which present patients with unique characteristics are Medicare, Workers' Compensation, and third-party liability for personal injury claims.

Because Medicare patients are over the age of 64, their age usually makes their medical treatment more complicated and time consuming. Paradoxically, Medicare reimbursement rates are often among the lowest, along with Medicaid recipients and uninsured patients. Workers' compensation and liability reimbursement rates are generally greater than Medicare and managed care, but sometimes they are less than commercial indemnity fee-for-service rates, and the fact that workers' compensation and liability patients have their legal claims as a secondary concern to their medical well-being can also complicate their treatment and consume

valuable neurosurgical time. Because reimbursement is procedure-based and, of course, because surgical procedures are reimbursed at much higher rates than evaluation and office charges, patients who require less of the surgeon's time in the office relative to surgery time are economically preferable. Consequently, when evaluating the economic profit potential of patient populations categorized according to payment source, the practice should consider the rate of reimbursement relative to surgical time consumption implicit in the characteristics of each population subset.

The practice should also attempt to maximize the yield of surgery cases derived from the total number of patients seen in the office. This can be done by tracking the surgery-to-patient ratio in different groups and then favoring the groups with the higher yield. For example, if Workers' Compensation patients tend to have a lower than average yield, the practice might restrict the numbers of these patients seen in the office unless the fee reimbursement rate is high enough to offset the lower rates. Likewise, it might be profitable to accept a managed care plan's lower rate of reimbursement if the surgery-to-patient ratio is relatively high.

Because so many of today's neurosurgical reimbursement rates are either negotiated with managed care plans or imposed by government, general pricing strategies are less relevant than they were before. In most places, however, there are at least some remnants of the old fee-for-service indemnity insurance health plans. As discussed previously, this type of insurance offers little reason to have lower prices. With respect to commercial indemnity insurance, profitability is maximized when prices are set near the high end of the applicable "usual and customary" charge. If your charges exceed the insurance company's definition of usual and customary, a compromise regarding the excess can be negotiated with the patient, if necessary. Routinely accepting only the insurance payment as payment in full, however, can provoke disputes with the insurance carriers, especially when deductibles and copayments are waived.

Finally, collecting as many practice charges as possible and collecting as soon as possible is critical to profitability. For a mature neurosurgical practice, gross accounts receivable should be less than 30% of annual gross billings; bad debts should average 6% to 7%; and collection-to-charges ratios could range from 70% to 80%. If your accounts receivable remain fairly constant and the collection-to-charges ratio stays below 70%, your prices may be too high. Likewise, if the ratio is consistently much higher than 80%, prices may be too low.

COST MANAGEMENT/DATA MANAGEMENT

Cost Management

The old days are most definitely gone. Yesterday, neurosurgeons worked, billed for their labor, and raised their fees as necessary to maintain their practices and incomes; today, however, the managed care industry controls over 80% of practice revenues (including Medicare, Medicaid, and Workers' Compensation), greatly limiting physicians' ability to control their own fee schedules. In order to survive in the current marketplace, neurosurgeons must not only carefully select the people with whom they do business, but also must be vigilant about the cost of doing business. Scrutinizing costs, line by line, has become vital to the successful management of a neurosurgical practice and will in large part determine how profitable this, or any enterprise, will be.

Costs can be measured in terms of *productivity—the value of output* relative to *the costs of input.* Any number of things can be considered to be an "input," the most obvious and valuable of which are the neurosurgeon's billable services. Consequently, the primary focus of most neurosurgical office administrators is to find cost expenditures that will facilitate maximal productivity from the surgeon, such as nonprovider salaries and benefit expenses; information services; occupancy expenses; insurance premiums; and supplies and capital expenditures.

Nonprovider Salary and Benefit Expenses

Neurosurgical practice management is no different from any other service industry, in that its greatest operating expenses emanate from nonprovider (personnel) salary and benefit costs. While each neurosurgical office requires different personnel in order to operate at maximal efficiency, such staff could include nurses, physician assistants, and nonprofessional medical assistants. Other employees might perform administrative functions, such as billing and col-

lections, patient registration and reception, appointment and surgery scheduling, precertification, data processing, transcription, accounting, personnel management, and many other management functions. Of course, in order to attract and retain quality staff members, it is necessary to provide them with excellent benefits, i.e., medical, life, and disability insurance, vacation time, sick leave, and retirement plans (which might include a profit-sharing program). Historically, the tax advantages associated with these benefits have allowed medical practices to provide quite generously for their employees' benefit packages; nonetheless, employee benefits can be a substantial business expense. Administrators should endeavor, therefore, to keep employee benefit plan funding requirements flexible and mandate at least some employee contribution toward payment of plan costs.

Information Services

Information services are of ever-increasing importance to most businesses, and medical businesses are no exception. Though the cost for such services has also increased, the advantages of excellent communication with others via sophisticated information systems usually outweigh installation and maintenance costs. Included in this cost category are telephones and facsimiles, computer hard and software, maintenance costs, and service bureau fees. Since surgery and all other medical specialty practices are dependent on referral sources, it is essential that these sources, as well as third-party payers, can *easily* communicate with the office at the appropriate time in order to ensure smooth flow of business and practice profitability. Information services, therefore, become quite crucial to the overall productivity of the practice.

Occupancy Expenses

If the neurosurgical practice is housed in leased office space, occupancy costs generally consist only of rent; if, however, a neurosurgeon elects to own the practice facility, these costs would also include depreciation, interest, property taxes, and maintenance costs. The most prudent course during these unsettled times favors leasing over owning, in order to allow for greater flexibility should circumstances dictate a change of status. In addition, real estate ownership and the accompanying responsibilities can be counterproductive and distracting to the physician.

One thing is certain: expensive and lavish offices should be avoided, as they are not only costly, but also offensive to increasingly cost-conscious patients who know that they are ultimately paying the bills. With this in mind, neurosurgeons' medical offices should be comfortable, spacious, and attractive, while conforming to a certain degree of modesty.

Insurance Premiums

Insurance premiums include not only employee benefit insurance, but also general property and liability insurance (which is usually not significant), professional liability insurance, and perhaps key-man life or business-continuation insurance. The advisability of key-man life or business-continuation insurance depends on the number of partners or associates in the practice and what their financial relationship is to one another. Professional liability insurance is very expensive, but because the risks involved in neurosurgical procedures are high, neurosurgeons should usually purchase the most coverage that is reasonably available. If a neurosurgeon is unable to receive group ratings because of previous litigation, asset protection strategies could be considered, but these are never substitutes for appropriate insurance protection. If the practice is separately incorporated, combined professional liability insurance coverage can often be leveraged by purchasing additional, rather than shared, corporate limits at reasonable rates.

Supply Expenses/Capital Expenditures

The final cost categories to consider are supply expenses and capital expenditures. Within the context of the neurosurgical office, medical supplies are generally few, since most procedures are performed in the hospital setting. Administrative supplies are more substantial, consisting of such things as printing and paper products, postage, and general office supplies. As far as capital expenditures are concerned, most neurosurgical offices require little in the way of medical equipment (with the possible exception of certain types of diagnostic equipment such as X-ray), though fixed assets such as furniture, fixtures, and office equipment might entail some cost burden.

In order to measure practice expenses, a common rule of thumb is to calculate the percentage of each cost component to the total practice revenue. In a typical neurosurgical practice, these averages should look like the following percentages: about 14% for nonprovider salaries; about 6% for office expenses; 6% for professional liability insurance; and 2% for fixed asset depreciation. Including other miscellaneous expenses, total nonphysician expenses average about 38%, with an average of 3.5 nonprovider support personnel per surgeon. The ratios of major expense categories to total revenue can serve as useful benchmarks for neurosurgeons attempting to determine the cost effectiveness of their practices.

All of the significant operating cost components in a typical private neurosurgical practice are virtually fixed over a wide range of business activities. The expense components that do vary with changes in the activity rate tend to do so in discrete increments, rather than in a continuous proportional manner. Take, for example, personnel costs, which generally constitute the largest single component of total operating costs. Because a private neurosurgical practice employs a whole number of full-time support personnel, this employment configuration remains constant over a wide range of practice activity. If, however, business increases or decreases beyond certain points, employment will increase or decrease in full-time employee increments accordingly.

In an effort to bring costs under control, some neurosurgical practice administrators are attempting to create cost structures that are more variable and flexible. These efforts generally involve the use of hourly or part-time employees, or even the practice of paying overtime for peak activity times, while keeping full-time employment to a minimum. Remember that the highest cost in neurosurgical practice is labor-based, so the practice must guard against exorbitant salaries, benefits, and perks for employees as well as physicians. Another alternative is to procure administrative contracts with MSOs or service bureaus, whose contracts are based on activity level, thereby converting relatively fixed costs to variable costs. It is even possible to lease professional services, such as nursing, from third parties, in order to provide for maximal flexibility.

Data Management

A critical aspect of controlling practice costs is how well you collect and manage data. This information management requires that data be accurately gathered and converted into useable information and that the information be analyzed carefully, in order to draw proper conclusions. Financial success could very well depend upon how well physicians and office staff master these tasks, two of which are to purchase a Management Information System (MIS) and to accurately analyze the data compiled by such a system.

Medical Information Systems

The importance of a good automated Management Information System is considered in detail elsewhere in this volume, but it should also be mentioned here as an effective tool for controlling costs. The best systems are those bought off-the-shelf, which have proven their value over time in many kinds of medical practices. In other words, avoid succumbing to the pressures of salespeople who claim to be customizing a system to fit your needs, but who are actually planning strategies for making high commissions. Small practices should expect to spend $15,000–$20,000 for an adequate in-house medical information system; larger practices may spend $100,000 or more. Regardless of what you spend for your system, it is vital that you analyze your data daily, as this information will control costs and overhead. Your system must be able to maintain patient accounts, bill and produce statements, file claims electronically with third-party payers, account for receipts, and analyze and summarize patient and managed care demographics and financial data. Adequate systems should include a general ledger package that handles accounts payable, payroll, and daily business costs. Ideally, these information systems will lead to such things as paperless electronic medical charts and voice recognition transcription.

Despite the many available technologies related to data analysis, the best set of data available is of no value if that data is not converted into useful management information, or if the manager fails to use that information properly. Data generally must be massaged in order to create information, and administrators must carefully consider all the possible implications of the resulting information, in order to draw the proper conclusions. Sometimes the simplest data analyses are the most valuable; sometimes, however, simple analyses can be simply wrong. The following are examples of simple data analyses which are frequently misinterpreted:

Collection Fixation

One simple management data equation is the ratio of collections to charges. For example, a 90% collection of gross charges may appear to be very good at first glance; a closer inspection, however, may lead to a very different conclusion. Indeed, the only important factor in this formula is the collection rate itself. Charges, on the other hand, are a function of *production* multiplied by *the price per unit of production*. But the price we charge for our services usually has little to do with the price we are paid, unless we are charging less than the contracted fee schedule for each procedure. This would constitute "marginal pricing," which, according to microeconomic theory, can significantly affect profitability. Marginal pricing means setting prices based on what the last (or marginal) customer paid for the service. For example, if a business charges $100 for a service, and 9 out of 10 of the customers of that business pay only $50 (say, as part of a contract agreement), while just one customer pays the full $100, then the total charges are $1,000, but only $550 is collected. This represents a 55% collection ratio. If, however, instead of charging $100, the business charges $50 for the same service, it will collect $500, representing a 100% collection rate. In spite of the 100% collection to charges ratio, the business would be $50 poorer than it would be with a 55% collection ratio. The point of this exercise is not to encourage price increases without regard for competitors' prices, patients' needs, or even some insurance companies' economic profiling calculations; rather, the point is to discourage the misguided assumption that a high collection ratio is always a good thing.

Account Aging Fixation

Another common error in interpreting management data involves the age of the accounts receivable. It is easy to assume that if the accounts receivable are relatively young (as measured in days over 100), it is a favorable financial indicator. As noted in the previous example, however, the quantity of collections is of even more importance than the timing. A very young set of accounts receivable may in fact mean that the business has written-off, or turned to collection, some receivables too soon. Older accounts receivable may eventually yield a high rate of collection with persistent in-house collection efforts, as some payers inevitably take longer to respond. This is especially true of workers' compensation claims and third party liability claims, since legal red-tape often delays the payment process. Again, the point is that a simple interpretation of management data may very well be wrong.

Employee Minimization Fixation

A final mistake that neurosurgeons frequently make is in calculating the appropriate ratio of full-time-equivalent employees to full-time-equivalent physicians. Although a low ratio of employees to physicians (i.e., 3 : 1) appears to be an indication of efficiency, studies have actually shown that many of the most profitable medical specialty practices have a higher ratio of employees to physicians (2). Perhaps these additional support staff enable the physicians to be more productive, or perhaps it is a sign that a practice, which is highly profitable for other reasons, has been able to afford excess personnel. Only a careful analysis of the data can produce the proper interpretation.

Although one must be wary of misinterpreting data, sometimes analyses can be simple and can lead to the most useful management decisions. For example, in calculating the cost of producing a unit of service, Medicare has assigned units of relative value for every medical procedure and patient encounter. Multiplying the *total annual number* of these procedures and encounters by their *relative value units* (RVU) yields the *total units* produced for the year. Dividing the *total costs* (exclusive of physician compensation) by the *total units* will produce a simple measure of the *cost per unit*. This number can be compared to a *resource-based relative value scale* or *RBRVS*-based fee schedule conversion factor to see how the practice costs compare to a particular rate of reimbursement (Fig. 2.2). The calculation yields a practice expense conversion factor, in this example, $21.44, which is constant across all payers. This number can be subtracted from the total conversion factor (e.g., $40 for Medicare) to calculate the remaining portion of the payment available for physician compensation (e.g., $40 − $21.44 = $15.66/RVU).

Another relatively simple calculation is determining the gross estimate of a practice's equivalent per-member-per-month (PMPM) subcapitation reimbursement rate (Fig. 2.3). In order to make this calculation, an estimate must be made of the size of the population the practice currently serves. For example, a solo practice in a city of 130,000 with two neurosurgeons in town and with practices of equal size, yields the estimated population served to be 65,000 (130, 000 ÷ 2). If the practice's annual revenue is $710,000, then the annual revenue per population member served is $10.92 ($710,000 ÷ 65,000). The equivalent PMPM subcapitation rate, therefore, is 91¢ (10.92 ÷ 12 months), assuming patients outside the city are not served by the practice. If patients outside the urban area are also served by the practice, the denominator is larger and the numerator (capitation rate) is smaller. Of course, this is a gross calculation and would be insufficient data with which to negotiate a subcapitated contract. Given, however, that few neurosurgery capitation rates today exceed 50¢ PMPM, the example illustrates that a careful analysis of the population served and the equivalent fee-for-service costs is necessary when accepting a capitation rate, to avoid inadequate payment, or discount below the fee-for-service equivalent (Fig. 2.3).

CONSIDERING THE FUTURE

The sky is not falling; the future is bright. Neurosurgical practices of the future, however, will be based on the dramatic changes occurring in the marketplace. Change is the only constant, rate of change the only variable. Neurosurgeons will have to be flexible, knowledgeable, and extremely creative to be successful; many may even decide to become employees. Over 50% of the physicians in this country, in fact, are now employees of corporations. Many neurosurgeons will become entrepreneurs and will merge with other neurosurgeons in order to obtain power in negotiating with managed care companies. Many will also, along with referring physicians, develop and own imaging centers and "centers of excellence," in order to ensure that businesses succeed. Still others will become the ultimate capitalists, developing and owning insurance companies with HMO, PPO, and Workers' Compensation products. Enterprising groups will develop and own integrated medical delivery systems, allowing control of patient flow into the neurosurgical practice. With these integrated medical delivery systems, the practice will also be able to control quality of diagnostic studies and treatment as well as control costs.

Neurosurgeons must keep in mind that the

JOHN Q. AVERAGE, M.D.
MIDDLETOWN NEUROSURGERY, INC.

	a	b	c	d	e
	#	RVU's Per	(a x b) Total RVU's	Revenue	(d / c) Conversion Factor
Primary Surgery Procedures:					
20661 Applic. Cranial Halo	4	8.74	34.96	2,200	
61107 Twist Drill Hole, Catheter / Pressure Device	10	11.18	111.80	8,900	
61154 Burr Hole(S) For Subdural Hematoma	5	34.44	172.20	9,800	
61312 Craniotomy For Hematoma, Intracerebral	7	49.13	343.91	19,700	
61510 Craniotomy For Glioma, Supratent.	8	55.33	442.64	26,700	
61512 Craniotomy For Supratent. Meningioma	5	58.56	292.80	17,900	
61518 Post. Fossa Craniectomy, Cerebellar Tumor	4	67.75	271.00	14,600	
61520 Post. Fossa Craniectomy, C / P Angle Tumor	4	78.09	312.36	16,900	
61548 Transsphen. Excision, Pituitary Tumor	5	48.96	244.80	16,100	
61550 Craniectomy Sagittal Craniosynostosis	3	27.16	81.48	6,100	
61700 Surgery Of Intracranial Aneurysm, Carotid	8	72.19	577.52	31,900	
61790 Stereotactic Lesion, Gasserian Ganglion	6	26.53	159.18	11,600	
62010 Repair Brain, Dura, Depress Skull Fx	3	41.02	123.06	7,700	
62141 Cranioplasty, Larger Than 5 Cm.	3	34.91	104.73	7,000	
62223 Ventric–Peritoneal Shunt	8	32.23	257.84	16,300	
62225 Revision, Ventricular Catheter Of Shunt	5	10.09	50.45	4,300	
62230 Revision Shunt Valve Or Distal Catheter	7	21.36	149.52	9,300	
63005 Lumbar Lam Decompression, <2 Segments	7	33.95	237.65	16,400	
63017 Lumbar Lam Decompress., 2+ Segments	11	40.14	441.54	29,600	
63020 Post. Cerv. Discectomy, Unilateral	7	31.95	223.65	16,900	
63030 Post. Lumbar Discectomy, Unilateral	51	30.42	1,551.42	115,000	
63042 Lumbar Lam, Re–Exploration	9	43.75	393.75	24,300	
63047 Lateral Facet Decompression, Lumbar	16	33.57	537.12	42,600	
63075 Ant. Cerv. Discectomy	25	40.55	1,013.75	60,900	
63276 Thoracic Lam, Excision Of Tumor, Extradural	3	51.69	155.07	9,100	
63280 Cerv. Lam For Excision Of Tumor, Intradural	2	59.79	119.58	6,600	
63706 Repair Myelomeningocele, Larger Than 5 Cm.	3	41.96	125.88	7,300	
64718 Neurolysis/Transposition, Ulnar Nerve, Elbow	3	13.33	39.99	2,900	
64721 Median Nerve Decompress., Carpal Tunnel	13	9.72	126.36	9,000	
Other Procedures:					
20660 Applic. Cranial Tongs	5	4.28	21.40	1,900	
22554 Ant. Cerv. Interbody Fusion	23	40.57	933.11	26,750	
22600 Posterior Fusion, Cervical Spine	3	37.42	112.26	3,650	
62270 Spinal Puncture	8	1.90	15.20	1,000	
62284 Injection Procedure For Myelography	60	3.86	231.60	15,900	
63035 Additional Interspace, Discectomy	10	7.95	79.50	6,300	
Total for Procedures	354		10,089.08	623,100	61.76
E & M Encounters:					
99204 New Patient Evaluation, Office	50	2.57	128.50	4,900	
99205 New Patient Evaluation, Office	150	3.22	483.00	17,900	
99214 Established Patient Visit, Office	400	1.48	592.00	20,100	
99244 Consultation, Office	50	3.57	178.50	6,900	
99245 Consultation, Office	150	4.81	721.50	23,100	
99231 Hospital Visit, Follow Up, Level 1	120	0.92	110.40	4,700	
99255 Consultation, Hospital	60	4.85	291.00	9,300	
Total for E & M	980		2,504.90	86,900	34.69
Combined Total	1,334		12,593.98	710,000	56.38

			Total RVU's	Total Costs	Cost Per RVU
Cost per RVU			12,593.98	270,000	21.44

Figure 2.2. Sample calculation of practice conversion factors and cost per RVU

JOHN Q. AVERAGE, M.D.
MIDDLETOWN NEUROSURGERY, INC.

Average Population Served:

1994 Population of USA	260,000,000	
1994 # of US Neurosurgeons	————————— =	65,000
	4,000	

Average Annual Revenue Per Person in Population Served:

1994 Gross Revenue	$710,000	
1994 Population Served	————————— =	$10.92
	65,000	

	$10.92	
Breakeven PMPM Capitation Rate:	————————— =	$0.91
	12	

Figure 2.3. Example calculation of practice equivalent PMPM subcapitation rate

changes occurring in the health-care industry are due to market forces which have been in place for hundreds of years in the business world; it is now time for the medical world to utilize the principles of business in a manner complementary both to sound medical practice and to sound practice management. There are tremendous opportunities available to those able to negotiate the changes and adapt to them effectively. It is essential to form strong groups. It is vital that small competitive neurosurgical groups merge so that they can develop more powerful positions from which to work with managed care companies.

It is also imperative to hire well-trained business personnel to assist in the technical aspects of managing surgical practices. An organization not previously mentioned, but comprised of such business professionals, is the Medical Group Management Association (MGMA). These professionals are trained to look at bottom-line numbers and to develop the strategies discussed in this chapter. These professionals assist neurosurgeons now, and probably will even more in

the future, by performing much of the routine day-to-day business, while the physician's time is freed to be productive in treating and operating on patients. It is also helpful when these professionals are well-versed in the intricacies and negotiations of contracts. They can accomplish significant improvements and changes in a contract with managed care company personnel, since the two speak the same language. They are often able to accomplish what neurosurgeons negotiating alone, or even within a group, are unable to do. These business professionals are experts in the development of communications and medical information systems within the office and oversee every area of the neurosurgical business, again helping to free physician time. It must be stressed, however, that no matter how well the practice is run by business professionals, the neurosurgeon's personality, communication skills, and marketing prowess are still the most important factors in a successful practice. Physicians cannot just blindly follow others; they must clearly see what the practice is doing and where it is going at all times.

Successful neurosurgical practices of the present and future will also have more room for professional physician extenders, such as physician assistants, clinical nurse practitioners, and Registered Nurse first assistants. These extenders will allow physicians to see more patients, resulting in easier access to the neurosurgical practice. Well-trained physician extenders will help interview patients, obtain histories, and assist neurosurgeons to efficiently evaluate patients in the office. In the hospital, physician extenders will be responsible for assisting with surgeries, admission histories and physicals, day-to-day routine orders, and operative discharges. They can also counsel patients regarding discharge instructions and follow-up information. Having a trained professional perform these time-consuming, but vitally important, duties frees neurosurgeons to be more productive and to see more patients.

Medical training will soon include more business-related courses. It is already possible to attend professional development programs sponsored by the AANS and CNS that address the socioeconomic issues affecting neurosurgery. In fact, national meetings are becoming a major source of socioeconomic information for neurosurgeons. Nationally, the Joint Council of State Neurosurgical Societies (JCSNS) allows transfer of such information, which is simply not obtainable elsewhere. Practicing neurosurgeons are urged to join their state neurosurgical society and to become delegates, alternates, or appointees to the JCSNS, in order to share important information and to become a part of this process.

There is no doubt that neurosurgeons all have the potential to lead personally fulfilling and financially rewarding professional lives, despite all of the confusing changes swirling about in health care. If neurosurgeons view such change as challenging, rather than defeating, while remembering that a physician's primary calling is to serve patients well, equipping themselves to do so with every resource available and becoming vocal when injustices surface, then they are already well on their way to a promising future.

REFERENCES

1. Pevehouse BC, Gary Siegel Organization, Inc. 1995 Comprehensive Neurosurgical Practice Survey. Park Ridge IL: American Association of Neurological Surgeons and Congress of Neurological Surgeons, 1996.
2. Margolis JW, Medical Group Management Association Survey Operations Department. Cost Survey: 1996 Report Based on 1995 Data. Englewood CO: Medical Group Management Association, 1996.

CHAPTER 3

The Computer Workplace

PHILLIP W. TALLY, M.D.

INTRODUCTION

Just as any neurosurgical resident now has the basic background needed to use a computer in the operating room, so it is becoming equally necessary to apply computer technology in the office. As much as neurosurgical techniques have evolved and become more exact with the aid of the computers, so too has the business of neurosurgery (and medicine in general) become more dependent on electronic information. Any scientific venture has to be financially viable in order to progress, and efficiency and expeditiousness are possible in today's health-care field only with the aid of computerization. This need exists for any medical practice, whether solo or group, single-specialty or multispecialty.

This chapter will describe how the computer has enabled us to streamline our practice, become self-sufficient with a minimum of outside expertise, and significantly decrease our overhead. Many of the concepts in this chapter will be obvious. There will be, however, some specifics that are less intuitive, but can make a difference between a practice surviving or folding in today's highly competitive health-care market. This description will dissect the basic operations of an everyday private practice. The use of the computers will be demonstrated in all phases of the practice: appointments; X-ray records; history taking; physician encounter; diagnosis and ordering of tests; surgical scheduling; hospital rounds; prescriptions; billing information; financials; record keeping and outcomes analysis.

PAPER RECORDS

Medicine has been the last major profession to embrace the technical age, particularly in the realm of word processing. By tradition, all encounters with a physician are recorded manually or dictated. Documenting patient encounters at the office requires fully 38% of an physician's time. Charts typically are hand-carried to the hospital by the physician to assist in patient admissions. When in need of patient information at the hospital, the doctor must call the office and have the information read off the chart, assuming the chart can be found. In personal discussion with other physicians or in correspondence, data must be summarized, frequently resulting in specific information being omitted. The typical system often leaves office personnel searching for a chart—e.g., the billing office looking for insurance information or a nurse trying to answer a phone call regarding medication. The chart may, for example, be sitting in the surgical scheduling area, or even in the physician's car! In fact, in the average practice for approximately 30% of searches made, the patient's chart cannot be easily located.

Billing traditionally has been done by hand, although this custom has changed on a large scale and increasingly is done electronically. Over the past decade, the CPT (Current Procedural Terminology) and ICD-9 (International Classification of Diseases-9) coding systems have dramatically altered the way billing is done. A large percentage of practices still bill and mail by hand. There is usually no tracking system available to check the aging of the accounts.

Medical records typically are filed by patient name only. There is no intrinsic system to retrieve data by age, procedure, or outcome. Retrospective reviews are nearly impossible, or at least extraordinarily time-consuming, and prospective studies require pulling charts out of circulation within the office, tagging them, and possibly making them even more inaccessible to other departments within the office. The chart itself typically is organized chronologically, with only two faces in a bifolding chart, displaying nonmedical information on the left face and medical information on the right side. Charts often have a mixture of hand-written and transcribed notes. This inconsistency generates mistakes when the record needs to be copied or read by someone else, and legibility may be a problem. X-ray and laboratory data get filed haphazardly between both sides, making it very time consuming to review the information at a glance. In this charting system, there is no way to see any category of results without wading through the entire chart looking for every related piece of data. This frustration may be most obvious, for example, in searching for how many prescriptions a patient has received before and after surgery, and for noting the type of medication and frequency.

SURGICAL SCHEDULING

Surgical scheduling is a function that is now being done electronically in many hospitals for the smooth operation of a heavy caseload. However, in the physician's office, it is still done by hand, and communication between staff and physician is prone to mistakes when staff is trying to inform the physician what procedure is scheduled, at what time, at which hospital, who is assisting, what special instructions or equipment are needed, and how much time is the allotted for the case.

FINANCIALS

Financial records typically are seen as two "buckets." How much money came in last month, how much was paid out, and what is the difference? The office may have a gross figure of accounts receivable, but has no way to determine how much of that account is "real" (i.e., collectable), how much has been adjusted by managed care plans (i.e., write-off), and how much is overdue. This uncertainty makes planning, and budgeting, for the future, difficult or impossible. In the current wave of health-care competition, with numerous plans ranging from private pay to capitated prepayment, keeping up with the financial health of the practice is a difficult challenge. Changing markets, widely varied and numerous third party payment methods and

schedules with providers participating in multiple health plans and patients shifting insurance coverage among different plans, all make the "business" part of neurosurgery complex and confusing. As patients are transferred from one "gatekeeper" to another, continuity of care becomes haphazard, even for neurosurgery. The ability to streamline and facilitate a physician's time and provide information about and for a patient has become a practice necessity. The ability to handle each patient's encounter (whether it is the physician, registered nurse, receptionist, or billing personnel) in the most efficient manner, utilizing the least amount of time with the greatest accuracy, is a challenge faced by every medical practice.

"To Err is human. But to really louse it up, it takes a computer."

THE COMPUTER WORKPLACE

What follows is a step-by-step (or window by window) description of the use of computers by our medical office with an individual patient. Even as this volume goes to press, we are continuing to evolve the programs and upgrade hardware. This information management system has eliminated duplicative effort by staff and increased their access to information on each patient.

Basic Hardware

When our office first acquired a financial and chart system (in this case, Medic®PM), it consisted of a basic server with slave or "dumb" terminals. This construct was the classic hub and spoke design, that only allowed us to use the programs installed in the server. The arrangement of the system consisted of a Medic®PM "box" or a RISC 6000 server using AIX software. That system is very good for database functions, because it can hold vast amounts of text and financial information. The system currently has a capacity of 400 megabytes (mb), and can easily be upgraded, if necessary. Because there were certain functions that this program did not provide, an additional database was developed using Microsoft® Access®. This system provides for tracking and storing X-rays, acquiring First Communication Information along with demographics and previsit insurance authorizations. The program is run on a WindowsNT® operating system, an arrangement

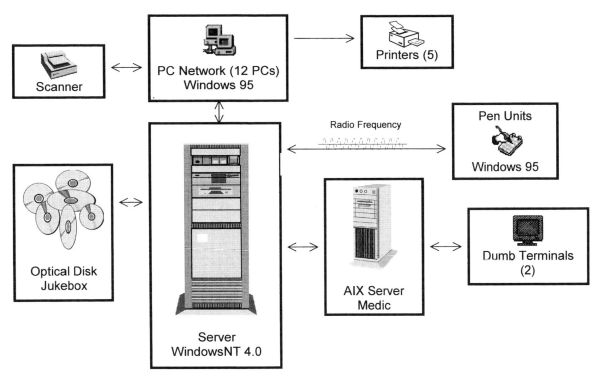

Figure 3.1. Schematic of office computer network.

that immediately created a problem, because the "dumb" terminals were unable to utilize the Windows® programs and made it necessary for the office personnel to have access to personal computers (PCS). PCS allow staff to access the Medic®PM server as well as have PC-based programs. Over the last year, we have almost eliminated all of the "dumb" terminals, going from eight to two, and are now up to a total of 12 PCS within the office. (See Fig. 3.1) With the addition of the Windows®-based Auto-Chart® and AutoImage®, all PCS have access to all Medic-based information stored on the RISC server, as well as to data stored in the ACCESS® program and in an optical disc reader ("Jukebox"). A bottleneck in the use of these two servers is the combination of Auto-Chart®, an AIX-based program, with the Auto-Chart® for Windows®. Currently, a VanGui, COBALT-based shell program is required to interface the two. While this format may be a little slow for now, in the near future it is to be converted to an INFORMIX-based language, creating a "transparent," and therefore much faster, interface between the two programs. Using mul-

tiple PCS (each containing the software programs and with access to the server working as a database) allows multiple personnel to access the same database simultaneously.

As the technology continues to develop, the capacity for information storage becomes more and more remarkable. Currently we have an optical disc reader ("Jukebox"), which holds 10 discs. These discs have 2.6 gigabyte (gb) capacity per side, for a total of 52 gb. This capacity is roughly the equivalent of 100 sets of the Encyclopedia Britannica! The advantage of this vast memory is obvious when storing records. Whereas previously our office kept a 30 to 20 foot room filled with boxes of records, we now put that same information in something smaller than a shoebox. This capability is expanded by the AutoImage® program, which allows us to scan all documents that enter the office. Each document is laser-scanned and then filed in the patient's computer chart by directories and subdirectories. The original is shredded, when possible. These electronically recorded documents can be cross-referenced for multiformatted access.

As an example of the efficiency of the system, all operative notes in the last 6 months can be called up for review within minutes. This feature would be useful for researching a particular third-party payer, e.g., an HMO's payment history, or determining how many Worker's Compensation files have been subpoenaed. One might expect to do similar research when determining time and expense related to a particular patient population. The Jukebox is a Windows-based operating system. No backup is necessary, because the information is on an optical disc, and therefore cannot "crash." Data can be directly filed, either on the optical disc, or it can be temporarily stored on the server. The server box itself has a 4.5gb capacity, which is "mirrored" with a hard drive of identical capacity as its own internal backup to avoid data loss. The active paper charts can be filed in the computer with ease. The laser scanner itself can read a 1-inch thick chart in under 2 minutes and can then be indexed and filed in another 10 minutes. Alternatively, the office can maintain a duplicate system, allowing old charts to diminish by attrition.

As in any charting system, security is an issue. There is a perception that, because of its "high tech" nature, an electronic system is easier to alter, when, in fact, it actually may be made more difficult to alter than a paper record. In addition, all access programs are password protected. For example, in the Medic® program, stored histories have an automatic lock, so that once the history has been "closed" at the time of the initial visit, it can never be reopened. Only addenda can be added to the history; no words can be entered in or deleted from the original without destruction of the entire record. Data stored on the optical disc reader can be deleted and reentered, but only by changing the chronological record numbers, so that if the document were deleted, a number out of sequence could easily be discovered. It is impossible to reenter the document under the same locator number. Also, the internal clock mechanism would have to be totally altered, and if that were done, a record is kept that the internal clock was changed as well. Under these circumstances, an astute computer operator would easily be able to detect that records had been altered. This system leaves the same trace as a "white out" paste on a regular document. On the whole, this system makes record altering considerably more difficult than any scheme using paper documentation.

Appointments

When a patient calls, the appointment secretary calls up a database that has been constructed through Microsoft® Access®, a database program designed for Windows® environment. Under a Main window, the appointment secretary Worklist is pulled up, and the patient is added to it. (Fig. 3.2.) The Worklist shows all currently active First Communication Sheets which contain basic information about the patients, such as date of birth, name, symptoms, and any testing the patient may have had. There is also a box for listing the patient's insurance. If the patient has insurance that requires authorization, such as Worker's Compensation, Motor Vehicle Injury, or Vocational Rehabilitation, the appointment secretary clicks on the corresponding button on the screen to enter information required for obtaining the authorization, as well as information necessary for filing the insurance. All HMO authorizations are entered into a standard generic form. In our current market, this process has become necessary to verify patient preapproval before the initial visit. As many patients require multiple visits, each of which have to be authorized, the secretary's ability to keep all the authorization numbers and the names of the individuals with whom she has spoken in chronological order has been very helpful to the staff.

Once the initial visit has been authorized, the patient is contacted again for the actual scheduling of the appointment. If no authorization was necessary, the appointment is scheduled immediately. This process is performed using the Medic® program that identifies the patient by a chronological identification number as well as by Social Security number. All demographic data is obtained over the phone, with the exception of specific insurance information, which is entered into the computer on the patient's arrival. With the name and the Social Security number entered, the computer allows any patient to be found by one of three identifiers: name, patient number, or Social Security number. The patient number becomes the account number, but this can also be duplicated with patients who have more than one account. For example, if a patient is first seen because of cervical pain from a motor vehicle accident, the computer assigns a five-digit number. If sometime thereafter the patient is seen because of a Worker's Compensation low-back pain, the same five-digit number is used with the addition of the appropriate let-

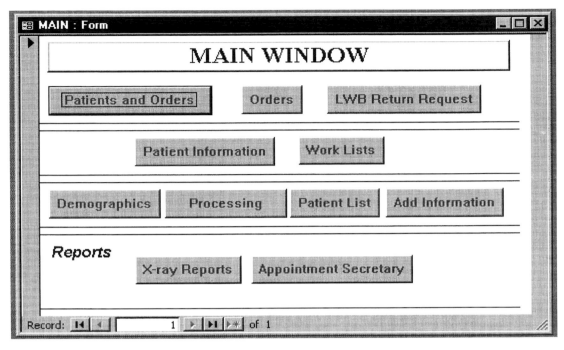

Figure 3.2. Screen showing Worklist with First Communication sheets.

ters, in this case "WMC." This identification method also becomes very helpful when legal costs are involved, as this ID will be a five-digit number followed by an "A" (attorney). Using this method, the staff can make sure that all bills go to the correct payer (e.g., a deposition fee is sent to the attorney's office), enabling the office to keep track of which bills are paid and which are delinquent by tracking payer rather than patient.

Even though the patient may have multiple billing accounts, all other records related to the patient, operative notes, office dictation, etc. are kept in one medical file, so the doctor has access to all the information in one location. Therefore, when scheduling, the appointment secretary enters the desired date and the physician the patient requests to see. This entry pulls up that physician's schedule for that date, and the patient is offered the next available appointment. The information is then entered in the First Communication Sheet. When the secretary has finished obtaining all information and the appointment has been scheduled, the information is automatically transferred to the film department with a click of a button.

X-Ray Supervisor

Review of imaging studies is often critical for accurate diagnosis and valid treatment recommendations. We find it worthwhile to have a dedicated person handle all films to ensure their availability and minimize any physician decision-making undertaken, with or without the patient, in the absence of necessary imaging studies. The films listed by the appointment secretary are noted for type, location, and date performed. Each film is placed in the "bucket" of the facility where obtained. The information also includes the appointment date, physician, and the reason (A for Appointment, R for Review, TR for a Test Result). A list is constructed for each facility that will be faxed or e-mailed each day. The facility then puts all requested films together to be picked up or delivered the following day. As the X-ray supervisor files the films on each patient, it is taken off the Worklist. This system allows the staff to modify appointments to minimize visits without films, and it also documents where the films are at any given time, avoiding confusion about film whereabouts, whether at imaging facilities, hospitals, or doctor's offices. The film program is also utilized for ordering tests, allowing us to keep a very accurate record of resource utilization. Recently for example, we needed to know how many MRIs were ordered on a monthly basis; the information was obtained within 15 minutes, including how many MRIs were done, which facilities were used, which physician ordered them, and even the type of MRI. This information is highly useful in documenting resource utilization for self-evaluation and contract negotiations.

With the above information completed, the office is ready for the patient's visit. The total time spent by the office staff on all information is approximately 15 minutes. By comparison, when this was done by hand and by telephone prior to and during the office visit, the time expended was over 50% longer.

Office Visit

The Patient Reception Area PC has a computerized schedule for that day's patients for all the physicians in the office. When the patient checks in, the receptionist clicks on his or her name. By this click, the computer logs the time that the patient arrived and is present in the waiting room. The receptionist confirms the patient's demographic information on a computer-generated form. The patient then signs a medical release and financial responsibility statement on an electronic signature board. The insurance cards and driver's license are laser scanned and stored in the patient's file. Currently we are planning to use a small digital camera to do an in-office full body image to be stored with the chart. This can also be used for unusual physical findings during the exam. The person who takes the history then sees the patient. This can be a nurse, physician, or an experienced paramedical person, and information can be taken on either the desktop PC or on a handheld pen-based portable computer (Fujitsu Stylus 1000–Fujitsu Corp.). The template for the chief complaint is located either with the pen or the mouse (e.g., headache, neck pain, back pain, etc.). This selection then calls up a full set of questions and answers and the history is taken using the template. This history can be as detailed as the physician desires; we are constantly refining our own templates. Two obvious advantages of this system are (*a*) the computer prompts the history taker in the same order for every patient; (*b*) the history can be done in advance over the phone if the staff perceives a heavy load for the following day, thus allowing information taken by telephone simply to be reviewed by the physician at the time of the examination.

Physician Encounter

The AutoChart® program is a Windows-operated algorithm. We have constructed templates for most major problems that we see in the office. These templates can be constructed for any type of practice, whether neurosurgical or other specialty. These templates are physician-specific, so that even particular phrases that a particular physician would use can be incorporated without disturbing the other physicians' history-taking patterns. If the templates are sufficiently well constructed, the can be done without dictation or typing a single word. The system, however, does allow a notation to be made at any juncture in the history and physical by handwriting on the portable pen-based laptop or tapping an icon notifying the staff that there is specific dictation to be inserted at that point.

Before the patient interview has started, the referring doctor, the patient's age, and pertinent demographics have already been entered into the template. The categories are presented automatically on the screen; choices are tapped with the pen and the history and physical (H & P) is constructed. What follows is a mere fraction of all the possibilities that have been constructed on the template.

1. Cause of Symptoms (7 of 13 Choices shown)—motor vehicle accident; driver; passenger; went to the ER; did not go to the emergency room; Workman's Compensation injury; no episode.
2. Low Back Pain—with radiation; to the knee; to the calf (currently there are 29 choices in this category); to the foot; without radiation.
3. Duration (18 choices)
4. Symptoms—worsen with (15 choices); improved with (16 choices).
5. Previous treatments the patient has received (17 choices)
6. Medications—medications taken for present illness; medications taken for other chronic conditions.

Currently we have a list of medications taken strictly for neurosurgical conditions. We have not made an attempt to list all medications for all chronic conditions, even though these lists are available. We have found that it is faster to type in the medication than scroll through the computer equivalent of the *Physician's Desk Reference*.

7. Allergies (20 categories)

The most common medications are listed with five choices as to type of reaction.

8. Past Medical History (Currently, 54 choices)

These are listed by categories, such as cardiac, pulmonary, GI, etc. This listing works best in our practice, and conditions are listed in the order most likely to affect a neurosurgical evaluation.

9. Past Surgical History (Currently, 33 choices listed)
10. Social History—marital status; children (16 choices); habits: smoking—alcohol 18 total choices); occupation (30 most common choices)
11. Family History (42 total choices for 4 categories)—immediate relatives
12. Vital Signs

Although there is a numerical keypad on screen to enter this data, we currently find it faster to enter this information by hand.

Up to this point, the history can be done by either staff or the physician. We currently have the staff do this initial part. Although the above choices seem somewhat exhaustive, the staff have actually become very adept at this history-taking, exhibiting a very short learning curve and able to perform the history portion in under 10 minutes. Once this history has been completed, the patient is seen by the physician. Again, there is no paper-chart to pass to the physician and the handheld computer tells the physician in which examination room the patient is located. If the history was done on the PC at the nurse's station, the data is transmitted via radio frequency to the handheld computer for immediate use by the physician. The physician then has the following neurological exam available to him. Once again, this format can be expanded or contracted according to practice, patient population, and physician style.

13. Mental Status (5 choices)
14. Speech (7 choices)
15. Cranial Nerves (Currently, 2 choices)

We currently use the icon for dictation if this is anything other than within normal limits.

16. Cerebellar (4 categories, each with 10 choices)

In any of these categories, if something is within normal limits, the computer immediately bypasses the choices and goes to the next major category.

17. Carotids (6 choices)
18. Motor Examination (25 categories or muscle groups, each with 19 choices)

Choices include, for example, left and right, different grades of strength, and conditions such as atrophy.

19. Straight Leg Raising (18 choices by various degrees)
20. Range of Motion (14 choices, again easily expandable)
21. Spine (8 choices, including spasm, scoliosis, etc.)
22. Sensory (20 categories, each with 10 choices)
23. Reflexes (8 categories, each with 18 choices)
24. Gait and Station (14 choices)

All of the above categories have free text as one of the choices. The physician has the option to draw alphanumeric figures on the screen, which are automatically entered as part of the text. Figures, such as a drawing of a hand with accompanying notations, will not print out as hard copy, but will be stored within the databank, so that the physician has access to it on the computer.

25. Studies (18 categories, each with 44 choices in the imaging file, such as X-rays, MRIs, etc.)

If the reports came with the patient, these are scanned and put in AutoImage, and the physician can immediately call up the report. He also has the choice of entering his own interpretation under these choices. Other diagnostic studies, such as electromyography/nerve conduction velocity studies, are also listed.

26. Diagnosis (16 categories)

Diagnosis can be as voluminous as one desires and can be practice-specific or physician-specific. In a large practice, where physicians tend to subspecialize, the number of categories per physician will be much smaller.

27. Recommendations (Currently, 18 categories with 18 choices per category)

Recommendations include our most common surgeries as well as the most common tests that we order. Again, this is highly specific to each individual physician. It is not necessary to list ICD-9 or CPT codes, since these are automatically included in the program and are placed in the patient's summary sheet, along with the financial records for billing purposes. When the history and physical is finished, the ''save'' icon is tapped to keep the history active and is not placed in temporary storage until the staff can make sure that there is no dictation to be inserted and there are no errors. Once the document is considered complete and correct, it is entered into AutoChart and cannot be altered in any form. If changes are to be made to this original document, they must be entered back under the patient's ID number as an addendum. The document can be in a cryptic or prose form, depending on the detail of the template construction. (Fig. 3.3)

Patient Check-Out

When the patient arrives at the check-out counter, the CPT and ICD-9 codes have already been determined and entered into the computer network by the pen-based unit. A bill is printed and given to the patient to keep for personal records. The automatic transfer of the physician's choice of codes for billing eliminates the manual entry of data from a superbill to the computer and avoids unnecessary error. The computer displays the amount billed and the amount that is to be collected, if payment is due at time of service . This routine avoids any confusion about differing payment procedures among different insurance companies, allowing any staff member to work the position with little training.

Test Scheduling

Any tests or orders that the physician has requested for the patient are scheduled at this time. Facilities are called, and the patient is either scheduled on the spot or called later by the facility to schedule the procedure. After scheduling, the information is entered into the computer for the general knowledge of the office staff. If imaging studies are ordered, the information is electronically transferred to the X-ray Supervisor for proper handling. This transfer is done through the Microsoft Access database discussed earlier. Electronic scheduling increases staff efficiency and eliminates paper correspondence, which at times results in lost information. It also allows instant access by any staff person to information about the date, time, and location of the patient's test, as in the instance when the patient may call, confused about where and when to go for testing. Physical therapy and laboratory orders are treated similarly. Films that were with the patient for the examination are directed to the X-ray department, with instructions for processing. Computer notation is made, showing if films are to be held for the next visit, returned to the original location, or returned to the patient. The processing instructions, determined by the physician's plan of care, are also transferred electronically.

Staff performance with this system has increased efficiency in the flow of patient information in these areas. Near elimination of handwritten notes has sharply reduced paper usage and room for error in records, orders, and billing.

Prescriptions

Prescriptions can be ''written'' either from the pen-based computer or on the regular PC programs. The screen pulls up all previous medications that have been prescribed by the office. Prior prescriptions can be quickly refilled. Schedule II drugs are printed out by the computer and the prescription then signed immediately by the physician. Other prescriptions are either faxed or transmitted directly to the pharmacy's computer, using an internal file listing all local pharmacies. Electronic signature for Schedule II drugs is possible, though some legal hurdles will have to be cleared before it is widely accepted. At the end of each day, an activities summary and report of all medication orders that were sent via the computer can be printed out as can confirmation that individual prescriptions have been received by the pharmacy and actually picked up. Because of computer codes, electronic signature, and passwords involved, the overall security of this type of prescription writing is exponentially higher than paper.

Billing

The patient's basic insurance information is entered into the demographic screen during the

Philip W. Tally, M.D.
James A. Tiesi, M.D.

Neuro/Spinal Associates
5949 17th Ave. W.
Bradenton, FL 34209
(941) 794-3118

Michael A. King, M.D.

6/11/97   PHILIP W. TALLY MD
INITIAL EVALUATION

REFERRED BY: James Jones, M.D.
COPY TO: Family M.D.

DEMOGRAPHICS:
    AGE: 46
    RACE: Caucasian
    SEX: Male
    DOMINANT HAND: The patient is right handed.

CAUSE OF SYMPTOMS:
    The patient states can remember lifting heavy weight just before the symptoms
    began.

PRESENTING HISTORY:
    LOW BACK PAIN: The pain radiates down the right leg to the foot. Complains
    of numbness and tingling with this. These symptoms are constant. DURATION
    OF SYMPTOMS: The patient has had present symptoms for six weeks.
    PROGRESSION OF SYMPTOMS: The patient's symptoms have been
    progressing over time. SYMPTOMS WORSEN WITH: standing and with
    walking. Coughing, sneezing and straining will cause the symptoms to become
    worse. SYMPTOMS IMPROVE WITH: Lying on left side. Symptoms improve
    with the use of heat. TREATMENTS: The patient has had physical therapy
    without benefit. Patient has had ESB's without benefit. MEDICATIONS TAKEN
    FOR SYMPTOMS: Medrol dose Pac, Cataflam prn pain. Flexoril 10mg muscle
    spasms. MEDICATIONS TAKEN ON DAILY BASIS: No medications on daily
    basis. ALLERGIES: No known allergies.

PAST MEDICAL HISTORY:
    MEDICAL: History of kidney stones.
    SURGICAL: Appendectomy. Hernia repair. Vasectomy.

SOCIAL HISTORY:
    MARITAL STATUS/NUMBER OF CHILDREN: Married. Has three children.
    SMOKING: Currently smokes 1PPD and has done so for 20 to 25 years.
    ALCOHOL: A moderate amount of alcoholic beverages. OCCUPATION:
    Professional businessperson.

FAMILY HISTORY:
    Mother living and healthy. Father is deceased. He died in his 60's, of cardiac
    disease. There is a family history of cardiac disease, hypertension. There is no
    family history of lung disease, diabetes, cancer.

PATIENT: TEST, TESTY T.   SS#: 000 00 0000   PAGE 1

Figure 3.3. Example of a History & Physical document.

Philip W. Tally, M.D.   Neuro/Spinal Associates   Michael A. King, M.D.
James A. Tiesi, M.D.   5949 17th Ave. W.
                                  Bradenton, FL 34209
                                    (941) 794-3118

6/11/97   PHILIP W. TALLY MD
INITIAL EVALUATION

VITAL SIGNS:
    HIGHT: 5'7
    WEIGHT: 185

REPORTS AVAILABLE FOR REVIEW AT THIS VISIT:
    There is a report of patient's EMG study here for my review. Report of MRI of
    the lumbar spine also present for my review.

NEUROLOGICAL EXAMINATION:
    MENTAL STATUS: Alert. Oriented X 3
    SPEECH: Within normal limits.
    CRANIAL NERVES: II through XII intact.
    CAROTID BRUITS: No carotid bruits.
CEREBELLAR:
    CEREBELLAR: Within normal limits.
MOTOR EXAMINATION:
    ILIOPSOAS: 5/5 throughout.
    QUADRICEPS: 5/5 throughout.
    HAMSTRINGS: 3/5 on the right.
    TIBIALIS ANTERIOR/EHL: 3/5 on the right.
    GASTROCNEMIUS: 5/5 throughout.
    STRAIGHT LEG RAISE SIGN: Positive, on the right, at 30 degrees.
REFLEXES:
    GASTROCNEMIUS: +2 on the right.
    QUADRICEPS: symmetric
    PLANTAR RESPONSE: Downgoing bilaterally.
SENSORY:
    HYPESTESIA: Moderate on the right, L5 distribution.
SPINE:
    RANGE OF MOTION: Moderate loss range of motion of lumbar spine.
    PARASPINAL SPASM: Present in the lumbar region, greater on the right. This
    is moderate.
GAIT & STATION:
    GAIT: Antalgic.
    HEEL WALKING: Mild difficulty on the right.
    TOE WALKING: Mild difficulty.

X-RAYS:
    AP/LATERAL LUMBAR XRAYS: Evidence of degenerative joint disease.
    LUMBAR MRI: Evidence of disc herniation L4,5 on the right.

PATIENT: TEST, TESTY T.   SS#: 000 00 0000   PAGE 2

Figure 3.3.   *(continued)*

Philip W. Tally, M.D.
James A. Tiesi, M.D.

Neuro/Spinal Associates
5949 17th Ave. W.
Bradenton, FL 34209
(941) 794-3118

Michael A. King, M.D.

6/11/97   PHILIP W. TALLY MD
INITIAL EVALUATION

OTHER DIAGNOSTIC STUDIES:
  EMG STUDY: Evidence of L4,5 radiculopathy.
DIAGNOSIS:
  1. Lumbar radiculopathy
  2. Right L4,5 disc hernaiation

RECOMMENDATIONS FOR SURGERY:
  Surgery is recommended to this patient as a last resort option. The indications,
  risks, goals and alternatives of surgery vs. continued conservative management
  have been explained in full. Patient states understanding. Currently considering
  all of the options and will return decision regarding surgery in the near future.

  Patient is to return for reevaluation in two weeks.

Figure 3.3. *(continued)*

initial evaluation. The insurance company is entered from a list in the Medic® program, with the list updated as often as necessary. Policy information is entered from the patient's card, which was scanned on the patient's arrival at the office. The charges are then filed with the insurance company. Most primary claims are submitted electronically to a clearinghouse, which in turn forwards the claims to the actual insurance company. Within 2 hours of transmission, an answer can be received from the clearinghouse confirming the transmission. The clearinghouse reviews the claims for any errors that may cause the claim to be rejected by the insurance company. If errors exist, the claim is sent back to the office for correction and resubmission. Electronic filing saves the time and expense wasted folding bills and stuffing envelopes, as well as postage and mail time. Currently, secondary insurance claims must be done on paper, because these require that an Explanation of Benefits to be attached. All printed claims are computer-generated on the standard HCFA1500 form. Increasingly, insurance companies require the physician's notes to be attached to the claim for their review, and these can be immediately downloaded by the department.

Patient billing is now handled in-house. Patients are a divided into two billing cycles, and statements are printed on the first and fifteenth of each month. At the end of each month, reports are run to provide statistical information as well as the financial status of the practice. Once the month is closed, these reports can no longer be run for that month. However, on Open Item Accounting, reports can be run at any time of the month for any period of time. These reports generate information such as the top 10 CPT codes and how reimbursements compare to charges.

Increasingly, third-party payers demand operative reports for justification of payment for procedures. This is particularly true for neurosurgery, because of its typically high dollar charges. The networking of our office system with the hospital has greatly facilitated this operative report acquisition. When the operative report is generated, usually dictated into the hospital's system, we produce a ''stand alone'' document. The preoperative diagnosis is listed in the same language as the ICD-9 code. The procedure is listed by both the CPT code and descriptors found in the workbook. A brief history is dictated indicating the reason for the procedure, followed by the operative note. This information is transcribed to the in-hospital computer system and can be electronically signed by the physician from his PC, either in the office or at home, and then can be downloaded to the office for filing and mailing when required. Similarly, if hospitalized patients were not seen in the office, the admission note, consultations, and discharge summary can be entered into the medical records for recall when the patient is seen for follow-up in the office. Conversely, H & Ps done in the office are immediately transmitted to the hospital as part of presurgical documentation requirements.

Payments are currently mailed directly to us. Electronic reimbursement is available, but we have found it to be impractical for several reasons. Many procedures in neurosurgery involve multiple CPT codes, making it risky to automatically assume that the insurance company has paid on each CPT code without doing a direct check. Currently, electronic reimbursement does not have an adequate system for listing each payment per CPT code, and, when it does, there is no way to check the amount per code. Visual confirmation of payment per code is done directly on the accounting programs. This problem is complicated by secondary insurance, which only pays once the primary insurance has reimbursed to its limit. In other words, one cannot bill the secondary insurance until all of the primary insurance money is received.

Within the Medic System, open item accounting, or payment by line, is done in such a way that any receipts are posted directly against a particular charge in a patient's account. For example, if a check is received for a patient who has been seen by two physicians at different times, the check is posted against the particular service and its charge as generated by one particular physician; it is not posted against a total balance of the patient's account. This program allows us to accurately assess which codes (services) have been reimbursed. If there is a discrepancy, the itemization allows us to be accurate when writing to the insurance company about a specific code, which was not reimbursed or was reimbursed at a significantly reduced rate. It then allows for refiling of that code only, thus facilitating the review process.

Most reports can be generated in any number of formats. As all information is entered, any combination can be combined to assess the data. The following is a sample of reports that we review every month:

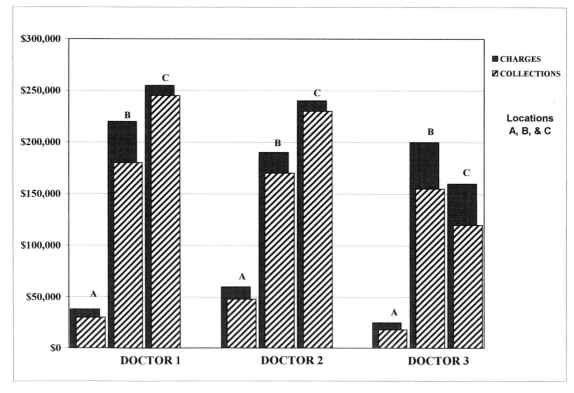

Figure 3.4.   1997 Charges and collections by doctor and location.

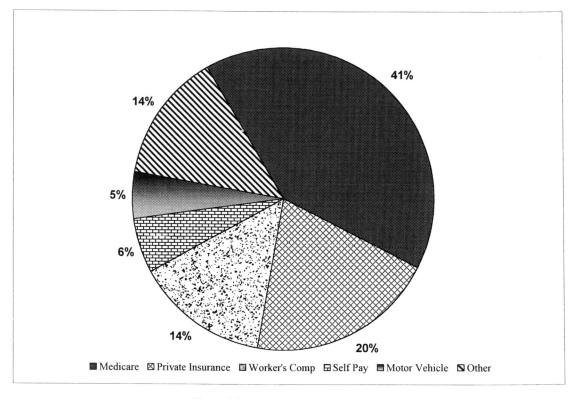

Figure 3.5.   Reimbursement by payer.

1. Reports for gross charges, gross collections, net charges, net collections. This category includes charge adjustments, or write–offs, either by contractual agreement or bad debt. A current cumulative total is generated, comparing year-to-year and month-to-month, to see if any of these categories are increasing or decreasing, reflecting market changes.
2. Reports for charges and collections by individual doctor, location (different hospitals versus office), specific procedure, department (new patients vs. return visits, inpatient surgery versus outpatient surgery)(Fig. 3.4).

In the ever-changing marketplace, tracking payer mix in our practice has become very useful. The computer can track the charges and receipts and the total accounts receivable (A/R) by payer. One can quickly get percentages of the A/R by the type of payer, e.g., Medicare, Workman's Compensation (WMC), Motor Vehicle (MVA), Blue Cross/Blue Shield, HMOs, and others. Plotting the mix by monthly receipts, one can assess how prompt the payments are by any individual payer, or who's "making the float" (Fig. 3.5). We find other information useful as well, e.g., charges and receipts by CPT code and which procedures are generating income in the practice. (Fig. 3.6)

Generating a listing of referring doctors is also possible along with the amount of charges and receipts contributed by their patients. This information is very helpful in marketing. It is also helpful in determining patient mix by zip code. The computer can also generate number and types of procedures by age. From such information one can predict new costs for future contract negotiations. Similarly, a graph of new patients, number of CPT codes, and receipts allows one to quickly assess practice performance over time. (Fig. 3.7) In multi-physician groups, primary surgeon and assistant charges by physician can also be tracked, and changes made accordingly by the practice. For example, surgical assisting and office charges can be plotted and used in determining where a physician's time is best spent.

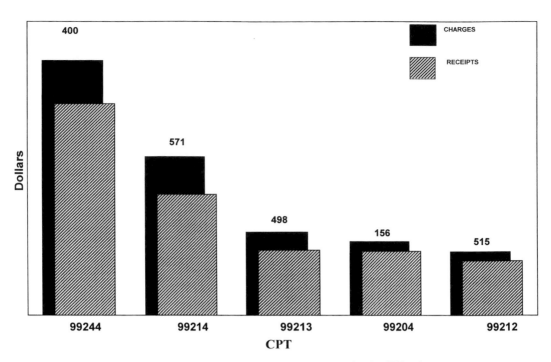

Figure 3.6. Year-to-date office charges and receipts by CPT code.

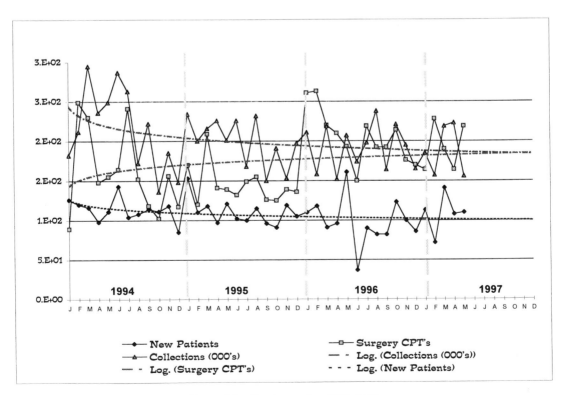

Figure 3.7. Practice trends—1994–1997

Practice Expenses

Currently, the practice is tracking all overhead expenses on PEACHTREE program. This software can generate both a balance sheet and an expense and income statement with ease, detailing monthly, year-to-date, and percentage reports. By tracking overhead expenses as a percentage of the revenue, the actual versus expected expenses can quickly tell the manager if overhead is within its budget for the year (Fig. 3.8). This program also generates the entire payroll and payables, and it automatically does the required tax reporting. All payables are immediately allocated to the proper general ledger account. Bills and checks are never lost, as the system can quickly locate all information. There are multiple safety features built in , so that misuse is extremely difficult.

Approximately 6 hours of the business manager's time are required to prepare 15 pages of statements and graphs for monthly reports. Quarterly reports, which are approximately 30 pages in length, require very little more.

What is the benefit to the practice? The total overhead expenses incurred by the practice decreased by approximately 30% in the first year. This expense decrease included the start-up expenses with the hardware and software acquisition. Personnel costs are on the decline. The computerization has allowed the staff to do more, and because it is user friendly, there has been less specialization of tasks by the staff. Because of this "cross-training," there has been a dramatic reduction in the "key-person" function. Practice operation is minimally disturbed when there are any changes in personnel. This improved efficiency also allows addition of more income-generating personnel, such as expanding the number of physicians, with minimal increases in support staff. Other "hard costs," such as printing, publishing, postage, and paper, have dropped dramatically. Copier usage has decreased by 75%. Total transcription costs have dropped by approximately 90% and record storage has been eliminated. For practices with more than one location, a PC and modem make virtually all aspects of the office portable.

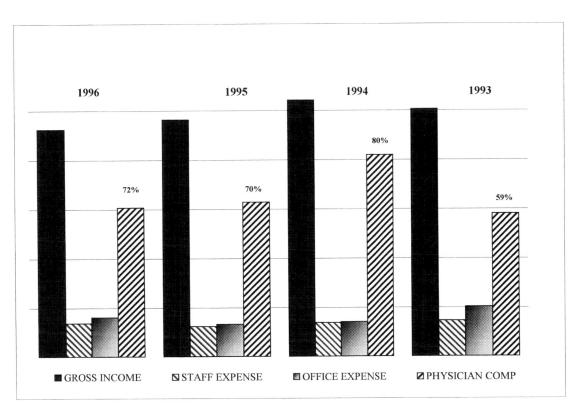

Figure 3.8. Annual income and expense comparisons.

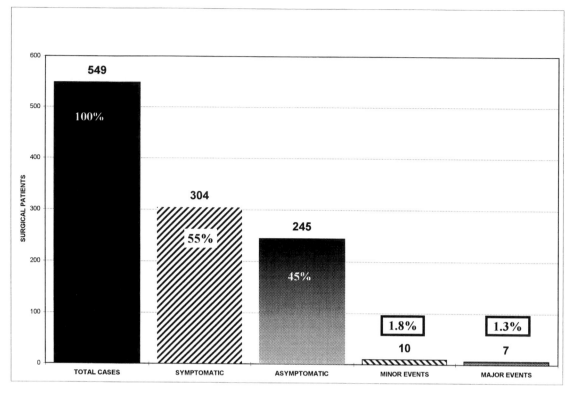

Figure 3.9. Carotid stenosis statistics for surgical patients from February 24, 1989 through December 31, 1996.

Outcomes Research

Usage of the data has already been mentioned for contract negotiations and budgeting. The outcomes research is also easily performed by diagnosis code. For example, in reviewing our carotid surgery data, it is simple to determine morbidity by follow-up codes after surgery (e.g., CVA), and the program can generate the data within a few minutes (Fig. 3.9). We combine this data with that obtained from the hospital, to calculate the average cost of procedure, length of stay, and other data and use this information for marketing brochures as well as contract talks. We are currently using similar data for spine procedures.

CONCLUSION

In the persistent drive toward leaner, more efficient practices, the computer allows the office to be much more systematized, allowing even the physician, with minimal additional effort, to perform functions previously done by specialized staff. This information system allows the doctor to see more patients efficiently with an actual reduction in overhead.

The computerization of the medical practice is inevitable. The sooner the transition is made, the better one's ability to adapt to health-care changes, leaving the physician to achieve the highest goal—serving patients.

"With computers doing all the thinking, all we need now is a worrying machine."

Acknowledgment

The author wishes to acknowledge the assistance of Amy S. Zuidema in the preparation of this manuscript.

CHAPTER 4

Changing Reimbursement for Neurosurgery

RICHARD A. ROSKI, M.D., F.A.C.S.

INTRODUCTION

This century has seen medicine in the United States evolve from a struggling young profession into a giant, highly technical industry. With health-care expenditures approaching a trillion dollars a year in the United States, health care has become one of this country's largest and fastest growing enterprises. Neurosurgery stands out as a notable example of the costly high technology expansion that has taken place in the practice of medicine. Magnetic resonance scanners, operating microscopes, surgical lasers, computerized navigational systems, and ultrasonic aspirators have all improved the ability to treat patients with neurosurgical diseases. These advances, however, have come at a high societal cost. The public today demands the highest level of health care, but they are ambivalent about how it should be funded. As the Federal government, corporate businesses, and individuals have seen their health-care costs rise, efforts to find ways to reduce those costs have increased. The focus of cost reductions has been on hospital costs, pharmacy expenses, and physician fees. All attempts to contain health-care costs have directly or indirectly affected physician reimbursement. Not only has payment altered, but neurosurgeons have been unable to preserve traditional practice autonomy amidst the evolutionary changes sweeping physician reimbursement This chapter analyzes the issues that have shaped the changing environment of medical reimbursement.

A review of neurosurgical reimbursement must encompass more than just the fluctuations in the monetary payments to physicians. It must also include changes in the health-care market, such as the growth of the health insurance industry, the enactment of Medicare and Medicaid, and the increasing expansion of managed care. These changes have caused other effects more serious than simple income reduction. They have dramatically altered the physician-patient relationship, changed physician relationships with their colleagues, and allowed for nonmedical administrative personnel to participate in medical decision making. Scorecards have been created to grade physician performance. With the development of the Resource-Based Relative Value Scale (RBRVS), an attempt has been made to place specific, itemized values on all aspects of work that a physician performs.

All of these issues must be considered when evaluating the changes that have taken place in the reimbursement for neurosurgical services. Many of these issues are addressed in more detail in other chapters of this book. This chapter will explore the impact, where appropriate, of related changes in health care, but will focus on the development of traditional fee-for-service reimbursement and how it has changed with the evolution of the health-care industry throughout this century.

TRADITIONAL REIMBURSEMENT— "The Old Days"

At the turn of the century, a physician had personal and relatively unencumbered patient relationships. Illness was considered a private affair and most medical care was delivered in the home. The only individuals involved in the decisions regarding treatment of an illness were the physician and patient or, at times, the immediate family. No third parties or outside agencies influenced the private medical decision-making process. From a reimbursement standpoint, the physician was able to charge whatever rates seemed appropriate and fair for his medical services. In determining charges, a physician was free to consider the patient's financial situation and whatever other factors he felt were significant. At times, money was not even exchanged. Payment was made in services or other goods in a form of barter. Most hospitals were charitable community institutions and in-hospital care was reserved primarily for the poor and the dying. During the ensuing several decades, medicine experienced a significant transition, as a higher proportion of medical care was delivered in hospitals, instead of in the home. Diagnostic studies, such as X-rays, and in-hospital surgical procedures became much more common. Within this transition period, in the early part of this century, neurosurgery itself emerged as a surgical specialty.

This period of transition and movement toward more in-hospital treatment did not adversely affect the physician-patient relationship. The increased use of hospital services and diagnostic testing did, however, place a larger financial burden on patients seeking medical treatment. It wasn't uncommon for a severe or debilitating illness to financially ruin a family. Several changes occurred to help ease the financial burden placed on the average worker by catastrophic health problems. The two most significant changes were the development of pre-paid health insurance and tax deductibility of health insurance premiums.

Initially, the insurance industry gained a foothold when employers wanted to provide a death benefit to families of workers who were killed while at work. This benefit was intended to provide money for little more than funeral costs. Eventually this insuring against the financial consequences of ill health developed into prepaid health insurance. The first prepaid health insurance plan started by Blue Cross in 1929 reimbursed patients only for hospital charges and did not include payment for physician services. Coverage subsequently expanded to include physician payment, and prepaid plans grew steadily in number and enrollment over decades into the large health insurance industry known today.

Health insurance became a business and labor negotiation issue when employee groups bargained for wage adjustments. Making this employee benefit option more attractive to the employer, the premiums for health insurance were made tax deductible after World War II. This evolution of private and employment-based insurance coverage greatly increased the number of people with the resources to pay for health related problems. Physicians initially strongly opposed the establishment of health insurance, fearing the interposition of any agent between the patient and the doctor. However, in the long run, physicians gained greatly from the spread of routine health insurance coverage. The physician was still able to charge whatever he felt was appropriate for his services, and the patient remained financially liable for whatever cost remained after health insurance indemnity coverage paid for part or all of the charges. Reimbursement to physicians during this period of history remained heavily under the control of the physician. It was not uncommon for a physician to write off bills to the indigent and to write off charges to colleagues and hospital workers as a *professional courtesy*. There was little, if any, regulation of the entire physician payment process.

As more money became available within the insurance industry, physicians prospered greatly. This *fee-for-service* environment is the reimbursement system that has been most familiar to practicing physicians today. The changes that came with the first generation of prepaid health insurance did not adversely affect the physician-patient relationship. The physician made decisions based on professional perceptions of what was best for the patient. Only the patient and the physician were involved in the decision-making process. Looking at subsequent changes in physician reimbursement, it will become evident that as cost containment methods were instituted, a change occurred not only in reimbursement, but in the relationship of the physician with his patient.

GOVERNMENT INVOLVEMENT

The federal government has played a very active role in American health care for many years. With the establishment of the National Institutes of Health following the Second World War, the federal government became directly involved in the financing of health related research, including selection of areas of preferential support. The federal Hospital Survey and Construction

Act (Hill-Burton Act), enacted in 1946, provided funding for the building of numerous community hospitals during the next 27 years. That federal support led to a significant increase in the number of hospitals across the country and, therefore, a greater availability of operating room facilities. This government funding made it possible for neurosurgeons to practice competitively in less populated communities, rather than limiting their practices to the larger metropolitan areas. This growing accessibility to hospitals clearly expanded the scope of neurosurgical care across the country.

MEDICARE AND MEDICAID

As health insurance became more available, two large groups were left out: the elderly and the poor. The rising cost of illness had a significant financial effect on the elderly. Those who had planned poorly or were unable to put much away found their life savings completely depleted when unexpected illnesses developed. The federal government made a dramatic move to solve the problem in 1965. The law enacted in July of that year provided for three changes under The Social Security Act. These included a plan for compulsory health insurance, known as Medicare Part A, and a voluntary insurance plan to cover physician charges, known as Medicare Part B. A final component, Medicaid, matched federal funds with state contributions to provide for the poor. Medicare and Medicaid were initially opposed by physician organizations, just as earlier physicians had opposed the establishment of health insurance. In retrospect, both the Medicare and Medicaid programs became a tremendous source of revenue for physicians, as well as the entire health-care system.

The money provided through the Medicare program also helped to pay for a significant part of the technological growth seen over the past three decades. Because hospitals were reimbursed based on their costs, it was advantageous for hospitals to increase their costs by buying new and expensive equipment. New community hospitals built with the help of the Hill-Burton funds could be equipped with the most up-to-date technology by passing those costs through to the federal government via their Medicare reimbursement. This new funding source continued to add to the availability of diagnostic scanners and sophisticated operating equipment in

many smaller hospitals. Neurosurgeons not only had available operating facilities within which to work in smaller communities, but these facilities were often as well equipped as many large teaching institutions. Through the Part A Medicare payments to hospitals, which included direct medical education (DME) and indirect medical education (IME) payments, the federal government subsidized most of the salaries of medical and surgical residents throughout the country. This availability of resident physicians led indirectly to higher reimbursements for neurosurgeons in academic centers, because academic departments did not have to use practice revenues to subsidize the salaries of the residents.

When the Medicare payment system came into being, the elderly were provided with only partial coverage for their health needs. The physician was offered the option of accepting the payment from Medicare as payment in full, or requesting that the patient pay the remaining balance of the physician's bill. The hospital charges were paid in full. A great deal of additional money flowed into health care, but few, if any, restrictions were placed on how physicians practiced. In the beginnning, there was no government or insurer interference with the physician-patient relationship.

MEDICARE COST CONTAINMENT

Medicare costs exceeded 25 billion dollars in 1980. This amount was five times the projection made at the program's inception. Total health-care expenditures for the United States in 1980 was 230 billion dollars and is projected to reach 1.7 trillion dollars by the year 2000. Facing rapidly escalating costs for the Medicare program, Congress made two fundamental payment changes, designed to control expenditures. The first change was the implementation of the prospective payment system in 1983. This hospital reimbursement system provided for bundled, per-episode-of-illness hospital payments, based on diagnosis-related groups (DRGs). The second change was the development of a physician fee schedule, which took effect in January, 1992 with a 4-year phase-in. These two congressional acts have had significant ramifications affecting both physician reimbursement and the relationship between patient and physician.

The DRG payment system to hospitals was the first major step by the government to oversee the specifics of inpatient hospital care. Designed as a means of decreasing hospital costs, it did even more to interfere with the physician's decision-making process when it came to questions of length of hospital stay and the necessity of diagnostic tests. Physicians had long been exposed to peer review of their work, but, with propsective payment, Medicare precipitated direct review of physician activities at an unprecedented level. The DRG system succeeded in decreasing the length of hospital stay for most Medicare patients and shifting many surgical procedures to the outpatient or ambulatory-care setting. These changes did not significantly alter neurosurgical reimbursement for surgical procedures. It did, however, decrease the reimbursement for nonoperative inpatient care, because patients were not approved for admission or were discharged from the hospital much sooner. Such problems as nonoperative low back pain seldom could be worked up or treated on an inpatient basis. This reduction in inpatient services produced a noticeable decline in neurosurgical reimbursement and an even greater reduction for many nonsurgical specialists, who were accustomed to treating a large number of patients in the hospital setting. The more important change produced by the Medicare DRG payment system was the increased involvement of nonphysicians and even nonmedical personnel in evaluating the appropriateness of medical care and second guessing medical decision making. The effect on the physician-patient relationship was detrimental, as the physician became caught in the middle in disagreements about the timing of patient discharges from the hospital.

RBRVS AND THE MEDICARE FEE SCHEDULE

The Health Care Financing Administration (HCFA) failed to significantly decrease Medicare expenditures with the DRG system. Congress had to develop other methods of controlling rising Medicare costs. An obvious target was the reimbursement paid by Medicare for physician services. To control physician reimbursement expenditures, Congress felt it was appropriate to establish a national physician fee schedule. The plan was to control physician reimbursement and thereby decrease physician costs. The plan failed to achieve the goal, but the physician fee schedule remains in place.

When physician work is billed to Medicare or nearly any insurer, the physician services are described by using a code to define the work performed. The most universally used coding system today is the Current Procedural Terminology (CPT) system, which is copyrighted and maintained by the American Medical Association (AMA). In order to develop a physician fee schedule, HCFA established a specific fee for each CPT code, taking into account regional variations in practice costs, liability insurance costs, and variations in physician charges. HCFA contracted with Professor William Hsaio at the Harvard University School of Public Health to develop a relative value scale relating all CPT codes and physician charges. The resource-based relative value scale (RBRVS) that resulted from this work was based on a concept of "resource" inputs by the physician for each billed service. Each CPT code was given a total "relative value" as it related to every other CPT code. Each relative value had three components: the physician work component, the practice expense component, and the malpractice liability insurance component. Each of the three components was multiplied by a geographical practice cost index (GPCI), which adjusted for regional variations in resource costs. The final relative value was the summation of the three components after multiplying each by its regional GPCI. Finally, the relative value units (RVUs) for each CPT code were multiplied by a dollar conversion factor to establish an actual fee for each CPT code. An important aspect of the entire RBRVS process was the assumption that there would be one relative value for each CPT code. That value applied regardless of who performed the service. No provision was made for level of training, experience, board certification, or any other differentiation between physicians.

There have been numerous criticisms of the Medicare RBRVS. The work done by Professor Hsaio focused on establishing physician work values for a select group of CPT codes. These values were then extrapolated to other similar groups of CPT codes to obtain relative values for the entire listing of CPT codes. The reference work values were obtained in cooperation with organized medicine and focused on the issues of physician time and work intensity. The other components of the scale, the practice expense component and the liability insurance component, were not based on resource input studies.

Those values were obtained using historical cost data obtained by HCFA. In 1993, Congress mandated that HCFA obtain resource-based values for the practice expense component of the RBRVS, to be implemented into the fee schedule by January 1998. There is growing concern that the proposed changes in the practice expense values will drop neurosurgery reimbursement by 10 to 30%.

Another criticism of the RBRVS is its adoption by payers outside Medicare. When changes are made by HCFA to physician work values, they are frequently made to maintain Medicare budget neutrality, not based on a new, valid change in the relative value of the actual work. This internal adjusting to fit Medicare budget needs progressively distorts the original, balanced relativity of the scale, a distortion picked up by private payers who also use Medicare's RBRVS. This adjustment usually means that other CPT work values are decreased to offset the change that is made for a new or altered work value. These adjustments may be important for Medicare to control its budget, but they progressively invalidate the fundamental relativity of the scale when used outside of the Medicare program.

Another consideration when analyzing the Medicare fee schedule is the establishment of maximum allowable fees for each CPT code. When Medicare payments were first established, physicians could choose to participate with Medicare. If they participated, they received their payments directly from Medicare and they accepted the payment as payment-in-full. If a physician did not participate, the patient could be billed personally for the portion of the bill not paid by Medicare. The physician had the choice of writing off the remainder of the bill if he thought the payment would produce an unusual burden for the patient. If the patient had adequate resources, full payment was expected. Since there were no restrictions on what could be charged by the physician, some Medicare recipients faced a significant financial hardship, despite their thinking that they had full coverage through Medicare. As the new RBRVS fee schedule was implemented, Medicare also began to limit what could be charged by physicians, even if they did not participate with the Medicare plan. The Maximum Allowable Charges (MAC) for the first time placed an actual ceiling on what a physician could charge for services,

even without a contractual relationship to lower fees. This process not only coerced many physicians to finally participate in the Medicare reimbursement plan, but it also set an important precedent for the government. Congress, in effect, established the upper limits of what could be charged to a Medicare patient. Free market forces were no longer at work in the health-care marketplace.

The importance of the RBRVS to physician reimbursement extended far beyond its effect of limiting payments to physicians for Medicare patients. The RBRVS provided a tool that was lacking for those who wanted to limit or control physician reimbursement in the private insurance sector. Armed with a relative value scale that was developed with the input of organized medicine, managed care organizations were able to use the scale to reduce physician fees. More importantly, it became ammunition for one specialty group of physicians to point the finger at other specialties that they felt were overcharging for their services. With the relative value scale, it was easy to argue that any physician group that was charging a higher conversion factor than others for their services was being unfair or greedy. By turning physicians against each other, it became much easier for managed care organizations to force physician groups to comply with lower fee schedules. The groups that were most affected were the surgical specialists who historically had been able to command higher compensation. Often those higher fees were based on the scarcity of certain specialists. In an open competitive market, one would expect the services of those physicians in scarce supply to be priced at a higher level. The implementation of the RBRVS on a wide scale negated many of those normal market forces which function in a free market economy.

Without question, the most significant changes that have affected physician reimbursement in this country have come about because of the actions taken by the federal government. Earlier in the century, those governmental changes were somewhat positive for physician reimbursement (tax deductibility of health insurance, Medicare and Medicaid coverage of previously uninsured), but, more recently, they have reduced physician, particularly surgical, income. The elimination of balanced billing for Medicare has flowed over into other insurance contracts as well. The development of a relative value scale for physician fees, which does not take into account differing regional market forces, has given insurance companies a strong tool to use against physicians when negotiating contracts. These changes limit the ability of physicians to price their services based on the value that they bring to their geographic area. That limitation conflicts with the standard concept of free-market competition. Whether a truly free, competitive market in health care ever existed is questionable; but price control by the Medicare Fee Schedule and Medicare's annual conversion factor makes the future liklihood of a free competitive health-care market even more doubtful.

MANAGED CARE AND THE HEALTH INSURANCE INDUSTRY

Corporations that wanted to protect their employees from the financial effects of catastrophic illness found their cost for employee health insurance premiums increasing at a rate similar to Medicare's experience with its rising program costs. Health insurance companies were not especially concerned, because they simply passed on the increased costs to employers through higher premiums. American industries realized that their increasing health costs were dramatically affecting their profits, making them less competitive in the international market. That loss of profitability created a substantial push to lower the cost of health care. Numerous methods were instituted by insurance companies to reduce the costs of medical care, the so-called "medical loss ratio." Discounts were negotiated with hospitals for their services. Preapproval became required for many operations and invasive diagnostic tests, and hospitalized patients were followed concurrently by insurers to control or reduce their length of stay. These methods produced some incremental benefits when they were first implemented, but they failed to produce the dramatic changes that were expected.

Insurance companies began to focus more on the people who had the most direct control over the utilization of health-care resources: the physicians. Contractual arrangements, or participation agreements, were used by the insurance industry in a fashion similar to that initially used by Medicare. The difference was that a specific fee schedule was not clearly defined in the early arrangements. Insurance plans asked physicians to accept as full payment the insurance company's fee schedule, which usually was not disclosed, but was described as *usual and customary* for the region. The fee schedules varied rather dramatically across the country. This nebulous definition often produced significant arguments about certain fees, because the basis for the usual and customary fees was difficult to substantiate. In effect, the insurance companies set fees to their liking.

As smaller managed care organizations developed, physicians demanded a more accurate listing of the fees they would be paid for their surgical procedures. It was common to negotiate a complete fee schedule for each physician or group of physicians who participated in a managed care plan. Physicians felt they had some negotiating power to control their destiny in the managed care market, because they had at least the ability to negotiate the costs of their services. From the managed care plans perspective, however, the situation was not workable. They faced two major problems. First, the use of a different fee schedule for each physician in the plan made it difficult to handle claims and to accurately predict changes in premiums. Second, there were no controls placed on other areas of health-care expenditures, such as medication costs, hospital utilization, and use of expensive diagnostic testing.

With physicians under tighter contractual control, managed care plans focused on how to *manage* the excessive use of hospital facilities, diagnostic tests, and pharmacy costs. Physicians were instructed to use generic drugs when writing prescriptions, or they were given formularies, which listed the approved lower-cost alternatives for all prescription drugs. These pharmacy policies were sometimes just suggestions, but, at other times, physicians were punished or sanctioned for not complying with the drug policies. Diagnostic tests, hospital admissions, and operative procedures not only required precertification before they could be performed, but the criteria were made much more stringent. Insurance companies have long monitored patient lengths of stay in the hospital. Those numbers were now used to grade and compare one physician's performance against another. Today, use of that data is referred to as *economic credentialing*, when physician participation in health plans depends on a financially favorable cost profile. Physicians have traditionally not been trained to evaluate the costs of their treatments, and, historically, cost consideration was not part of their clinical decision-making process. Managed care organizations, therefore, had little difficulty cutting out some of their costs, or ''excess fat.'' What was not considered, however, was how these external controls affected the physician-patient relationship, or how they might affect the appropriateness of a physician's medical decisions. They are a matter of concern that haunts the medical profession today.

As managed care organizations became more competitive, it became more difficult to squeeze additional savings out of the system. They turned next to tighter controls on physician payment. The first strategy was to simplify the reimbursement to physicians by eliminating variation in fee schedules. It was much easier to deal with one fee schedule for the whole plan. With various specialties unable to agree on a common fee schedule, the appearance of a national relative value scale in the health-care market filled an obvious need. There had been earlier attempts to develop relative value scales with the California relative value scale and later with the McGraw-Hill relative value scale. The purpose of the relative value scale was to help bridge the gap between different specialties and to help to squelch arguments about levels of reimbursement. Because the AMA printed changes to the CPT book each year, there were always gaps in any relative value scale until numbers could be developed for the new or revised CPT codes. The federal government helped solve the problem when HCFA published the RBRVS in 1992. Although designed for use by the Medicare program, it was intended for adoption in the private health-care sector according to the 1992 Physician Payment Review Commission (PPRC) Annual Report, and it spread quickly throughout the insurance industry.

By design, the RBRVS addressed the questions of how a particular medical specialty's work related to the work of other specialties. To remain current, it has been updated annually as new and revised CPT code changes have been developed. This standardized fee scale provided the tool that managed care plans needed to address their own problems with negotiating physician fee schedules. Since 1992, the use of the RBRVS by the private insurance sector has grown steadily and will continue to grow dramatically in the coming years.

Along with the positive aspects of the RBRVS have come some unfavorable effects. When HCFA makes changes to the Medicare Fee Schedule, those changes are often dictated by Congressional budgetary constraints. HCFA has also worked through the RBRVS to increase reimbursement to primary care physicians relative to, and, at the expense of, specialists. These two important factors will continue to determine future changes that will be made in the RBRVS. They will also continue to produce distortions in the RBRVS that fail to reflect the true relativity that was present when it was originally developed. Although these changes may work well for the Medicare system, their distortions will be multiplied even more as the use of the RBRVS grows outside of Medicare.

A criticism of the RBRVS is the absence of a method for accounting for a physician's level of expertise or training. All practitioners submitting a bill for a CPT code are reimbursed the same amount, regardless of differences in skill, knowledge, or experience. Another flaw is that it does not recognize the actual market forces regarding the availability of certain health-care providers in different regions. For the only neurosurgeon within a 500 mile radius, the RBRVS eliminates the ability to capitalize on that market scarcity (a true shortage of neurosurgical practitioners).

What has been the result of the federal government and managed care influence on reimbursement to neurological surgeons? The influence has been both a monetary decrease and a loss of autonomy in the decision-making process regarding the treatment of patients. The principles of managed care have placed an additional barrier between the patient and the physician. Precertification and other similar utillization control processes have attempted to supplant the physician in treatment decisions. These influences have had a worrisome influence on the ethics of patient treatment. Closed physician panels have served to limit patient access to, or choice of, the physicians they are able to see for medical services. This limitation has several effects on the individual neurosurgeon. If a patient is not permitted to see a neurosurgeon for consultation, the neurosurgeon loses that opportunity for reimbursement. If the neurosurgeon is not allowed on the panel of approved neurosurgeons, the loss in potential revenue is even greater. In markets such as California's, where there is a significant excess of surgical specialties, the growth of managed care has been devastating to many specialty physician practices.

The development of the Medicare Fee Schedule has allowed Medicare to decease the reimbursement to surgical specialists and to progressively divert money toward primary care physicians. This shift has produced a gradual reduction in the reimbursement to neurosurgeons. By dramatically limiting what nonparticipating physicians can charge Medicare, the federal government has all but forced most physicians to accept their fee schedule. These reductions alone could probably be adequately tolerated by most neurosurgeons. Medicare reimbursement provides about 16% of the revenue to an average neurosurgeon's practice. A gradual drop in Medicare reimbursement, therefore, could be tolerated, were it not for the extensive use of the RBRVS outside of Medicare. As more insurance companies have shifted to using the RBRVS as the basis for their fee schedules, physicians total reimbursement has drifted closer to Medicare levels. Some insurers are already reimbursing *lower* than Medicare rates in selected parts of the country. These fee reductions have been quite difficult for neurosurgeons in solo practice or small-group settings to overcome. The widespread use of an RBRVS-based fee schedule will continue to drive reductions in income for neurosurgeons until an as yet undetermined floor is reached.

CAPITATION

Medicare, and many managed care organizations, have found over the years that reducing physician fees does not decrease overall expenditures, as hoped. A fee-for-service, or even a discounted fee-for-service environment does not control how physicians utilize other health-care resources. As managed care plans struggled to decrease the utilization of expensive health-care resources, they sought ways to share the financial *risk* for those health-care costs not included in the direct physician reimbursement. The justifying rationale was that shifting financial risk for medical decisions to physicians would make them more conscious of medical costs and more cautious in creating health-care expenditures by their medical decisions. Health plans offered to share that risk with physicians by several strategies. Managed care plans began to share risk by

developing risk pools for pharmacy, physician, and hospital costs and then allowing physicians to share in the savings, if expenditures for those pools fell below projected targets. This type of risk sharing is common in many relationships between health maintenance organizations (HMOs) and independent physician associations (IPAs). Under this arrangement, physicians could share in some of the savings from their prudent use or nonuse of specific services. This provided another source of revenue for physicians as the revenues from individual patient care services fell. The end result of this trend has been the development of *capitated* contracts with physicians.

The first capitated contracts involved gatekeeper primary care models. The primary care group was paid all of the budgeted money for physician services for a defined group of contracted patients. This was usually paid monthly for each insured life. This per-member-per-month payment (PMPM) was paid whether or not the insured patient population needed or used medical services. If the patient needed the services of a specialist, the primary care group paid the specialist for those services from their PMPM allocation. Primary care physicians would obviously attempt to contract with specialty providers who would agree to markedly reduced fees for their services. Many specialties, such as neurosurgery, found themselves in the position of having to accept dramatically reduced fees just to get contracts from gatekeeper primary care groups. With some parts of the country experiencing 70 to 80% penetration by capitated plans, specialists have found fewer and fewer indemnity-insured patients to treat. Capitated plans have also produced a strong incentive for primary care physicians not to use specialty care. By avoiding the use of other physicians, the primary care physician keeps more of the capitated payment. By not treating their patients with the help of specialty physicians, gatekeepers could potentially make much higher incomes in such a capitated arrangement.

Specialty subcapitation has become a growing trend among managed care organizations in attempts to further reduce costs. Recognizing that much of the cost of care is still generated by patients who pass the first filter of the primary care gatekeeper and reach the specialist or hospital, the subcapitation strategy is to reproduce among specialists the same incentive to reduce or conserve expenses as that experienced by capitated primary care physicians. Capitated specialists in a single group are paid the entire monthly capitation payment for all the patients covered in the plan. For multiple groups on a specialty panel capitated by a health plan, each specialist draws from a pooled fund, paid out based either on discounted fee-for-service claims (often with a withhold), service relative value unit claims, or a fixed uniform payment per new patient encounter. Only the third payment method reduces the financial incentive to perform unnecessary surgical services. There is a growing trend to return primary care physicians to fee-for-service when specialists are capitated, giving them an incentive to retain patients and be paid for services that might otherwise be sent to capitated specialists. The forms and permutations of capitation are numerous, and continue to evolve.

Most important for neurosurgeons facing capitation is the ability to accurately calculate the practice costs and the effect a particular capitation rate will have on the practice's income. Regional average rates are available through actuarial firms, such as Milliman & Robertson or Towers Perrin. These are averages, however, and do not reflect the makeup of the individual managed care plan. The best method for calculating an initial capitation rate with a health plan is to calculate the fee-for-service equivalent. This calcualtion requires accurate data from the practice or the health plan for all the neurosurgical services provided to that health plan's enrolled population over at least the preceding year. At a minimum, all neurosurgical CPT codes reimbursed, all payment amounts, and total enrollment must be known. The assistance of an actuary experienced in capitation is invaluable to a neurosurgeon first confronting a capitation contract.

Concerns have been raised about the ethics of medical decision making in capitated arrangements. In markets with a large number of the insured covered under managed care plans, growing numbers of neurosurgeons face capitated neurosurgical care contracts. The same ethical concerns faced by capitated primary care physicians confront neurosurgeons signing specialty capitation contracts. If neurosurgeons will receive the same reimbursement whether or not they perform a difficult surgery, will they tend to recommend against surgical treatment, even

if beneficial? These kinds of questions will continue to arise as specialty capitation increases across the country. There has been a great deal of publicity about the anger expressed by the public when medical services are denied in managed care plans. Because of contractual arrangements, many physicians have not been allowed to discuss with their patients treatment options not covered by the managed care health plan. These *gag clauses* raise the most serious questions regarding the ethical treatment of patients. Current state and federal legislation, or ''patient protection acts,'' are reactions against the perceived abuse of patient welfare by managed care health plans. In the future, society will look with even greater scrutiny at the role physicians play in highly managed or capitated health plans. Physicians must always consider patient needs first, not allowing outside financial forces to influence appropriate medical decision making.

THE FUTURE OF REIMBURSEMENT

What does the future hold for neurosurgeons in this depressing stage of downwardly spiraling reimbursement? Despite some estimates of an excess of neurosurgeons, there may not be an oversupply of highly qualified neurosurgeons in the United States. Patients today are very well informed about options for treating their medical problems. Television programming and the World Wide Web both provide access to current medical information, educating the lay community and helping to make them well-informed consumers. Although managed care plans sell themselves on the promise of improved quality in health care, they have not yet been able to provide or even to define quality health care. As patients become better informed about health care issues, they will demand better quality and will want an even greater say in their choice of treatment and provider. There is an ongoing effort by many specialty medical societies to develop quality and outcome data, so that physicians can be evaluated and compared in a equitable way. As patients have greater access to meaningful data about physicians, they will likely demand access to those physicians, placing quality physicians in a better position to negotiate favorable reimbursement for their services. That change will not come about overnight. Physicians today must be much more aware of their clinical outcomes and they need to know how to market their skills. Medical schools today are just begining to teach students about socioeconomic issues. Physicians have always been regarded with great respect in this country. Reputations have been tarnished, however, as physicians have been required by managed care plans to enforce health plan policies. Physicians must again become the advocates for their patients and not for the insurors. Once at-

tention has been refocused on improving individual patient care, the issue of appropriate reimbursement for neurosurgical services can again be addressed.

SUGGESTED READINGS

Starr P. The social transformation of American medicine. New York: Basic Books, Inc., 1982.
Siegel MJ, Heald RB, eds. Medicare RBRVS: The physicians guide. Chicago IL: American Medical Association, 1997.

CHAPTER 5

The Role of Quality in Neurosurgical Practice: The Objective Basis of Accountability

ROBERT E. FLORIN, M.D.

INTRODUCTION

An understanding of quality of care by physicians is rare. Most neurosurgeons in practice more than a few years had no encounters with quality as an explicit concept during training. As an issue of increasing importance in the past decade, it has become both a challenge and a mandate to comprehend and use the ideas and implications of quality in the daily interface with the health-care delivery system. No longer do physicians have an exclusive right to judge the quality of a service or an outcome by implicit means. The Era of Accountablity for such decisions, founded on explicit criteria, publicly acknowledged, has arrived and cannot be ignored. This chapter outlines the relevant history of these changes, identifies the components of quality, and offers advice on how this information can be applied to render assessments of the quality of the many parts of an intervention and its consequences. Finally, some comments on where and how neurosurgery and its practitioners can adapt to this changing environment are offered.

THE HISTORY OF QUALITY IN HEALTH CARE

In 1934, Ernest Codman, a surgeon in Boston, proposed systematic collection of data on outcomes to analyze what we do and with what results. He collected data, planning to use the information to provide analysis of the actual results of surgical operations to the profession and public as a method of self improvement. He stated that such ''comparisons are odious, but are necessary in science. Until we freely make therapeutic comparisons, we cannot claim that a given hospital (physician, procedure, drug) is efficient, for efficiency implies that the results have been looked into.'' He was a true prophet of the need to critically examine the outcomes of interventions that were intended to improve the health of his patients. Unfortunately, his zeal and persistence failed to attract a following and his early work in this field lay untouched for over 5 decades before it was rediscovered.

In 1988, Arnold Relman (23) announced the ''third revolution in medical care.'' This came on two previous revolutionary eras. The first started in the 1940s and continued into the 1960s, with rapid growth in hospitals, physicians, new advances in medical treatments, and coverage of most of the people with health insurance. He called this the Era of Expansion. The second revolution was termed the Era of Cost Containment. With many more specialists and hospital beds plus an open-ended health insurance system that paid for almost anything, accelerating costs precipitated a response that placed restraints on cost inflation, which had reached 11% of the gross national product. Concurrently, the efforts at cost control by third-party payers generated increasing worry about the effects of cost containment on outcomes and quality of care.

The third revolution was called the Era of Assessment and Accountability. This change was based on a perceived and growing sentiment that decisions on future funding and the organization of health care required a better understanding of the relative costs, safety, and effectiveness of what physicians do, while trying to understand the variations in performance between equivalent providers and hospitals.

More recent concerns that have rekindled interest in quality are analyzed in the following sections, which offer insights into how providers can and should respond to concerns over quality of care. The way that medical services are currently changing obliges physicians to understand how the systems of health-care delivery affect quality. This change, in turn, has a direct influence on understanding how the interaction of providers, the system, and the patient influence the outcomes of any intervention.

Quality in the Health-care Marketplace

The changes in the health system in the past can be assumed to reflect the values accepted by our society in its relation to our health-care delivery system. Government efforts at system-wide reforms in 1994 were rejected and have been replaced by managed care as the driver of marketplace reform. With the current dominance of the health plans, attention is turning to the effects of their competition for market share. In advanced markets, this has driven down costs to a point where genuine concerns about the quality of their services come into question. In response to these concerns, both purchasers and consumers are beginning to broaden their role by comparing the plans for indications of differences in the quality of their services. However, this is notably difficult to do, because of the paucity of broadly based, valid, reliable, and risk-adjusted data on outcomes, which are the foundation of quality.

Employers want this type of information to assure themselves and their employees that providers in the health plan are not cutting corners on cost to the detriment of quality of care. Groups of large employers in several markets are forming purchasing coalitions to improve the value of the services from the health plans with whom they contract on a competitive basis. This trend reflects a demand for the best knowledge about quality for the patients, providers, and the employers.

A number of quality assessment tools have been developed in response to this demand. Short of good data on patient outcomes, they include various procedural criteria developed as accreditation and measurement tools for evaluation of the health plans. The National Committee for Quality Assurance (NCQA) is one of the larger organizations utilizing this strategy. The Joint Commission on Accreditation of Hospitals Organizations (JCAHO), the Foundation for Accountability (FACCT), and the Health Plan Employer Data and Information Set (HEDIS) are all busy generating report cards on the quality of services provided by the plans. Although these measures have differing orientations, they do overlap and serve the function of initiating systematic examination of some basic elements of quality within health plans that address process and performance questions. With wider use, it seems likely that these and other tools yet to be developed will begin to provide data on quality and cost that can more effectively guide purchasing decisions to more optimal combinations of cost and quality that yield increased value.

How Did These Changes Occur So Rapidly?

The rather sudden rise to prominence of quality dates back about 4 years to the debate about the Clinton reform plan. At that time, the emphasis was on how to provide universal access to health care within a national system designed to contain costs. Access has become much less of an issue, although 40 million people remain uninsured. Costs have been ratcheted down by many health plans to substantial discounts below Medicare local rates, and, in some markets, the cost competition among different plans is leading to use of various measures of quality as their only remaining factor differentiating one from another. Hence, the rise in quality and its cousin, accountability as the present focus of concern.

The basic reason for this change in focus is that the quality of health care is now seriously threatened by the rapid shift to managed care as the way to contain costs. These plans contain an inherent conflict of interest between their agreement to provide care for the enrollees and their dependence on providing as little care as possible for financial success. Other factors contributing to this change include the role of consumer that is now played by payers, who function as proxies for individual patients, and an emphasis in managed care plans to deal with the whole population of generally healthy enrollees, rather than the sick individuals that physicians encounter. Finally, the current focus of quality measures remains on the processes of care rather than outcomes.

All of these factors serve to emphasize the depth of the conflicts involved in these issues. Since most doctors in the present system are trying to deal with the conflicting demands of the system and the financial interests of the health-care plans, it is important to consider methods to counter the incentives of the health plans to ration care. This is where monitoring of quality measures can be applied with tangible benefit for patients.

The "Outcomes Movement"

In 1990, Arnold Epstein (9) characterized the changes that were in progress as an "outcomes movement." By this, he referred to the remarkable growth in activity directed at outcomes assessment, analysis of effectiveness, and the general issue of quality. Signs of this movement were seen in the change by the Joint Commission on Accreditation of Hospitals and Organizations (JCAHO) from an evaluation of structural measures to planned use of formal assessments of quality, based on risk-adjusted outcomes as a key element of its strategy to monitor hospitals. The Agency for Health Care Policy and Research (AHCPR), with federal funding (22), has been engaged for the past 8 years in programs directed at examining the effectiveness of various medical interventions and in developing guidelines through the assessment of patient outcomes. Other signs were posted by Paul Ellwood (8), who in 1988 called for a national program termed "outcomes management," in which clinical guidelines were to be based on carefully developed patient outcomes. He recognized the need to deal with an ever increasing amount of information in health care, for "a central nervous system that can help us cope with the complexities of modern medicine." This observation translated to the need for an information network that would permit more efficient analysis and management of the large amounts of data needed in outcomes research. This need for a system of information management came at a time when small computer capabilities were emerging as a tool for management of large volumes of data.

The Loss of Physician Power and Autonomy

The present state of physicians in the "pecking order" of health care is the topic of this section. The reasons for the decline in power and autonomy, with the consequent impact on reimbursement, relate to the events outlined below. This decline in status is relevant to a discussion of quality, since quality is the only tool that the profession can employ to regain their lost influence and respect.

How physicians came to their current state of loss of autonomy and power to influence the evolving arrangements for health care and reimbursement needs emphasis here. George Tyson (26) has given an historical perspective on how the medical profession arrived at a position of power and influence and maintained its autonomy into the late 20th century. Private medical practice has been a cottage industry for a small segment of the population that maintained control over a substantial and growing percentage of the national economy for decades. He attributed the basis for this privileged position of physicians to the effects of political organizations and corporate consciousness under the direction of the AMA. With the sellers' market that followed World War II, with an expanding economy, advances in medical science, and a growing population covered by health insurance as an employment benefit, physicians enjoyed their prosperity, while the AMA protected their turf from competition and governmental intrusions (18). The interests of organized medicine were accommodated as a matter of political expediency.

In the 1970s, after the inauguration of Medicare, medicine gradually became less well unified, and federal grants and subsidies increased the rank and power of academic medicine at the expense of the authority and influence of private practitioners. This had the effect of shifting the agenda of organized medicine away from issues of private and clinical practice. Rapid growth of medical specialties led to narrower loyalty among physicians, and the political unity of medicine became hard to maintain. Increased numbers of medical students and the rapid growth in hospital beds followed, laying the seeds of our current oversupply of both physicians and hospitals. This excess supply, coupled with the growth of voluntary medical insurance and the fee for service system that failed to chal-

lenge the prices doctors charged, led to an escalation in health-care costs that gradually exceeded inflation by double digits. Hospitals also
thrived in the environment of a cost-plus-fee
structure subsidized by the government and the
insurance industry. However, the continued escalation of costs to the clients of both hospitals
and providers created increasing public and private complaint, resulting in a commitment to
control the costs of health care by businesses
and taxpayers. These combined forces were able
to exert far more political influence than organized medicine could muster. As a consequence,
the balance of power has shifted towards the purchasers and consumers of health care signaling
the sundown of the so-called ''golden age'' of
medicine.

The new health-care arena will no longer support and insulate private practice in a fee-for-
service environment. The distress that these
changes are generating do not make it any easier
for physicians to relinquish their autonomy or
consider participation in a redesigned health-
care system. Many of them are caught somewhere between anger and denial, while a few
have passed beyond to bargaining and acceptance. These latter-day explorers of the new
health-care terrain have accepted the need to
abandon the balance of power structure in favor
of a collaborative approach to managing a spectrum of services, while sharing common professional values with their colleagues. The basic
tradeoff, therefore, is between autonomy and the
stability of physician practices. Only a few organizations have made a successful transition to
this new operational state, and both Mayo Clinic
and the Cleveland Clinic come to mind. Professional survival is at stake, and the need to adapt
to the changes in progress is increasing at an
accelerating rate.

Obstacles to a More Rational System

Society has placed an unrealistic demand on
the health-care system to maximize quality
while minimizing costs, without actually considering costs. This is what David Eddy (7) calls
the ''cost taboo,'' which results from at least
two factors. The first is the public demand for
sparing no effort—and no cost—in trying to
achieve the best possible outcomes. The second
factor is that, due to insurance, prepayment, and
taxes, many of those receiving care are not directly paying the costs of that care. This effec-

tively isolates the patients from one measure of
the value of care, i.e., the cost.

Eddy feels that the biggest threat to both cost
and quality in health care today is the unrealistic
cost taboo. The only way to break the cost taboo
is to change public expectations. People must
understand that when participating in a system
that shares resources, they cannot expect to receive everything they might want or that
squeezes out the last bit of benefit. He suggests
that the leadership for getting by these barriers
can come from the professional societies, by emphasizing the distinction between fee-for-service insurance and managed care.

The HMO Backlash of 1996

A combination of reactions brought together
patients who complained of denied services and
physicians experiencing loss of income and autonomy. The common reaction of the two groups
was to strike out at the HMOs blamed for these
actions that are felt to affect the quality of care.

A litany of abuses attributed to the HMOs
appeared as the balance of power shifted towards
these organizations. Some of the examples cited
include gag rules, termination-without-cause
clauses, selective contracting, denials of appropriate care, use of less well qualified gatekeepers
to restrain specialty referrals, and, worst of all
(from the patient's perspective), the inability to
see the physician of the patient's choice.

These accusations have resulted in a great deal
of media exposure of alleged abuses by HMOs
for impacting the quality of care that was expected by their customers as well as the public
at large. Reactions to these stories have spread
across the nation and into Congress as well as
state legislatures. Almost a 1000 pieces of legislation proposing either regulation or control of
HMO policies were introduced in 1996, and 56
such laws were passed in 35 states that same
year. Other reactions include lawsuits against
HMOs, state electoral initiatives to curb abusive
practices, physician-run HMOs, and proposals
to establish Medical Savings Accounts to compete with HMOs on terms of price.

THE CONCEPT OF QUALITY IN HEALTH CARE
Definitions
- Quality is a degree of excellence, such as grade
  or caliber, a degree of conformance to a standard.

- Assessment is an appraisal or evaluation, as of merit.
- Assurance is the quality or state of being sure or certain, of having freedom from doubt.
- Outcome is something that comes out of, or follows from, an activity or process or something that is arrived at on the basis of logic or reason, as a conclusion.
- Guidelines are an indication or outline of future policy or conduct.
- Accountability is subject to giving an account; answerable; responsible; or to furnish substantial reasons or a convincing explanation.
- Standards of Quality can be a minimum level of acceptable performance or results; the range of acceptable performance or results; or excellent levels of performance or results.
- Value is the amount of a service, a commodity or medium of exchange that is equivalent to something else; or it may be relative worth, utility, or importance. The synonym of value is worth, which suggests more lasting, genuine merit resting on deeper, intrinsic, enduring qualities; worth contrasts to value in that value suggests an evaluation made from an individual or specific point of view.

Health-care quality should be defined in terms of benefits to consumers: high quality health care is care that best maintains and improves beneficiaries' health and satisfaction. Since health care is the primary product of the health-care system, how can that system be designed and operated rationally unless the quality of that product is measured, understood, and controlled? Does knowledge of cost matter, if the quantity or quality of the product is unknown?

The Institute of Medicine (IOM) defined quality as ''the degree to which health services for individuals and populations increase the likelihood of desired health outcomes and are consistent with current professional knowledge (17).'' In general terms, quality consists of the ability to achieve desirable objectives using legitimate means, where the goal specified is an *achievable* state of health. The concept of quality is a social construct which includes the idea and valuation of health, expectations of the provider-patient relationship, and views of the roles of different players in the health-care enterprise. Quality assurance reflects an attempt to oversee individual and public responsibility, and reflects the degree of commitment to equal access to and the enjoyment of health. A simple but persuasive definition of quality in health care is care that meets or exceeds expectations (14).

These definitions of quality illustrate the complexity of the concept and the need to consider it from a variety of perspectives. One example is through the eyes of various stakeholders.

Perspectives on Quality

The perspectives of key stakeholders in the system need to be considered, as the concept of quality differs when viewed by different parties and is related to the expectations and values held by different groups.

Physicians' views are already tainted by apprehension due to measurements of quality being developed outside of organized medicine. These measurements often challenge the belief of many physicians that professional judgment should be authoritative in matters of quality of care. This belief is further threatened by the reduced importance of physician judgment and autonomy resulting from the intrusion of third parties into decision making. When patients' values are included in the selection of a treatment plan, the physicians feel a loss of their professional status and control.

Patients evaluate quality in terms of responsiveness to their own needs. Medical and other technological advances have led to expectations of the ability to solve almost any health problem. The traditional fee-for-service system that paid physicians for doing everything possible for the patient has influenced the patient's perception of quality and sometimes inflated their expectations to unachievable levels.

For purchasers, quality represents a way of evaluating how well premium dollars are being spent for the clients of the purchaser. In considering the value of services for their employees or members, they are gradually shifting from quantity measures to measures of the efficiency and appropriateness of the care delivered. While this approach focuses on unneeded services, it should also examine and guard against underuse or lack of access to needed and appropriate services.

OUTCOMES

The Foundations of Quality

Outcomes can be defined simply as the result of doing the right things well. They are essential components of quality, in that outcomes judged as good or beneficial support the definition of quality as measuring up to a standard of excellence. Accountability represents another key component of quality, assigning responsibility for an outcome that results from an intervention in an episode of care. Finally, appropriateness of the care is an important component of quality by its guiding of choices that avoid misuse of services and resources, while helping to identify the right mix of risks versus benefits.

How Do Outcomes Relate to Quality?

Medical care has been measured and evaluated based on three factors in the delivery of care: structure, process, and outcome of care. Emphasis on the structures and processes of care in the evaluation of quality has diminished, shifting to practice guidelines, outcomes assessment, and patient-oriented measures, such as satisfaction, function, and quality of life.

Outcomes can be considered at several levels. The first is the level of process elements, such as morbidity and mortality, unexpected returns to surgery or the emergency room, nosocomial infections, or treatment-related complications. A second level is outcome measures, such as patient satisfaction, functional status, ability to return to work, and other patient-oriented measures. The third level couples the first two levels to create the concept of value, i.e., better proven outcome at a lower cost. This third level highlights the importance of the distinction between process measures and outcomes. The important observation is what happens to patients, rather than whether the processes meet some arbitrary threshold. Given that the medical evidence linking an intervention to an outcome is frequently poor, the connection between quality and improved outcomes of care often is uncertain. Self-evaluation, review of the processes of care, and reliance on data rather than anecdotal information all are involved in total quality management. They can improve outcomes, but have not been used widely, even in academic centers, because physicians have not been stimulated to pay attention to quality improvement and outcomes.

Physicians do understand that wide variations in practice exist, but they have not been provided with trustworthy guidelines concerning what treatments within the range of variation are the most effective. Many fear that practice guidelines and total quality improvement are but one more assault on physician autonomy. As a consequence, the use of appropriate guidelines is rare, in part due to the fact that well developed and reliable guidelines are not widely available.

Why Are Outcomes Measured?

A number of factors have emerged during the past decade that explain the need to examine outcomes in health care. The first of these factors is the need for cost containment—exemplified by the growth of Managed Care Organizations (MCOs) and government payment policies designed to control increases in medical services and costs. In the context of cost containment, outcomes are an index of relative effectiveness of different interventions. Outcomes measures allow recognition of ineffective care and elimination of unnecessary services and expenditures and help to detect potential deterioration in health status, while, at the same time, directly improving quality of care.

A second factor is a renewed sense of competition among MCOs for patients and contracts. This competition has been based almost wholly on price, despite concern that price alone is an inadequate basis for competition. Purchasers should "buy right" as advocated by Walter McClure (15) to compare outcomes and quality, as well as price, when making a buying decision.

Finally, John Wennberg's (27) work on the unexplained variations in care delivered to comparable populations in different geographic areas raise questions about whether they reflect unnecessary costs in overuse or suboptimal care and underuse. Application of outcomes assessment is the first step in answering this question.

Advocates of outcomes measurement believe it will increase understanding of the effectiveness of different interventions, allowing better decisions by physicians and patients. Understanding effectiveness can, in turn, lead to development of valid guidelines that aid physicians and others in the optimal use of available resources. Use of outcomes-based guidelines in clinical decision making is a form of basic clinical research and is based on the evidence of what works and what doesn't.

Another aspect of outcomes measurement is analysis of the appropriate use of services and recommendations for interventions based on the results of such analysis. In a now classic study, Chassin et al. (4) found that one-third of patients that had a carotid endarterectomy were felt to have had an inappropriate surgery, based on a review of their cases by a consensus panel convened by the RAND Corporation. Even if the proportion of inappropriate surgeries was overstated, the fact that a significant amount of inappropriate surgery was provided illustrates the magnitude of the problem of appropriate care.

The need for cost containment, coupled to the growth of managed care programs and governmental prospective payment systems, has created concern that administrative and payment policies, designed to control the increase in medical services, will have harmful effects on the quality of care. Furthermore, the intensity of cost competition in markets with high penetration of MCOs has left little to differentiate one plan from another, aside from issues of quality. This concern with cost has resulted in a heightened awareness that the issue of quality needs much more attention, and it has been addressed in a variety of ways by different plans, usually in a very limited fashion.

How Are Outcomes Measured?

The following Table 5.1 outlines the categories of measures most often used for outcomes assessment.

Note that several common patient-related factors are included under Structure, although they are not strictly structural elements. However, they need to be considered somewhere, and the variance contributed by one or more that deviates from the average will need to be considered in the final appraisal.

Who Uses Outcomes Data?

Application of outcomes measures, once collected and analyzed, can have a direct impact on clinical and policy decisions that are intended to improve the value for the money expended for health-care services. The audiences for use of this information include the following:

- Policymakers, who need information on quality to determine whether value for money is being provided under Medicare reforms or within a specific MCO.
- Providers, who need some measure of the quality of their services to compete for market share, saving costs by improving efficiency rather than sacrificing quality.

TABLE 5.1
Quality-Related Measures of Care[a]

Structure	Process		Outcome
Characteristics of the setting and recipients of the delivery of care	Elements of the encounter with the patient		Effects of care on the health and welfare of individuals and populations
Defines Environment in Which Care Occurs	Technical Measures	Interpersonal Process	Defines the Effects of Care on the Health Status of Patients
Physical plant	Consult with provider	Access to provider	Disease-specific health status
Healthcare personnel	Choice	Info about Rx	Patient-Reported Status and Satisfaction
Organization of the system	Proficiency/skill	Communication	Functional status: 1—physical function
Credentials of facility	Rx ease	Concern/caring	2—Social function
Qualifications of providers	Rx complexity	Status of symptom	3—Role function
Access to services	Rx discomfort	Patient preference	4—Psychologic function
Comfort, convenience and privacy	Rx convenience		Health-related quality of life General health status
Patient-Related Factors			Procedural End Points (Intermediate Outcomes)
Demographics Comorbidity Severity of illness	Disease-specific technical measures		Mortality, morbidity, complications, unplanned returns to OR, ER, ICU, charges, LOS

[a] OR, operating room; ER, emergency room; ICU, intensive care unit; LOS, length of stay.

• Beneficiaries, who need the ability to judge the relative quality of their providers in order to choose the types of coverage and providers that best suit their circumstances and resources, such as in the Federal Employee Health Benefits Program (11).

Important aspects of clinical performance that determine health outcomes and satisfaction are: access; appropriateness; safe, timely, and trouble-free implementation; and communication with providers that is acceptable to beneficiaries. Defining health care quality should be undertaken in terms of benefits to consumers and should represent care that best maintains and improves beneficiaries' health and satisfaction.

How Are Outcomes Adjusted to Improve Accuracy and Reliability?

Comparisons of health outcomes require stratification for case mix, comorbidity, severity of illness, patients' tolerance for symptoms and risk, and patients' preferences concerning therapies. The goal of risk adjustment is to account for pertinent patient characteristics that may modify the effect of an intervention before making inferences about the effectiveness of care. This allows for more accurate assessment of the outcomes of care.

Modifying factors include age, sex; acute clinical stability; primary diagnosis and its severity; the extent and severity of comorbidities; physical functional status; psychological and cognitive functioning; cultural, ethnic, and socioeconomic attributes; patient attitudes and preferences; health status; and quality of life.

Examples of several systems of prepackaged severity measurements include:

• Diagnosis Related Groups (DRGs), which include total hospital charges and length of stay
• Acuity Index method, using Length of Stay (LOS) within DRGs
• Acute physiology, age, and chronic health evaluation (APACHE) that measures in-hospital mortality for adults in intensive care units
• Medis groups, using clinical instability as measured by risk of in-hospital death

The Changing Scope of Outcomes Measurement

Recent outcomes studies have taken some specific directions that affect the types of data collected and used, the types of studies per-

formed, and the types of outcomes assessed. Use of large computerized databases has allowed access to data collected by state commissions, by third-party payers, and even by the Health Care Financing Administration (HCFA) on Medicare beneficiaries. These large collections of data offer the potential for assessing efficacy of a procedure using a nonrandomized study with some ease and accuracy. Use of large-volume databases allows comparisons of different interventions using statistical techniques like matching, stratification, and structural modeling. Absence of data on coexisting diseases and the severity of illness hamper this type of analysis, but efforts at including these have begun.

The scope of outcomes measurement has broadened beyond rates of mortality, readmission, and complications to include subjective data from patients on functional status, degree of disability, social interaction, and other parameters. Supporters of this increased emphasis on outcomes believe this approach will help achieve increased understanding of the effectiveness of different interventions. This, in turn, will improve decision making by both physicians and patients and support the development of guidelines and standards to optimize the use of resources.

The process of developing guidelines from outcomes is fairly direct. First, large databases are used to establish monitoring systems. Then variations in outcome and differences in procedures or interventions associated with a different outcome are identified. Next, nonrandomized trials, meta-analysis, decision analysis, or randomized controlled trials are used to assess the results of the different interventions. Then the results of the data analysis are incorporated into appropriate guidelines. Finally, the guidelines are used for education and feedback to modify physician behavior in the appropriate direction.

Outcomes Management

The need for a system of response to the apparent chaos in medicine was identified by Ellwood (8) with a call for a new technology which he named "outcomes management." This method reflected a need to better understand the relation between medical interventions and their outcomes in terms of the patients health and the costs.

The health-care system has become unstable and unable to deal with the interests of all the parties involved in delivery of care to patients. The basic problem is an inability to measure and understand the effect of the choices of patients, payers, and physicians on the patient's desires for a better quality of life. The result is uninformed patients, skeptical payers, frustrated physicians, and health-care executives threatened by regulatory restraints.

Uninformed patients are still forced to judge medical care on the basis of the quality of the amenities, such as the physician's manner, their waiting time, and their ability to communicate with the doctor. Consumers believe that the only power they have is to choose a physician, hospital, or health plan, yet they still have no way of making an informed choice among interventions, because they have no way of knowing which choice will yield the best results.

Skeptical payers for medical care ask "What value do we get from the mounting expenditures on medical care?" The wide variations in practice style between geographic areas, without corresponding differences in health outcomes, supports the payers' skepticism about "buying right" to attain value for the price paid for services.

Frustrated physicians are concerned about the ability of primary-care gatekeepers to perform the gatekeeping function well along with an apparent lack of recognition of the broader needs of the patient. Physicians are also troubled by the sharing of decision making and power with patients and others, and they are concerned that nonphysicians simply do not have the information necessary to make rational decisions about medical care. The physician's capacity to make sound decisions is also jeopardized by the increasing complexity of medical practice, the cascade of medical information, and the growing number of chronically ill patients.

Health-care executives need a management tool that calculates health outcomes for the patient as a bottom line of greater importance than the economic wealth of the organization.

Ellwood's proposed "outcomes management" is a program of collaborative action based on the good of the patient. It is a technology of patient experience designed to help patients, payers, and providers make rational medical, care-related choices based on better insight into the effect of these choices on the patient's life. Outcomes management consists of a commonly understood language of health outcomes; a national database containing information and analysis on clinical, financial, and health outcomes that estimates the relation between medical interventions and health outcomes; an estimate of the relation between health outcomes and money; and an opportunity for each decision maker to have access to the analyses that are relevant to the choices they must make. Outcomes management would draw on guidelines, measures of function and well being, clinical and outcome data on a large scale, and analysis made available to all the parties involved.

OUTCOMES RESEARCH

Outcomes assessment and research is very much a part of the larger health-care reform taking place in response to a demand for greater accountability. This demand originates from policy makers, health-care payers, purchasers, consumers and the health-care community itself.

Research in outcomes, like manufacturing and industry's research and development or "R & D," is research designed specifically to support clinical operations. Like "R & D," outcomes assessment must be part of a comprehensive strategy that starts with one project and then integrates into the overall organization's functions.

Outcomes research deals with two aspects of treatment, i.e., appropriateness and effectiveness. It seeks to relate the type of medical care received by typical patients with a specific condition to a range of positive and negative outcomes in order to identify what works best and for whom.

The field of outcomes research includes development and testing of methods for measuring the process and outcomes of care, for identifying and quantifying the structural characteristics of the setting in which care is provided, and for obtaining the information needed to accomplish these tasks. The effects of deliberate, controlled changes in system characteristics on quality would also be included, as would methods for initiating organizational and behavioral change in response to demonstrated deficiencies in the quality of care.

Outcomes research evaluates medical and health services and procedures to determine whether particular procedures or services, such as surgical techniques, diagnostic tests, or therapeutic interventions, work as intended; i.e., whether they are effective in identifying a source of illness or disability, relieving symptoms of illness, curing a disease, or preventing illness. The term "outcome" indicates that the focus is on the success or failure of a service in producing a desired outcome for the patient.

Outcomes research can offer a database for deciding what works and how and when to use it. However, this is not yet a well developed process; the study of effective medical and surgical care is still in its infancy. Only a small proportion of medical services have been subjected to rigorous testing to determine their actual effectiveness or relative merit compared to alternatives.

A second problem lies in defining what is a "desired outcome." This can range from the observable and objective to a subjective impression by the patient.

A related problem lurks in the "benefit" concept, since a study of outcomes alone may miss important elements in the process of care that have a dominant influence on the particular outcome. A good outcome may occur in spite of inappropriate care, and a poor outcome may occur even if outstanding care is provided. Inclusion of evaluation of the process of care and the effects on patient satisfaction with the intervention is important in deciding what actually works for the patient.

Finally, translating the results of outcomes research into effective medical care depends in part on how the research is used. This relates to the utility of the information to different consumers, ranging from policy makers, providers, and payers to patients. It is not clear that providers or payers are best armed to make judgments on what kinds of risk will be accepted and how much uncertainty among alternatives can be tolerated. The results leave undecided the question of which patients receive what care, although the current trends favor patient-based decisions, provided the patients are given sufficient information on which to base their choices.

Dissemination of the results of outcomes research should provide better information to practitioners in making clinical decisions, which should help them achieve a more consistent, better quality of care while avoiding treatment that is less effective.

Patient satisfaction has also entered outcomes research as a critical measure of the quality of care, since the recipients of the medical services deemed effective need to be party to the decisions regarding their application and effects. It will be impossible to know "what works" for patients unless the effectiveness of care is measured partly in terms of patient values. This kind of measurement is the rationale for including issues of patient satisfaction into the research product.

The legitimacy of outcomes research and the conclusions that result from the research are based on their accuracy. The validity of research results depends on the integrity of the study design, including whether the right research questions are asked, the appropriateness of the data selected for study, and the objectivity and accuracy with which the data are collected and analyzed. A flaw in any component of the study may produce erroneous results. Thus, it is important to ensure that research is conducted properly to generate valid and reliable results.

Outcomes research is an evolutionary extension of clinical research with several important differences: its analysis of large databases; its organized or structured reviews of the literature, known as meta-analysis; its small-area analysis of health-care utilization; its prospective clinical studies emphasizing patient oriented outcomes of care; and its development of decision making analytical models, cost effectiveness studies, and practice guidelines.

Appropriateness and Effectiveness

There is a balance between appropriateness and effectiveness and the value of services. Such value will include not only considerations of the cost, but also the judgments of patients on such things as what kinds of risks will be borne, how much uncertainty can be tolerated, and which people should receive what care.

Efficacy and Effectiveness

A central theme of quality improvement is that quality is proportionate to the attainment of achievable improvements in health. Efficacy is used to indicate what we consider to be achievable, while effectiveness is what is actually achieved, relative to what is achievable.

Knowledge of efficacy will result from testing clearly specified strategies of care under standardized circumstances, since the purpose is to reveal the strategy of care that produces the best results under a set of fixed circumstances that the clinician may face. The effort to make a cost/

benefit valuation as part of this process should be limited to the clinical situation that was assessed.

Efficacy can be equated with the results of controlled clinical trials, which are usually performed under ideal conditions. Effectiveness is more akin to what happens when a physician performs a procedure in an average hospital without controls or collection of such data. This distinction is important in improving the understanding by all practitioners who participate in clinical research directed towards providing relevant data on efficacy and effectiveness of our interventions.

Cost Effectiveness

Outcomes assessment does not necessarily relate the effectiveness of a medical service to its cost, although it may. Cost effectiveness research can compare the effectiveness of alternative therapies with their respective costs to determine which therapy achieves the desired result at least cost. But the judgment whether the benefits of such services outweigh their costs is a question of economic and ethical policy. Outcomes research can provide the data to consider, but, by itself, does not make the policy choice.

Technology Assessment

Technology assessment is considered by some to be part of quality assessment. However, more precisely, it represents the knowledge that guides clinical practice as determined by testing efficacy under standardized conditions. In comparison, quality assessment is concerned with investigating the degree to which the knowledge contributed by technology assessment is implemented in actual practice.

QUALITY ASSESSMENT AND MEASUREMENT

The terms *quality measurement* and *quality assessment* are frequently used interchangeably. This does not mean that they are always equivalent in the context of judging quality in health care. The ability to actually measure quality, defined as the degree of conformance to a standard, requires that such a standard exist and be available for comparison to the component of quality under examination. The role of outcomes now comes clearly into focus as the basis for identifying those components of quality amenable to

measurement and capable of serving as a standard or benchmark. Assessment represents a somewhat looser judgment about the component with an overtone of gestalt in the appraisal. Perhaps it even implies that precision in the measurement of process and clinical outcomes is not mathematically exact, but conforms more realistically to the operation of biologic systems with their inherent, residual uncertainty. Consequently, assessment is more probabilistic than its cousin, measurement. If the term *assurance* is then added and defined to imply a degree of certainty about the appraisal, it becomes clear that the term is misleading, since it would be rare indeed to reach that state of confidence regarding most components of quality. Relative certainty would be as close as one could approach this goal of assuring the quality of an outcome. Therefore measurement and assessment are the yardsticks to use when evaluating how well a component of quality approaches some standard of reference.

Measuring Quality in Industry Compared to Health Care

A comparison between the efforts to measure quality in health care and quality in industry may be useful. In industry, quality is defined as a defect-free product at a competitive cost. Traditional quality assessment has been guided by the theory that poor quality is caused by incompetent workers (Bad Apple Theory). Industry in Japan has developed an orientation that is based on the Theory of Continuous Improvement, in which quality depends on understanding and revising production processes based on data about the process itself. Quality is then defined as meeting quality standards in the process as well as the product. Workers are assumed to be competent, and the system is at fault if quality is lacking. This is basically the system that Ed Deming exported to Japan during their industrial restructuring, and implementation of that system has resulted in efficiencies of production and levels of quality that have made their products world market leaders.

Historically, reliance on professional judgment has been the method employed to ensure high quality health care. In the new marketplace, the nature of quality assessment with its focus on comparing components of care to some specific point of reference tends to be criticized because of the emphasis on identifying outliers (Bad Apples) as the cause of substandard quality. This is viewed by many, especially physicians, as a punitive rather than a corrective process, which may explain the lack of general acceptance of quality assessment by the medical profession. In contrast, quality improvement focuses on the performance of the system of delivery of care, and attempts to improve quality by identifying how to improve the processes of care relative to outcomes, with less attention to specific outliers.

In health care, there has been no widely accepted definition of quality. However, when the components of quality are examined, we are able to identify three categories that help to define the scope of the concept. The three are as follows: structure—defining the environment in which care occurs, including physical plant, personnel, and system organization; process—involving elements of the encounter between the patient and the provider and including the technical components of the physicians skill and judgment, plus the interpersonal relationship that has generally been encompassed in ''bedside manner;'' and outcomes—referring to the effects of care on health and welfare of individuals or populations.

For assessments of quality to be credible, the variation in structure or process must be shown to lead to differences in outcome. For outcome criteria to be credible, a difference should result if the processes of care are altered. Process data are usually more reliable measures of quality than outcome data for assessment of quality, because a poor outcome does not occur every time there is an error in provision of care.

Parameters of Quality Assessment

The scope of an assessment of quality must be tied to the context for assessment and must address the concerns pertinent to each level. These adjustments are necessary because, as the scope widens, our view of quality changes.

When an assessment of quality is done to judge the performance of practitioners, it involves the identification of two components: the technical care and the management of the interpersonal process (6). This fits into the second component, which is characterized as process.

When the scope includes the performance of an institution (hospital, clinic, office, surgery center) the view of quality expands to the amenities of care, including privacy, comfort, and con-

venience of access and use of the services. These factors match the structural component.

If the scope widens to include the care actually received by patients, the assessment of what the patient and family members contribute to their care is added. If the assessment encompasses care received by a population group, all of the aspects of care mentioned above need to be included. At this level, quality depends on the following parameters:

- Access to care;
- The performance of providers in diagnosis and treatment;
- The performance of patients and family through their participation in care;
- Evaluation of the patient's satisfaction and health status.

Standards represent thresholds above or below which quality is declared to be excellent or to some degree less than excellent. These can be developed rather simply or with great complexity. An example of a simple standard that could be used for case review is setting a threshold for the use of blood replacement during lumbar diskectomy. If the threshold for excellent quality excluded transfusion, then a quality judgment could be made rather easily, based on that simple standard. Affirmation of the basis for the standard would be a necessary precondition to its use, and the information should be provided to all involved physicians. Standards can be developed in this way to measure care provided in a variety of ways, and the thresholds can be tailored to local needs and circumstances. They can also be used to identify exemplary providers to act as local benchmarks for other providers.

Outcomes judged in the context of quality assessment represent a change in status that can be traced to some antecedent care. When other contributory factors, such as case-mix or study design have been incorporated in the analysis of cause and effects, the relationship between the intervention and the results will become clear. The residual uncertainty about the cause of the particular outcome studied can then be identified in its true context and that information used in the assessment of the quality of the intervention. This highlights the role of outcomes as the only reliable measure of quality. Outcomes serve as cues that guide the assessment of process and structure in a search for interventions than can actually be improved.

Satisfaction with Treatment

Treatment satisfaction is the patient's rating of aspects of the process and result of the treatment experience as measured by predetermined criteria. There is a difference between general satisfaction with outcomes and the patient's health status as an outcome. The latter includes five types of measures: biological and physiologic variables, symptom status, functional status, general health perceptions, and overall quality of life. In treatment outcomes, patients bring their expectations about treatment as well as preferences for a treatment, while the duration of the disease and the treatment provided are the remaining treatment variables.

Patient Assessments and Satisfaction

Health is one of the most important determinants of quality of life. The health-related components of quality of life include disease-specific symptoms, general health perception, somatic discomfort, physical, social, and role functioning, cognitive functioning, and psychological well-being.

Why has patient satisfaction been so little used in quality assessment? The answer is that practitioners are biased in favor of technical care, and that attitude has been inbred as part of their training. Acknowledging that patient satisfaction counts in this assessment represents a difficult adjustment for many, especially for older physicians set in their ways and attitudes.

HRQL—Health-Related Quality of Life Outcomes

There is accumulating evidence that measures of "health-related quality of life" (HRQL) are valid and reliable in showing that outcome measures are responsive to important clinical changes (28). The goal of developing this tool has been to describe health status comprehensively with valid measures of the components. These include dimensions of physical functioning, social, and role functioning, mental health, and general health perceptions, including vitality, pain, and cognitive functioning. The model used includes five levels: biological and physiological factors, symptoms, functioning, general health perceptions, and overall quality of life.

Reporting of Quality of Care

Report Cards

The rationale for the measurement and reporting of quality is based on the belief that public release of data on performance will lead to changes in behavior and improved quality. The intent of such reports is to guide the choices of patients, purchasers, and other physicians in their choice of provider services.

Public reporting of health-care provider performance is becoming commonplace. Reporting of data on the quality of health care has taken the form of report cards, and many rely on quality measures taken from the Health Plan Employer Data and Information Set (HEDIS). Others simply use data from patient satisfaction surveys obtained within various health plans. Even the print media have entered this field, with reports appearing in Consumer Reports. The Health Care Financing Administration (HCFA) is working with the National Committee for Quality Assurance (NCQA) to develop report cards that address the needs of the Medicare and Medicaid programs.

Reporting of quality measures is becoming an important feature of the new health-care system, largely due to the perceived need for the data to better inform purchasers and Managed Care Organizations (MCOs) about their choices among different plans and providers. The lack of an accepted form for such reporting is causing much concern among providers, who are worried about potential errors in case mix or severity of illness adjustments that could contribute to an adverse rating. Physicians are especially concerned about report cards that focus on performance that comparing them to their peers and to other groups. Generally, physicians favor indicators of technical quality ("the hundred best Doctors in your area"), which may include disease-specific measures of the processes of care. However, physicians remain very concerned about the potential for the report card offering an unfavorable rating due to flaws in data or the inability of lay readers to appreciate technical measures of quality assessed. In contrast, consumers support use of such data on the performance of individual physicians, since they believe their doctors determine the ultimate quality of the care they receive much more than does their health plan. Consumers will generally depend on measures of satisfaction with the physician encounter, such as convenience, access, and amenities to a greater degree than the technical measures of physician proficiency. It appears that there will be little relief from these trends examining physician performance and quality by measures unfamiliar to physicians.

ASSESSMENT OF QUALITY IN HEALTH PLANS

Early efforts at monitoring quality in public health plans began with federally sponsored Professional Standards Review Organizations (PSROs), which have been transformed into the present version called peer review organizations (PROs). The primary role of PROs has been to prevent the inappropriate use of services by utilization review and to identify individual instances of poor quality for focused corrective or punitive actions.

The purchasers of health care are presently relying on report cards to assess quality of care, since the cost reduction efforts of Managed Care Organizations (MCOs) have reduced reimbursement to marginal levels in a number of markets, with the worry that quality of care will suffer as a consequence. Also, the fact that wide variations in practice patterns persist supports concern about the scientific basis for what we know and how we know it.

The National Committee for Quality Assurance (NCQA) was formed in 1991 as a nonprofit organization to measure and report on the quality of care provided by MCOs. Its leadership includes representatives of health plans, employers, consumer and labor groups, quality experts, regulators, and organized medicine. To date, NCQA has reviewed process measures believed to have an impact on outcomes in their accreditation process of the MCOs. Many large employers are relying on NCQA accreditation when considering which health plan to contract for their employees.

A second activity of NCQA has been the development of the Health Plan Employer Data and Information Set (HEDIS), which focuses on performance and outcomes measures to supplement the NCQA evaluations. Recent versions have issued report cards on the health plans based on clinical quality, access, satisfaction, utilization, and financial performance of the plan.

NCQA—The National Committee for Quality Assurance

The quality of medical care provided in managed care plans traditionally has been measured by professional judgment. Greater accountability is being imposed on the health plans by government and corporations (i.e., purchasers) as the growth of the MCOs accelerates with an increasing proportion of the population enrolled. The key concern is that economic motives may reduce services or prices, or both, to a degree that quality of services deteriorates. Many health plan managers have felt that some type of approval would increase their share of the health insurance market.

Initially, the managed care plans declined participation, since their competitors in fee-for-service medicine were not challenged by suspicion of a risk to quality. As the plans enrollment grew, it became evident that the NCQA had to become an independent organization to sustain its credibility. The suspicions of undertreatment within the system of prepaid care, where the providers are at risk, required that the HMOs be subject to review by an independent quality assurance organization.

The NCQA became independent in 1991 with a grant from the Robert Wood Johnson Foundation and funds from the HMOs. As an independent organization, the NCQA became a watchdog that could apply pressure to health plans to raise their quality levels. The technique is similar to that of the accreditation of hospitals by the JCAHO, and NCQA now accredits all types of health plans on a contractual basis. This is a voluntary process and utilizes an evolving set of performance indicators that cover quality of care, access to and satisfaction with the care, use of services, finances, and management of the plan. The nine indicators that deal with quality focus on process measures, especially on preventive services. Only two outcomes are assessed in the quality appraisal, and these are low-birth weight and hospitalization rates for patients with asthma.

Despite the uncertainties inherent in the measurement of quality, the NCQA has become a prominent purveyor of several forms of quality assessments. It has substantial support among employers, purchasers, and even federal and state governments, which have an oversight obligation to protect people who rely on publicly funded medical care. They hope that NCQA will be able to keep pressure on the health plans to ensure and improve the care they provide even in this era of cost containment and down-sizing.

HEDIS—Health Plan Employer Data and Information Set

The Health Plan Employer Data and Information Set, or HEDIS, appears to be leading in the fight among a variety of report cards that have appeared in the past two years. HEDIS was developed by NCQA. It attempts to evaluate the validity and reliability of a health organization's capabilities in managed care. Using a standard format, it uses a group of procedural criteria intended to enable employers and other purchasers to hold an MCO accountable for its performance in providing care to specific populations, i.e., employees.

Initially, the report cards generated were suspect because of the inability of most MCOs to collect and record patient information accurately. HEDIS has been more a measure of service delivery than of quality or outcomes of care, due to these constraints.

HEDIS is undergoing continual refinement with version 3.0 released last summer. This includes components that will extend its application to Medicaid and Medicare as well as the MCOs already covered. The most significant change is a new emphasis on medical outcomes and patient health status, compared to the former predominance of performance measures. Accreditation by NCQA is becoming increasingly important as one criterion that major private and public employers require for bidding to take place on contracts to cover their employees. Since the shortcomings of performance measures are generally well understood, employers and purchasers who use those measures realize their decisions are now based on better information than was available before NCQA.

However, the effects on the provider community are beginning to surface. The need to improve the credibility of the process with providers is critical due to the inevitable involvement of providers in the evaluation process. Risk adjustment mechanisms have been a provider concern, but even more important is the refinement of the criteria to make them relevant and clinically meaningful. Physicians who have examined HEDIS have concluded that it did not look at things that were important.

FACCT—The Foundation for Accountability

The Foundation for Accountability (FACCT) was formed recently by Paul Ellwood and includes representatives of large employers, consumer groups, and government. Its purpose is to promote use of a common set of patient-oriented outcomes measures, using the purchasing power of its members to speed up adoption of these measures. The measures include an outcomes-based report card and are just beginning to be used. FACCT's basic goal is to develop standardized measures of outcome for health-care entities that can be used to hold them accountable.

AMAP—American Medical Accreditation Program

In 1996, the American Medical Association (AMA) decided to develop a quality assessment program for physician practices. This has been characterized as the American Medical Accreditation Program (AMAP) and is based on a self assessment of the physician's clinical skills and performance measures. The program is couched in terms of an AMA-endorsed accreditation of the surveyed physicians' practices, provided they meet certain criteria that address some of these same report card issues, along with several quality-of-care criteria. Apparently, many physicians have felt harassed by the repetitive surveys of their credentials and performance conducted by the contracting health plans. Unfortunately, many specialists view this program as a threat to their specialty board certification. The feeling is that this represents an effort by the AMA to provide noncertified members with a tool bearing the AMA emblem that imputes accreditation of board-equivalent training and experience.

QUALITY IMPROVEMENT

The outcomes movement motto of ''proving and improving quality'' highlights continuous quality improvement as a key goal of outcomes assessment and research. The key to quality improvement involves a complex process, with detailed and careful examination of the entire process and dissection of the components of care that may yield opportunities for improvement.

By measuring and collecting information on the direct effects of medical care on patients, as reported by patients and clinicians, quality improvement committees have empirical evidence of what programs and services result in the best care. New services and treatments, like a new drug or surgical technique, can be evaluated in a comparison with more traditional treatment that looks at which treatment results in better patient outcomes. Process measures can help detect redundancy and inefficiency in the treatment process. Clinics may also use patient satisfaction instruments to focus on improving efficiency, access, and other problems patients experience during the episode of treatment.

Problems in Quality Improvement

Quality problems in health care are widespread and predate the growth of managed care. These problems take three basic forms and deal with the balance between the risks and benefits of the intervention. *Underuse* is the failure to provide a service whose benefit exceeds its risk; *overuse* is the opposite, i.e., occurring when the service provided has more risks than benefits; *misuse* happens when an appropriate service is provided poorly, with a resultant complication that reduces the net benefit received.

Underuse of services of proven effectiveness is widespread; such underused services include immunizations, detection and treatment of hypertension, and the comprehensive treatment of heart attacks. In the latter example, one study showed that only 21% of eligible older patients received treatment with beta blockers, and the subsequent mortality rate for those who did not receive this treatment was 75% higher than that for the treated patients (25).

Overuse is frequent, and it includes overuse of medications, diagnostic services, and surgical interventions. One of the most famous examples was the RAND study of the appropriateness of coronary angiography and carotid endarterectomy. The study reported that 17% of coronary angiographies and 32% of carotid endarterectomies were performed inappropriately in 1981 in a large sample of Medicare patients (3).

Misuse reflects avoidable complications that result most commonly from errors in use of medications and from complications of diagnostic and surgical procedures. The supporting data is found in the reports of higher rates of postoperative morbidity and mortality among patients who have procedures from low volume surgeons and

in hospitals that perform low numbers of these procedures (13).

Quality Improvement Tools

Clinical Information Systems

Some health plans publish information collected from their claims information to generate ''report cards'' that have been praised for giving consumers better market information. Unfortunately, this data is hard for the physicians to use when negotiating with MCOs, because they are not familiar with the data source, cannot verify the numbers offered, nor understand why a physician may fall ''outside the norm.'' Outcomes assessment and research offer an important source of data that can counteract such report cards or profiles that are based on claims data analysis.

Collection of data in a systematic fashion for outcomes assessment requires the ability to handle large amounts of information from a variety of sources in a rapid manner, with flexibility in the way that data can be examined and analyzed. This requires an information infrastructure that is based on computerized data. In situations where the patient record has been computerized, the ability to do outcomes assessment is greatly enhanced. At present, the majority of practices and hospitals are still not using an electronic medical/hospital record that is integrated to include most of the data relevant to outcomes research.

Ellwood envisioned the computerized record as the basis of a system of outcomes management from which outcomes research data is drawn. In the 1988 Shattuck Lecture for the Massachusetts Medical Society (8), Ellwood described a computerized database that would link the outcomes of millions of patients to the observations and actions of thousands of health providers. Unfortunately, the adoption of a computerized patient record that includes elements useful in outcomes assessment is still the exception. Most patient information is still chart bound, covering only parts of an episode of illness and giving only erratic snapshots of the changing status and functions of patients.

An example of the advantages of using such an electronic record system occurred when the Allina Health System of Minnesota was negotiating a new contract. Their integrated system utilizes a fully electronic, computer-based record system, and they were able to develop outcome measures from their medical records in their clinics. They used this information in the contracting process to gain competitive advantage with purchasers of their services.

Analytic Processes

A technique called *meta-analysis* is a method of analyzing a number of reported series to systematically summarize research data on efficacy and effectiveness. However, the number and scope of studies employing meta-analysis are still small and can provide guidance to few treatment decisions at this time. Combining such a systematic assessment of the data with expert clinical judgment in a formal process of consensus can result in statements that are reliable as well as authoritative. They can guide practitioners as well as patients in making treatment decisions. These steps are the essence of the current guidelines process, putting as much reliance on explicit evidence as is possible. Employing well-developed guidelines in practice can increase the likelihood of providing an effective, rather than a marginal or ineffective intervention, that will have a direct impact on improving the quality of care.

These tools of quality measurement have already improved patient care in some instances (5). Practice guidelines, combined with feedback on performance measures and guidance through education by respected peers have been shown to improve both the process and the outcomes of care in randomized trials. An example is the Asymptomatic Carotid Atherosclerosis Study (10). When surgery for carotid endarterectomy was performed by surgeons with a stroke/mortality rate of less than 3%, the survival rate of patients with asymptomatic carotid stenosis of 60% or more was shown to improve. Surgeons were carefully screened in order to participate in the project with participation screening based on past performance (20). A low complication rate for the surgeon is key; yet, because of lack of information, community physicians are unable to identify the local surgeons who meet or better this 3% threshold and would be more likely to achieve the good outcomes predicted by the study. Practitioners currently do not have access to such data, but they must in the future in order to make informed decisions.

Quality Improvement Strategies

A number of strategies for improving quality can be identified, and the task of developing an approach to quality improvement that includes components of each of these strategies is appropriate, since reliance on any single strategic alternative is unlikely to do the job.

Regulation is unpopular and largely ineffective in achieving quality improvement, except on a broad scale. Certain functions, such as removing demonstrably poor or dangerous providers and setting rules that specify minimum levels of acceptable performance for all providers, is clearly a function of regulatory oversight. It could also be applied to regionalization of services that are shown to have clearly better outcomes when the services are provided in settings with generally larger volumes and broader experience. For example, Grumbach reported the risk of dying after a coronary artery bypass graft operation was reduced by half if the surgery was done in a hospital that performs over 500 such operations per year, as compared to a hospital that performs less than 100 annually (12).

Competition remains an attractive motivating force to drive better quality. However, this assumption is still theoretical, since almost all of the competition in the marketplace revolves around price. The theory remains unproven, despite the enthusiasm of supporters who believe that differences in quality will actually sway purchasers to favor the plan with better quality measures. Skeptics doubt that this will happen, with the intensity of attention presently focused on price. Given the many obstacles to production and dissemination of data on comparative quality, it seems probable that the skeptic's view will prevail into the near future.

For quality measures, it seems unlikely that any one hospital or clinic would be rated as "best" for more than a few measures. That will pose a problem for patients and purchasers in their deliberations about selecting a plan and a place for their service. It seems more likely that competition based on quality measures will continue to rely on process data and intermediate outcomes such as mortality and morbidity. This does allow for some degree of differentiation between one physician or group from another, and it guides the health plan to direct certain patients with specific problems to particular providers and facilities. This selection option could be called a boutique-type of referral system for specific conditions, in which one provider or institution has shown better outcomes than the competition. Use of more comprehensive and specific outcomes measures for competitive purposes will have to await their production and validation.

Continuous quality improvement (CQI) is another strategy for improving care that reflects the application of industrial management techniques to health care. In the effort to improve outcomes, CQI analyzes how systems permit errors, then seeks to measure and reduce them along with inappropriate variations in practice. To date, this technique has been limited to a few hospitals, and determining the effect on patient outcomes is largely indirect. There is greater potential for use of CQI in integrated delivery systems to provide rapid feedback on quality, where information is available and coordination of services better organized.

Financial incentives have powerful effects on behavior, and the potential use of such incentives to reward excellence in quality is a tool that could have far reaching consequences. However, the key operational problems involved in using an incentives tool for that purpose remains unresolved at this time, due to lack of reliable information on provider performance measures.

Several new sciences and techniques are integral to achieving progress in quality measurement and improvement. Some of them are described briefly here. *Clinical epidemiology* uses the statistical tools of classical epidemiology to interpret differing patterns of clinical practice. This method was utilized by Wennberg and Gittelsohn in identifying wide variations in the processes and outcomes of care among patients receiving routine treatment for the same health-care problems in different places and health-care settings. The challenge is to identify which variations produce the best outcomes. *Outcomes research* has produced new quality measures that can be applied to improve treatments, including assessments of functional status and satisfaction. *Information systems, computer technology, and communication techniques* have achieved remarkable progress to make the research collection and analysis of data essential to quality measurement easier, faster, and cheaper. *Industrial techniques of quality management* have been used to improve performance as well as reduce errors and inappropriate variations in care. These techniques can also safeguard the processes that ensure continuity of care. Finally, *Models of Excellence* can be used as benchmarks

against which to compare or model systems of organization of health-care delivery. They also offer benchmarks for providers to use in judging the relative quality of structural or process measures.

ADAPTATION STRATEGIES FOR THE FUTURE

Predictions of Change in the System of Health-care Delivery

Changes occurring in health care can be examined from the perspective of reengineering and restructuring of the system. Like a number of industries that have undergone deregulation in the past decade, such as energy, transportation, and defense, health care is undergoing a painful transformation based on changes in underlying economic value. This shift in economic value is bringing everything else along with it (hospitals, physicians, academic medical centers, and health-care insurers); it is recognizable in shifts from high utilization toward low-cost settings and lower utilization. Non–value-added components of health care have been dropped, and the excess capacity of the system, both of structure and manpower, will be trimmed or disappear. Consumers are coming into control as purchasers of health-care services and forcing down costs in a steady spiral. As costs have come under control, quality has assumed increasing importance.

Business and the federal government have demanded better value in health care. HMOs have been the primary force driving the reform of value. They have forced a realignment of the various value-added components that make up health care's chain of value. Survival of the HMOs depends on their ability to balance cost control against quality, clinical outcomes, and patient satisfaction.

Increasing pressure to do more with less will force large-scale reengineering in the system. Initially, individual organizations will improve workflow and reduce waste. The non–value-added steps will be removed, and new information systems will link together new and improved workflows. This internal shuffling will serve for a time, but will not last, since shifts in economic value, i.e., what the customer will pay for, quickly exceed the capabilities of individual organizations to keep pace with the rising performance and cost requirements. The final adaptation will require overhaul of the entire industry-wide value chain. An example of such an overhaul is the aerospace industry after the Cold War collapsed; the changes that followed required industry-wide layoffs and extensive restructuring.

It is important to figure out where value is shifting in the new environment and to shift with it. This transition will require elimination of excess capacity, improved quality, lower costs, new information platforms, all in an integrated management strategy. In health care, price leadership alone will not be sufficient to assure success in a deregulated market. A blend of quality and products tailored to the market will prove more attractive than simply low prices.

New team skills will be needed to overcome the old paradigm of friends and enemies that cripple so many organizations that invent ''integration strategies'' simply to preserve the old order and resist change. Real integration will require a major shift in applying team-based methodologies to health care and will require overcoming the notion of ''separateness'' and elitism that has lasted for so many decades. Trust will need to be developed to overcome the schisms that separate so many health-care professionals, including physicians, who distrust even their colleagues. Large-scale clinical integration will come only after team building and team-based behaviors become the norm. Real integration into effective teams will allow for coordination of the many elements in delivery of care into a model of quality/cost that equates to value, and such value will be recognized and rewarded in the new market.

Systems integration and information technology are pivotal to success in this adaptation process. Only with access to timely, accurate information is it possible to keep the patient moving through the system, while utilizing the lowest-cost settings to achieve the highest quality results—this is an information driven game. Poor information or inaccessible information is not only inefficient, but also dangerous. Work should be designed to reduce reliance on short-term memory and to have ready (even bedside) access to patient-related clinical information. An electronic medical record and appropriate use of bar coding with bedside display of patient information are two areas of high priority.

Standardizing treatments would be extremely valuable; standardization should include medical procedures, drug doses, and the timing of drug administration. Such protocols could be integrated into a comprehensive program of disease management, thereby reducing the risk of inappropriate and ineffective interventions. Standardization could offer a set of predetermined steps for treatment of a patient's symptoms after reviewing the current health status and history. Columbia HCA is currently developing an information system that will be able to integrate the mountains of data necessary for the management of such a complex system of care. Such innovation has made Columbia a leader at the forefront of change.

Finally, the attitude to reengineering the existing system requires a new mind-set in the larger context of the industry-wide value chain. Many still view integration as a defensive strategy to protect the status quo. They still don't understand that for integration to work, the total system must be rationalized and restructured. When the smoke clears, the overall system must be faster, cheaper, more convenient, and deliver consistently higher quality outcomes. Anything less will be rejected by consumers and payers. An insight into the motivation for change lies in a comment by Richard Scott, CEO and President of Columbia HCA who noted that ''change happens when the status quo becomes more painful than making a change (24).

How to Improve Accountability

It seems clear that containing the cost of medical care should be a high priority. As previously noted, making changes in the system of health-care delivery to contain costs while ignoring clinical issues may save money but at the expense of quality. To ensure that the health-care system, both public and private, does not sacrifice quality for cost, physicians need to change their responsibility to their patients in a number of ways.

First, physicians need to be encouraged to work with multiple specialties to develop specific clinical guidelines that define necessary (appropriate) care and evaluate the impact of such guidelines on health and costs.

Second, physicians need to demand the public release of data that links quality and cost to providers and individual health plans in order to improve accountability within the health-care marketplace. This should include details of the incentives built into the contracts with providers in capitated plans. Disclosure of this type of information would act to restrain incentive systems from inducing serious underuse of services, and it would provide some feedback in the system that is presently missing. This disclosure could also serve to bolster the trust between physician and patient in capitation plans.

Third, physicians need to participate in clinical studies to provide information on effectiveness and outcomes to the research community.

Fourth, measures to identify and promote physicians with experience and expertise in complex procedures or techniques should be implemented, similar to what was done in the Asymptomatic Carotid Atherosclerosis Study (ACAS). In this way, the chances of choosing a service and a surgeon with the best record of outcomes for a specific problem would be increased, and the prospects of a satisfied consumer improved.

Fifth, the link between clinical training and patient outcomes needs attention, since the traditional credentials that imply that physicians "know best" have lost much luster during the revelations of the past decade.

Finally, the way providers operate in delivery of their services needs attention. Improved communication and collaboration should be promoted to develop a team approach to management of patients, which would gain from the input of different perspectives and a wider range of experience. This collaborative approach encompasses some of the re-engineering concepts of Ed Deming, but it is an approach that seems appropriate in this climate of competition.

The Changing Role of Physicians in Quality Management

Quality of care cannot improve without the knowledge and willing participation of physicians and other health-care professionals in the work of redesigning the processes that make up our present system. However, physicians cannot act alone since they have little ability to influence the decisions of large organized health plans or providers of health-care services. The role of physicians should be based on the success of this applied science as demonstrated by both Brook (2) and Chassin (5) in the development and use of tools to measure and improve the quality of care.

Physicians still have unique attributes that makes their advice authoritative, including their training in science, their understanding of medical practice, and their understanding of patients' personal circumstances. The patient remains a primary ally in this arena due to the interests shared between the physician and patient. This alliance is based on the patient's trust that derives from the physician's ethical and professional commitment to hold the patients' welfare first, as well as from the ongoing personal relationship between doctor and patient. This confluence of interests between physician and patient has the potential to grow into a political and economic force of major consequence. However, it is highly dependent on the ability of physicians to gain perspective on quality measurement and improvement that will help overcome the conflict and fear that the release of clinical performance data generates. This problem will be further aggravated by the rapid growth of capitation and risk-bearing contracts that increase public doubts that physicians still place their patients interests first.

Physicians need to develop new skills, attitudes, and partners in order to advance their perspective on quality measurement and improvements. They owe it to their patients and themselves to master the issues in quality of care. Without such involvement by physicians, the prospects of improvement of quality will remain an elusive dream, rather than an achievement

The Effects of Applied Outcomes Management

As noted above, Ellwood in 1988 recommended that the medical profession establish a common national technology that measured the effects of medical care on health outcomes, which he called "outcomes management." He made a strong case for the imperative that the profession work together with all the stakeholders, including the government, foundations, business groups, insurance companies, and consumer groups. The role of the patient was emphasized, with a focus on the quality of life from the patient's point of view. But outcomes management is dependent on the participation and cooperation of the entire health-care enterprise, so that everyone can understand how it reaches conclusions. For physicians to remain in control of their profession, they must track and evaluate health outcomes routinely and systematically.

Ellwood speculated that this technology might take up to 10 years to have an effect on the system and that payers would need evidence of success, (as in lower costs and favorable health outcomes) to be persuaded that an intervention was worthy of payment. He cited the example of carotid endarterectomy, which was costing about $1.5 billion annually in 1988. Despite the large number of operations done, the benefits, such as better function through prevention of strokes, had not been established at that time, because the surgical intervention had not been shown to have a reliable connection to improved outcomes in patients.

This deficiency was subsequently addressed in a multicenter study by the North American Symptomatic Carotid Endarterectomy Trial (NASCET) group (21). Their results showed surgery to be superior to the best medical therapy for patients with symptomatic high grade (70% or greater) carotid stenosis. This study was followed by a multicenter, randomized, controlled trial of asymptomatic patients with $60+\%$ stenosis of the carotid artery under the Asymptomatic Carotid Atherosclerosis Study (10). This study showed an aggregate risk reduction of 53% in patients treated surgically by surgeons screened for their past performance as an eligibility criterion, as compared to patients with the same degree of stenosis treated medically.

The missing link for this carefully targeted group of patients was forged with the technology Paul Ellwood recommended 9 years ago, a fact which highlights the benefit of applying the techniques of outcomes management to actual clinical problems.

Changes in Health-care Contracting

Contracting decisions are related to key drivers of change in each health-care sector. Employers/purchasers in the private sector have become key drivers of health system change by shifting their purchasing power from paying for open-ended fee-for-service health insurance benefits to buying health care on a capitated basis from managed care plans. With the rapid growth in enrollment in MCO plans, employers have come to expect and demand that the premiums fall or only rise slightly, and they have succeeded in slowing the rise in health care costs to the lowest level in 30 years (16).

Some health plans have discovered that improved disease management can benefit from actively managing clinical care quality. Concurrently, they are still reducing specialists' fees

and use in oversupplied fields, such as neurosurgery.

As better risk adjustment methods are developed to appropriately pay providers that deliver effective services to the chronically ill and other high-cost patients, the health plans will become more efficient in their cost-to-benefit ratios for the more difficult cases. Ultimately, direct contracting between purchasers and providers seems a probable choice to facilitate continued development of such methods.

Providers will face continued pressure both on pricing and for downsizing (as a reaction to a market oversupplied with resources) from aggressive purchasers who have no basis for distinguishing among competitors in terms of quality or value of provider services.

There has been a rapid rise in the number of physicians who are organizing to take on clinical management and risk. This could alter the course and speed of health system change. Physicians used to control about 70 to 80% of health-care decisions, but they have been moved down the pecking order by well-capitalized insurance companies and hospital-backed ventures. Physician-organized systems could shift the balance far more toward competition among providers and away from competition among health plans, and such systems could foster organizations based on treatment of various conditions.

COMPETITION FOR NEUROSURGERY
Sources of Competition

Neurosurgeons have lost bargaining power to third parties that have improved their contracting position by consolidation and controlling a significant fraction of the practice's referral base. MCOs can obtain neurosurgical services without dealing with most of the neurosurgeons in practice. Due to this lack of bargaining power, MCOs have been able to bid down neurosurgeons services, with the result that neurosurgeons have discounted their fees steeply in order to retain a share of their market. Some have also been induced to accept the economic risk of their care under capitation contracts.

Hospitals involved in downsizing, mergers, and networks for contracting are gaining control of the referral bases of neurosurgeons and other specialists.

Other competitors include surgeons in other specialties who offer the same services and practitioners who offer alternative forms of treatment that substitute for a procedure that neurosurgeons are trained to provide. One of the reasons for this intrusion into a market previously held tightly by neurosurgeons is because neurosurgeons have not been interested in specializing in many of these services, while competitors have trained, promoted, and secured referrals for their efforts.

How to Improve the Competitive Position of Neurosurgery and Neurosurgeons

Ausman (1) examined the reasons for the loss of many neurosurgical referrals in the recent past. He found it is due in large part to the training and marketing by other specialists for the same patients neurosurgeons have managed in the past. Orthopedics has promoted the idea of "spine specialists" with effective marketing and have taken many of the patients with spine problems previously managed by neurosurgeons. The disinclination of most neurosurgeons to provide a comprehensive program of care for back-pain patients explains the offices of orthopedists that are filled with such patients. Packaging of care and marketing it to MCOs is an effective way to gain market share by attracting patients from the competing provider. Targeting specific types of neurosurgical services that others are providing, then creating a plan to develop expertise on a specific problem with additional training for its management, and finally marketing the new product will serve to recapture some lost patients.

Another difficulty regarding competition relates to the problem of the oversupply of neurosurgeons and the resultant competitive bidding for greatly discounted contracts in some markets. Virtually all students of the supply of physicians agree that there are too many neurosurgeons for the present market. When possible remedies for this problem are considered, attention usually focuses on issues of too many residents, too many foreign graduates, and fear of an antitrust investigation threatening any effort to regulate physician numbers. None of these potential actions would be effective or affordable in the present climate of pervasive litigation, and it would take several decades for training reductions to have significant impact on the market supply.

A long-term approach focused on the quality of the residents, rather than on their numbers, would enhance neurosurgery's position among medical colleagues and support the image of neurosurgery to purchasers. This strategy would require that the program directors standardize the qualifications for admission to training programs limiting candidates to those who meet explicit standards. Setting standards at a predefined, optimum level would act as a quality-related filter for the training programs, while providing a public affirmation of the specialty's commitment to maintaining the highest quality providers.

A strategy for community neurosurgeons would be to merge into groups that included previous competitors, thereby enabling the group to increase the product line and to develop special expertise or packages of service with better marketing potential. This could also include joining a multispecialty group with a broader base of service and a larger number of contracts to support specialists with a narrow draw on the market.

In some settings, considerable pressure has been applied to the local neurosurgeons to join hospital-sponsored (and controlled) programs of "integrated care" that contract with a variety of MCOs. Current trends suggest that this may be a short-term strategy, since the market place has demonstrated that the real source of revenue in health-care plans is the government or the employer, not the health plan. The plan simply serves as an administrator, while taking its 15 to 30% off the top before passing on what is left to the contracted providers. A move toward direct contracting coupled with global fees may be poised to replace many of the MCOs currently operating. As this happens, many of the vertically integrated hospital systems will face competitive pressures that they may not survive.

The type of program that offers global fees is based on a predetermined price structure and on specified packages of services. Their scope is variable but they are based on a contracted discount. This approach has strong appeal and may come to prominence in the next several years because it offers the most incentives for efficiency, quality, satisfaction, as well as more reasonable pricing. Employers retain control of the cost and flexibility to contract with any or all groups of providers, while the competition among providers should keep prices lower. At the same time, the ability of consumers to have their choice of physicians can be preserved.

How Can Neurosurgeons Adapt to the New Marketplace?

The response to this question needs to be addressed in several parts. The first part deals with neurosurgeons at the local level and with the changes they can effect in their own practices to begin their transition to this new environment. Some initial steps are addressed, both with regard to cost management and to the bigger issues of quality management and improvement. Increasing pressure to do more with less will force large-scale reengineering in the practice. This will include changes to improve workflow and reduce waste. New information systems that link and help control new workflow patterns will serve for a time but will not last since shifts in economic value, i.e., what the customer will pay for, will exceed the capabilities of the practices to keep up with rising costs and performance requirements. The next step in adaptation will require that the entire value chain for the specialty be overhauled, and this, in turn, will require an integrated strategy reaching beyond a single practice or even a single region. National neurosurgical organizations and their leadership need to take interest and action on these problems, since the issues affect all neurosurgeons.

This second part deals with the elements of an integrated strategy that should be developed for neurosurgery at the national level by neurosurgical organizations . It is becoming clear that price leadership alone will not be sufficient to assure continued success in a deregulated healthcare market. Consequently, cost control measures and initiatives will provide only a limited amount of relief from the continued pressure on price competition. A combination of quality and ''brand'' leadership are more likely to prove durable than low prices, and such a combination can provide competitive advantages. The problem is how to achieve identifiable quality and brand leadership. Strategies for achieving these goals will include elimination of excess capacity, improved quality, lower costs, new information systems, and overall integration of these components into a workable whole.

The idea of differentiating neurosurgical services from competitors is one way to approach the promotion of neurosurgical services as superior and something that can be associated with the concept of ''brand.'' Items such as Coke, Kleenex and Porsche all have market advantages because of the association of the name with the product, and the implicit quality of the product. The core question is how can neurosurgeons differentiate their services from their competitors? This question is the most difficult, since it requires a set of strategies that are largely undeveloped. Some of the solutions require that standards and guidelines be developed for neurosurgical practice, and then that performance be measured against these references. Benchmarking should be promoted in order to identify the best practices, and then other neurosurgeons should be encouraged to use the benchmarks as goals for improvement of their own practices. Benchmarking of training programs would also provide an opportunity for the adoption of policies and techniques of training from the best programs to all of the others.

One of the biggest challenges is the problem of measuring and improving quality. This has proved an elusive goal, due in part to the complexity of the issue, but also to the variable nature of the concept as viewed by different audiences of consumers. Neurosurgeons need to develop new skills, attitudes, and partners in order to advance their perspective on quality measurement and improvements.

Evidence-Based Practice

David Eddy, in considering this problem, said ''the greatest potential for improving quality is by a closer examination of the science-base of medicine.'' Examination of the processes of care and connecting their results to outcomes is the essential task before neurosurgery. This examination needs to be done for almost all neurosurgical care, since the outcomes of care have not yet been examined systematically or extensively enough to permit demonstration of the benefits of one treatment as compared to another. There are examples of the successful application of this methodology, such as the carotid endarterectomy trials, but the number is embarrassingly small. Clinical research focused on the quality of services and based on carefully designed and implemented outcomes studies are the way to that goal. The use of intermediate steps, such as comparisons of the performance measures, as in the report cards generated by MCOs from administrative and billing data, are in vogue, but do little to address the real issue of comparative value of the services. Nevertheless, the tools are needed to produce report cards from neurosurgical practices for comparison with those produced by third parties and competitors.

One of the roles for neurosurgical organizations will be to help make measurement of performance, effectiveness, and outcomes a part of neurosurgical culture. This will require initiation of not only residents, but academic as well as practicing neurosurgeons, into the rationale and methods of quality measurement and improvement. Application of such clinical research will lead to development of comprehensive and explicit standards and guidelines for neurosurgical practice. This development can be advanced even further by establishing national and regional benchmarks of the best practices, and then identifying them as goals for the rest of us to emulate. Comparison to benchmarks encourages people to excel, while meeting minimum standards simply encourages a passing mark.

How to Change Physician Behavior

The problem of influencing physician behavior on this broad a scale is daunting. Many neurosurgeons are still practicing in an environment with relatively low penetration of managed care and with stable or growing volumes of patients. The threats posed in other areas with less managed care have not yet impacted them to the degree that their attention has focused on survival strategies, rather than managing their profits. To gain the attention of those neurosurgeons not yet threatened by declining practice revenues will take the leadership of national neurosurgical organizations to sound the alarm and mobilize the membership to begin the long task of organizing and developing these measures of comparative value in the provider market. This process will involve the whole system of care, and the system must be rationalized and restructured, much like the model of industrial reengineering that has been so effective in the adaptation of the auto industry in the new market. Our new system needs to be faster, cheaper, more convenient, and able to deliver consistently higher quality outcomes, lest it be rejected by consumers and payers.

The problem of convincing neurosurgeons of the need to change their behavior in this enterprise will be large. Many neurosurgeons have chosen to play ostrich regarding the changes swirling around them. Others have added an MBA degree to their accomplishments and are poised to survive as managers, if their practices continue to decline. Most are aware of the threats and know of friends or competitors who have been impacted to some degree by the changed market for their services. However, to assume that neurosurgeons will respond in a rational and analytic manner to this problem would be folly. Only the behavioral model of decision making, in which behavior and decisions are influenced by social norms, cues, and culture, is likely to have a timely influence on changing their attitudes and behavior. This model is predicated on social science research (19) that has found that the social influence of the behavioral model is most applicable in the presence of uncertainty, ambiguity, and strong interdependencies, all of which certainly typifies the present situation. The model also predicts that behavior change will result from changes in norms, beliefs, and values. Some of the most effective agents for promotion of such behavioral change are ''academic detailing'' and the influence of opinion leaders. Participation in group-based performance reviews as well as continuous quality improvement programs is also effective. Neurosurgical leaders are the logical choice to promote this message and to induce the necessary changes in norms, values, and beliefs among their organization's members.

This is a multi-year project that will require a team approach, with commitment to developing a system and methodology to produce instruments of evaluation and to incorporate the results into ''standards of neurosurgical care'' in the form of guidelines, standards, and options. In this way, neurosurgeons can be positioned to track and evaluate health outcomes routinely and systematically, and thereby remain in control of our specialty. Ultimately, integration into effective teams of providers will allow for coordination of the many elements in delivery of care into a model of quality and cost that equates to value, and such value will be recognized and rewarded in the new market.

REFERENCES

1. Ausman JI, A strategy for your future. Surg Neurol 1966;46:304–307.
2. Brook RH, McGlynn EA, Cleary PD. Measuring quality of care. N Engl J Med 1996;335:1146–9.
3. Chassin MR et al. Does inappropriate use explain geographic variations in the use of health services?: A study of three procedures. JAMA 1987;259,18:2533–2537.
4. Chassin MR, Kosecoff J, Park RE, et al. The appropriateness of use of selected medical and surgical proce-

dures and its relationship to geographic variations in their use. Ann Arbor, MI: Health Administration Press, 1989.

5. Chassin MR. Improving the quality of care. N Engl J Med 1996;335:891–4.

6. Donabedian A. Quality assessment and assurance: Unity of purpose, diversity of means. Inquiry 1988;25: 173–192.

7. Eddy DM. Balancing cost and quality in fee-for-service versus managed care. Health Aff 1997;16:162–173.

8. Ellwood PM. Outcomes management: A technology of patient experience. N Engl J Med 1988;318:1549–56.

9. Epstein AM. Sounding board: The outcomes movement—Will it get us where we want to go? N Engl J Med 1990;323:266–270.

10. Executive Comittee for the Asymptomatic Carotid Atherosclerosis Study. Endarterectomy for asymptomatic carotid artery stenosis. JAMA 1995;278:1421–8.

11. The Federal Employee Health Benefits Program. Wall Street Journal April 2, 1992.

12. Grumbach KK et al. Regionalization of cardiac surgery in the United States and Canada: Geographic access, choice, and outcomes. JAMA 1995;274,16: 1282–1288.

13. Hannan EL et al. Investigation of the relationship between volume and mortality for surgical procedures performed in New York State hospitals. JAMA 1989; 262,4:503–510.

14. Hungate RW. Whither quality? Health Aff 1996;15: 111–113.

15. Iglehart JK. Competition and the pursuit of quality: A conversation with Walter McClure. Health Aff (Millwood) 1988;7(1):79–90.

16. Levit KR et al. National health expenditures: 1994. Health Care Financ Rev 1996;(Spring):205–242.

17. Lohr KN, ed. Medicare: A strategy for quality assurance. Washington, DC: Washington National Academy Press, 1990

18. Millenson MI. Miracle and wonder: The AMA embraces quality measurement. Health Aff 1997;16:183–194.

19. Mittman BS, Tonesk X, Jacobson PD. Implementing clinical practice guidelines: Social influence strategires and practitioner behavior change. Qual Rev Bull, 1992;18,12:413–422.

20. Moore WS, Vescera CL, Robertson JT, Baker WH, Howard VJ, Toole JF. Selection process for surgeons in the Asymptomatic Carotid Atherosclerosis Study. Stroke 1991;22:1363–1367.

21. North American Symptomatic Carotid endarterectomy Trial Collaborators. Beneficial effect of carotid endarterectomy in symptomatic patients with high-grade carotid stenosis. N Engl J Med 1991;325:445–453.

22. Public Law 101-239. The Omnibus Budget Reconciliation Act of 1989.

23. Relman AC. Assessment and accountability; The third revolution in medical care. N Engl J Med 1988;319: 1220–1222.

24. Sharpe A, Jaffe G. Colulmbia/HCA plans for more big changes in health-care world. Wall Street Journal, May 28, 1997.

25. Soumerai SB et al. Adverse outcomes of underuse of beta blockers in elderly survivors of acute myocardial infarction. JAMA 1977;277,2:115–121.

26. Tyson GW. Competition in neurosurgery: Part 1. Surg Neurol 1996;46:516–518.

27. Wenneberg J, Gittelsohn A. Small area variations in health care delivery. Science 1973;182:1102–8.

28. Wilson B, Cleary PD. Linking clinical variables with health-related quality of life. JAMA 1995;273:59–65.

PART II

Neurosurgical Training

CHAPTER 6

Clinical Practice Parameter Development in Neurosurgery

BEVERLY C. WALTERS, M.D., M.Sc., F.R.C.S.C., F.A.C.S.

INTRODUCTION

Medicine today is in the middle of a revolution. It reflects major intellectual and social change, and is based on the alterations in both the delivery and financing of health care. Relman called this the "third revolution in medical care" (1) and suggested that we must examine the costs, safety, and effectiveness of physician services, since society can no longer afford to pay for a steadily expanding delivery system.

The guidelines movement is a child of this revolution, a result of the need to examine the effectiveness as well as the costs and appropriateness of care provided to our patients. The underlying theme is to try to assure that the services delivered are likely to have the best chance of achieving an acceptable outcome, while reducing the wide variation in treatment options that may be used for any given condition. This focus on outcome and reduced variation is intended to have the effect of reducing the costs of delivery by avoidance of unproven treatments or ineffective therapies. Further, the choice of a treatment strategy should carefully balance the risks, benefits, and costs, while involving the patient in the selection process.

In its simplest form, the driving question is "What works?" Vibbert's monograph with this title, subtitled "How Outcomes Research Will Change Medical Practice" (2), reviewed the various interests and agencies involved in guidelines and outcomes and pointed out that continuation of the status quo with more utilization review, no consensus on the best practices, and antagonism between physicians and payers simply won't work.

The interest in clinical practice guidelines comes from several synchronous, but sometimes divergent, movements. Patients—now known as health-care consumers—want a greater role in decision-making and more involvement in the health-care encounter. Physicians—dubbed "providers"—are interested in the quality of care and guidance in the treatment choices, which may—or may not—benefit their patients. Payers—usually insurers—want more value for health-care dollars spent, as well as fewer dollars spent.

Although these motivations differ, all parties can potentially benefit from a careful examination of data available on treatment regimens and their ability to achieve desired outcomes. Patients can continue to be offered treatments that insurers may not want to pay for, physicians can offer scientific support for their treatment recommendations, and payers can eliminate costly and useless strategies in management of health and disease.

Historically, preferred treatments came out of the published experience of well-known experts in a given field. Those lesser—or, perhaps, clinically less busy—practitioners could then benefit from the clinical successes and failures of these experts. Thus, the art of medicine was transmitted from practitioner to practitioner through published reports. This promulgation of expert opinion continued for literally thousands of years, until the introduction of the scientific experiment in the form of the randomized controlled trial in the middle of this century. This method of scientifically examining a hypothesis applied to a clinical problem represented a clear departure from the subjective to the objective in developing information about what works.

The exponential growth of medical technology has been accompanied by a concomitant explosion in medical communications. Unfortunately, this information explosion has not been matched by a similar growth in the use of the scientific method applied to true human experimentation, and anecdotal case series still abound in the literature. However, the quasi-experimental nature of this form of evidence is becoming widely recognized, along with a desire on the part of clinicians to have more solid scientific grounds on which to base their practices.

The development of guidelines based on evidence, rather than expert opinion alone, has spread through most medical societies, while simultaneously attracting the interest and attention of government and the insurance industry. At this writing, over 1800 guidelines have been listed with the American Medical Association (AMA) (3), most of which are based on consensus of varying certitude. The Agency for Health Care Policy and Research (AHCPR) of the Department of Health and Human Services has also developed guidelines that are rather broad-based and focused on conditions of high frequency and cost and have the potential for reducing unexplained variations in the services directed at the condition. Using the National Library of Medicine's computerized database, one finds that the MESH subheading ''Practice Guidelines'' has only been present since 1993. Using this rubric, a search for the years 1970–1990 reveals no documents, but there were 2 in 1991, 118 in 1992, 374 in 1993, 592 in 1994, 815 in 1995, and over 1300 in 1996.

The insurance industry has taken a rather different tack, and, while purporting to base their internally developed guidelines on the issue of quality, some have had an agenda of applying their information to contain costs and limit access to certain services previously covered. These three examples cover a part of the spectrum of what already exists in the realm of guidelines. Unfortunately, the marketplace at present is rather full of guidelines on a wide range of conditions that, more often than not, are based on expert consensus alone, rather than a methodical review and analysis of the scientific evidence that pertains to the problem. A major reason for the paucity of sound evidence-based guidelines is that they are time and labor inten-

sive, and the funds required to develop such a product are considerable. It may take up to 3 years for a team of physicians and others to cover the steps in such a project, outlined below, and at a cost of hundreds of thousands of dollars.

THE PROCESS OF GUIDELINE DEVELOPMENT

The steps in guideline development include:

- Clearly identify and define the major questions regarding the clinical condition.
- Collect, review, and analyze the relevant scientific literature for each question.
- Assess the clinical benefits and risks of each intervention considered.
- Review estimates of important patient outcomes for each intervention considered.
- Examine the current and potential costs associated with the guideline, and, when possible, compare to the costs of alternative strategies for the same condition.
- Involve participation and comments on the topic(s) from other professional specialty organizations that may have an interest in the recommendations.
- Develop a table of evidence that ranks the quality of evidence ascribed to each citation in the final reference listing that would permit a reader to reproduce the results of such a critical examination.
- Prepare recommendations based on the evidence assembled; when scientific and empirical evidence is lacking on a particular aspect of the condition, professional judgment and group consensus are used and acknowledged.
- Provide an explicit description of how the evidence was abstracted from various sources, compared, and combined. Explicit documentation of any assumption is required.
- Rank the recommendations based on the quality and consistency of the supporting evidence, as well as on the magnitude of the benefits, risks, and costs of the intervention.
- Prepare a draft of the guideline and submit for peer review.
- Revise the guideline after peer review and comments received.
- Prepare the guideline in formats appropriate for use by the intended audience.
- Plan for the publication and dissemination of the guideline.
- Review, revise, and update the guideline pe-

riodically to reflect new scientific evidence or changes in professional consensus.

CLASSIFICATION OF EVIDENCE AND STRENGTH OF RECOMMENDATIONS

The American Association of Neurological Surgeons has taken a leadership role in establishing evidence-based guidelines for neurosurgery. In an attempt to avoid any proprietary disputes regarding the content of guidelines, a policy of strict adherence to the AMA's levels of evidence and subsequent strength of recommendations has been adopted. In this paradigm, therapeutic recommendations are divided into practice *standards,* practice *guidelines,* and practice *options.* Practice *standards* are recommendations based on strong experimental evidence such as randomized controlled trials. As described by Rosenberg and Greenberg from the American Academy of Neurology (4) , these reflect a high degree of clinical certainty. This is referred to as **Class I evidence**.

Practice *guidelines* reflect a moderate degree of clinical certainty and are based on less robust comparative studies such as nonrandomized controlled (cohort) studies or case-control studies. These study types are classified as **Class II evidence**.

Case series and expert opinion, considered **Class III evidence**, are placed together in the least compelling evidentiary group, namely, practice *options.* These categories are summarized in Table 6.1.

This classification ranks the treatment strategies fairly, according to how convincing the evidence is, depending on the methodological science used in its production. It also incidentally reveals gaps in the literature of supportive evidence for practice standards or guidelines, thus identifying future areas of needed research.

The process of scientifically producing guidelines from the data available is far more exacting and tedious than convening a consensus panel of experts. Using the methodological recommendations of the Institute of Medicine of the National Academy of Sciences (5) , the process begins with a search for all available medical literature on the clinical question. The products of this search are then evaluated carefully and classified by study type. In many instances, no Class I or II evidence is found, and, therefore, only practice options can be delineated. Within the categories of evidence, a qualitative review of the studies is undertaken according to well-recognized epidemiologic criteria (6) to reveal any methodological flaws which might lead to erroneous conclusions on the part of the study's authors. The evidence thus examined is then used to produce standards, guidelines or options.

The widely used evidence-based methodology described above and featured in several publications about evidence-based guidelines (7–10), applies only to therapeutic effectiveness. Any guidelines which pertain to diagnostic tests or prognosis are not covered by these recommendations. These need to follow similar *principles* of clinical epidemiology for strength of evidence as those for therapeutic effectiveness, though the *application* of those principles is different.

For diagnostic tests, the strongest recommendations come from studies that have been carried out in a diverse population, including patients who are known to be free of the target disease (11), i.e., true negatives, as well as those who are known to have the disease, e.g., true positives. In addition, the diagnostic test in question should be compared to a ''gold standard'' that provides proof of the presence of the disease or condition of interest. These have been formalized into a classification system similar to that devised for therapy, as outlined in Table 6.2.

An example of how this classification would work for diagnostic tests can be demonstrated using the example of plain radiographs used in trauma for clearing the cervical spine (C-spine). The guideline question being posed is: What radiographs are necessary to clear the C-spine? The questions posed of the relevant papers selected to help in formulating a guideline would include the following questions. Is this a pro-

TABLE 6.1
Classification of Evidence on Therapeutic Effectiveness

Class I:	Evidence provided by one or more well-designed, randomized controlled clinical trials, including overviews of such trials.
Class II:	Evidence provided by one or more well-designed comparative clinical studies, such as nonrandomized cohort studies, case-control studies, and so forth.
Class III:	Evidence provided by case series, comparative studies with historical controls, case reports, and expert opinion.

TABLE 6.2
Classification of Evidence on Diagnostic Tests

Class I: Evidence provided by one or more well-designed clinical studies of a diverse population using a ''gold standard'' reference test in a blinded evaluation appropriate for the diagnostic applications and enabling the assessment of sensitivity, specificity, positive and negative predictive values, and, where applicable, likelihood ratios.

Class II: Evidence provided by one or more clinical studies of a restricted population using a reference test in a blinded evaluation of diagnostic accuracy and enabling the assessment of sensitivity, specificity, positive and negative predictive values, and, where applicable, likelihood ratios.

Class III: Evidence provided by expert opinion, studies that do not meet the criteria for the delineation of sensitivity, specificity, positive and negative predictive values, and, where applicable, likelihood ratios.

TABLE 6.3
Classification of Evidence on Prognosis

Class I: Evidence provided by one or more well-designed clinical studies of a population completely followed from a uniform point in their disease, without bias, and with adjustment for extraneous prognostic variables (e.g., multivariate analysis).

Class II: Evidence provided by one or more clinical studies of data on a restricted population, collected prospectively, with complete follow-up and adjustment for extraneous prognostic variables (e.g., multivariate analysis).

Class III: Evidence provided by expert opinion, studies that include only three of the criteria for practice standards, but data must be collected prospectively.

spective study of a diverse population of patients who had cervical spine radiographs taken, with variable injury scenarios, and thus, a wide spectrum of presenting cervical spine complaints? And were these radiographs compared to some other proof of bony or ligamentous injury that could act as a ''gold standard'' of diagnosis, such as other imaging or operative findings?

Now, if we take two examples from the literature of citations that might be used to help in the development of guidelines, (12, 13) and that have been found through a computerized search of the literature, we can see how this might work. The first citation is characterized is Figure 6.1. From it we can see that, although the paper appears promising, it actually comes from a limited population of patients and does not provide enough data for us to be able to derive the characteristics of sensitivity, specificity, positive and negative predictive values, or likelihood ratios. This paper would only give us a practice option, at the most. However, the second citation, shown in Figure 6.2, was carried out in a diverse population (everyone admitted with a diagnosis of trauma of variable injury severity), and it used a gold standard of all ultimate radiographs done on the patient, as well as follow-up for patients who returned with subsequent problems. This latter paper provides more useful information regarding the value of the test, as depicted in the figure. A proposal has been made that available literature be combined to construct metaanalyses of the literature and use the combined data, where available, to determine characteristics of accuracy of a given test (14). The really important information regarding diagnostics tests, however, never appears in the literature. That information centers around the cost-effectiveness of the test and whether it makes a difference in patient outcome. As our literature improves, so will our definitions of Class I, II, and III evidence for help in determining strength of recommendations.

There is a similar problem for literature on prognosis. Literature on this topic has to be evaluated differently from that for therapeutic effectiveness, since patients can never be randomized to having or not having a disease. Such evaluation must, once again, embrace the principles espoused by clinical epidemiology. The main thrust of these principles is the avoidance of bias in the study population that would systematically influence the conclusions of the study. For this reason, only data that have been collected prospectively with a view to subsequent examination can be utilized. An example of this prospective data collection would be a computerized database including all patients with a given condition in a single or several collaborating institutions. This method is in contradistinction to retrospective studies, in which a population of interest is identified and an attempt made to locate its members, usually through a medical records system which has been set up for other purposes (Table 6.3).

The next issue for consideration concerns whether the patients are at the same point in their illness. For example, brain tumor patients at first diagnosis, aneurysm patients at the time of subarachnoid hemorrhage, and trauma patients at

		GOLD STANDARD		
		Patient has injury	Patient has no injury	
TEST RESULT: C-SPINE FILM	Positive: Appears to have injury	True Positive: ? (a	False Positive: ? b)	a + b
	Negative: Appears to have no injury	(c False Negative: ?	d) True Negative: ?	c + d
		a + c	b + d	

Figure 6.1. Evaluation of a published article that does not provide adequate data. From Ringenberg BJ, et al. Rational ordering of cervical spine radiographs following trauma. Ann Emerg Med 1988;17:792-296. This retrospective review included 312 hospitalized patients with cervical spine injuries. The main questions were, ''what are the presenting signs, symptoms, and coexisting conditions in patients with C-spine injury, and are any such injuries not diagnosed in the emergency department?'' This study was carried out in cervical spine-injured patients only, providing no ''true negatives,'' thus it cannot be used to evaluate C-spine x-rays as a diagnostic test in patients presenting to a trauma room.

the time of transfer to a Level I unit. In addition to the patients being similar, the reporting institution should also serve a variety of patients with a wide spectrum of disease. Appropriate endpoints or outcome measures should be used, and should be assessed in a blinded fashion or should be so objective as not to require blinding (e.g., patient testimonials, such as found in survey instruments.)

The study design should adjust for prognostic factors that may strongly influence the outcome, but are extraneous to the illness of interest. Examples of this would be cardiac disease in a trauma patient, coagulopathy in a subarachnoid hemorrhage patient, and previous stroke in a brain tumor patient. Adjustment is carried out using appropriate statistical tests, usually multivariate analysis.

		GOLD STANDARD		
		Patient has injury	Patient has no injury	
TEST RESULT: C-SPINE FILM	Positive: Appears to have injury	True Positive: **76** (a	False Positive: **18** b)	a + b **94**
	Negative: Appears to have no injury	(c False Negative: **16**	d) True Negative: **665**	c + d **681**
		a + c **92**	b + d **683**	**775**

Figure 6.2. Evaluation of a published article that provides adequate data. From Macdonald RL, et al. Diagnosis of cervical spine injury in motor vehicle crash victims: how many x-rays are enough? J Trauma 1990;30(4):392-397. This retrospective review examined 775 motor vehicle crash victims. The main question was, ''how many x-rays are enough to clear the cervical spine of injury in trauma patients?'' Gold Standard (i.e., further tests, e.g., CT scan, tomograms, flexion/extension) = accuracy of 741/745, 96%; sensitivity of 76/92, 83%; specificity of 665/683, 97%; positive predictive value of 76/94, 81%; and negative predictive value of 665/681, 98%.

RESPONSIBILITIES OF THE SPONSORING / DEVELOPING ORGANIZATION IN GUIDELINE DEVELOPMENT

A guidelines development project, such as that set up by the American Association of Neu-

rological Surgeons (AANS) and the Congress of Neurological Surgeons (CNS), has the responsibility of being both proactive and reactive. In the former circumstance, the general need for guidelines development within the various subspecialties arises from questions regarding reimbursement, wide variation in daily practice for common problems, controversy among experts with respect to "standard of care" recommendations, and frequency of treatment needed for certain conditions. In addition, guidelines developers must be prepared to be reactive to recommendations put forth by colleagues in other specialties who are interested in the same disorders. In both cases, the sponsoring or developing organization must have a mechanism for dealing with the situation at hand promptly and appropriately. According to Hayward and Laupacis, programs must equally be involved in planning, developing, validating, reporting, disseminating, implementing, and maintaining guidelines (15).

Within organized Neurosurgery, the role of planning and developing guidelines is taken on by the joint subspecialty sections of the American Association of Neurological Surgeons and the Congress of Neurological Surgeons, through the Guidelines Committee and the Joint Committee on the Assessment of Quality. The evidence-based approach outlined above has been adopted and the committee provides quality assessment as well as resources for guideline development. During specially designed guideline development tutorials, participants are taught the concepts of evidence-based guideline development and, throughout the development process, ongoing feedback and advice is provided.

Guideline dissemination may take several forms. The most extensive guidelines developed in neurosurgery to date are the "Guidelines for the Treatment of Severe Head Injury," and they have been distributed in loose-leaf format (with accompanying CD-ROM disc) by the Brain Trauma Foundation to members of the AANS. In addition, they have been published in their entirety in a special issue of the Journal of Neurotrauma (16). Neither of the official publications of the AANS (*Journal of Neurosurgery*) or the CNS (*Neurosurgery*) has published any guidelines.

Publication is only the first step in guidelines dissemination, albeit an extremely important one. After publication, many presentations at scientific meetings typically take place, at local, national, and international levels. In addition, special courses and seminars may be held to further educate physicians and allied health-care personnel in the use of the guidelines.

Implementation of the guidelines is controlled at a local, (hospital, city, county) or regional (state or province) level. If hospital administrations or government officials accept the scientific validity of evidence-based guidelines, they may insist on adoption as a local "standard of care." Insurance companies, on the other hand, will often use either consensus documents which have not been validated or "management review criteria" based on actuarial data without inclusion of patient outcome information to deny services to patients or determine aspects of care. Presumably, patients ultimately will insist on care if known to be beneficial, even if only some of the time, and insurance companies will have to show that cost-saving measures do not compromise patient outcomes.

Maintaining guidelines must be an integral part of the commitment to the process. Technological advances and new knowledge demand that guidelines be revisited on a regular basis. This review must be ensured by the developing or sponsoring organizations at the outset by a plan, such as the establishment of an oversight group whose responsibility it is to bring the needed revisions about. There are many ways in which this can be done. In the case of the Severe Head Injury Guidelines, a Governance Review Committee made up of representatives from the sponsoring organization (Brain Trauma Foundation), the professional organization(s) most heavily involved (AANS/CNS), and the authors' group oversees additions and revisions to the guidelines. Because the methodological standards for creating the guidelines have already been set, these do not have to be negotiated at each subsequent iteration of the document. However, the Review Committee can only make recommendations to the Boards of Directors of the AANS/CNS for acceptance. The final decision is in the hands of the leadership of these organizations, whose responsibility it is to be (or to become) well-versed in the tenets of evidence-based guideline development.

With respect to worldwide acceptance, the path for review and recommendation has been through the appropriate organ of the World Health Organization. In the case of the Severe Head Injury Guidelines, this has been done, after careful consideration, through the Neurotrauma Committee. Although the guidelines have been developed through critical review of the literature, there is a recognition that the recommendations may not be able to be implemented as developed, because of cultural, religious, or economic exigencies.

LEGAL ASPECTS OF GUIDELINE DEVELOPMENT

Although physicians, individually and collectively, may be appreciative of, grateful for, and desirous of practice parameters, there are concerns regarding legal implications. In response to this, the American Medical Association (AMA) instigated a study into the legal aspects of practice parameters, particularly as applied to malpractice liability exposure (17).

The primary purpose of practice parameters is to assist physicians. However, these guidelines may be used to judge appropriateness of care by risk management groups, quality assessment committees, or insurers or other payers. This use may be translated into criteria used for practice review, even when the level of evidence is relatively low, e.g., expert opinion or consensus. With respect to malpractice liability, the question is what happens if a physician chooses to ignore practice parameters, in the interest of his or her patient, and there is an unintended outcome?

The study by the AMA establishes that not all treatments can or should be applied to all patients and that the law allows for variability. There is no change in the law in its requirements of physicians to provide care, or of plaintiffs to prove that a physician owed a duty of care to a patient, that the physician failed in his or her duty by not exercising reasonable care, that whatever injury the patient suffered was caused by such failure, and that the injury is compensable. Provided the physician can demonstrate that he or she chose not to follow published guidelines as an integral part of providing good care because of doubts about the applicability of the guideline to a particular patient, the guideline would then not be considered the "standard of care" for that particular patient. In addition, using the terminology suggested by the AMA and adopted by the AANS and CNS (as well as related organizations, such as the American Academy of Neurology), will serve as a reminder of the level of certitude—with respect to the supporting scientific evidence—reflected in the designation of options, guidelines, or standards.

In spite of warning cries of potential harm to patients because physicians may abandon their own good sense and expert judgment out of fear of malpractice litigation, others feel that practice parameters "will likely assist in improving the fairness and uniformity of the malpractice litigation process (17)."

At the very least, practice guidelines that are evidence-based serve to summarize the pertinent medical literature in a critical and constructive way. This separates strong beliefs from scientific evidence, as well as identifying gaps in current knowledge and indicating areas for future research.

There will naturally be resistance to the use of the guidelines if they are at variance with an individual practitioner's current (and often long-held) clinical practice. However, the recommendations offered in evidence-based guidelines have the major advantage of being derived from carefully examined and weighed evidence that has been judged of good quality and sufficient to support such recommendations, even in the face of criticism. Part of the adaptation required of physicians faced with this conflict is captured in a paraphrase of comments by John Brockman (18) on the "Third Culture and the History of American Literary Intellectuals:"

"In a culture shaped by truly critical thinking and scientific method, being proven wrong, being constantly challenged to prove your most cherished concepts, is understood as part of intellectual evolution."

One would ideally hope that this same assumption would reach deeply into the nature of medical practice, but this is not necessarily the case. Indeed, those whose expertise has been developed and recognized as being built on repeated experience with a given clinical entity are often reluctant to adhere to scientific principles, lest their expertise be challenged. This personalization of practice is contrary to scientific advancement, and impedes learning. Rather than recognizing that medical education is a life-long process which involves—increasingly—acquisition of new knowledge (including computer skills), medical informatics, use of technological advances, and critical evaluation of the medical literature, a defensive stance is taken upholding the "tried and true." Those who attempt to promote this move into the future are then sometimes exposed to a rather high-level "kill the messenger" phenomenon, and they may despair of advancing the knowlege of those who are primarily clinicians, rather than scientists, or who believe that science is practiced only in the laboratory. This emotional, rather than intellectual, reaction needs to be abandoned if medical practice is to escape victimization by those who would develop guidelines for their own ends (e.g., for cost-saving), rather than for the benefit of patients.

Fortunately, there is growing evidence that health-care providers will voluntarily change their practice patterns if they are made aware that they deviate significantly from regional or national norms. Examples of such self-correcting changes, with consequent effects on both quality and cost, are numerous and increasing. The key step is dissemination of the information and guidelines to the interested providers in order to influence their behavior toward reducing inappropriate variations in patient management and resource use. When this has been done and monitored, it has produced some remarkable results. The Maine Medical Assessment Foundation has facilitated reviews of hysterectomy rates and of variations in use of prostatectomy for benign prostatic hypertrophy. In both instances, involving physicians on a local level and providing information on their differences in practice compared to well developed norms or standards was sufficient to effect beneficial changes in their practices regarding both conditions. A study by Grimshaw and Russell (19) in 1993 found 59 published clinical guidelines that were scientifically developed. In all but four of the groups studied, significant improvements in the process and/or outcomes of care were confirmed. They concluded that explicit guidelines do improve clinical practice when introduced in the context of rigorous evaluations, although the size of the improvements did vary considerably.

There is reason, then, to be optimistic about the direction neurosurgery is taking with respect to a commitment to evidence-based guidelines. This places neurosurgery in the forefront of this movement and affirms an intent to use available scientific information as an infrastructure for decision making for patients.

Acknowledgments

Grateful acknowledgment of the support and advice of Robert Florin, M.D., Chairman of the Joint Committee on the Assessment of Quality of the AANS/CNS throughout the writing of this document is made here. Thanks go also to Jay Rosenberg, M.D., of the American Academy of Neurology for promoting collegial collaboration between our professional organizations. Without the forbearance and understanding of George Buczko, M.D., Greta Florin, and Judy Rosenberg, the guidelines movement in neurosurgery and neurology would not be at its present point.

REFERENCES

1. Relman, A. Assessment and Accountability, The third revolution in medical care. N Engl J Med 1988;31(9): 1220-1222.
2. Vibbert S. What works: How outcomes research will change medical practice. The Grand Rounds Press, Whittle Direct Books, 1993.
3. American Medical Association. American Medical Association directory of practice parameters: Titles, sources and updates, 1995. Chicago: American Medical Association, 1995.
4. Rosenberg J, Greenberg MK. Practice parameters: Strategies for survival into the nineties; Neurology. 1992;42:1110–1115.
5. Field MJ, Lohr KN. Guidelines for clinical practice, from development to use. Washington DC: National Academy Press, 1992.
6. Sackett DL, Haynes RB, Tugwell PX. Clinical epidemiology: A basic science for clinical medicine. Toronto: Little, Brown, 1985.
7. Eddy DM. Designing a practice policy: standards, guidelines, and options. JAMA 1990;26(3): 3077–3084.
8. Sackett DL. Rules of evidence and clinical recommendations on the use of antithrombotic agents. 2nd ACCP Conference on Antithrombotic Therapy. Chest 1989; (Suppl) 2S–4S.
9. Woolf SH. Practice guidelines: a new reality in medicine, II: Methods of developing guidelines. Arch Intern Med 1992;152:946–952.
10. Woolf SH, Battista RN, Anderson GM, Logan AG, Wang E, the Canadian Task Force on the Periodic Health Examination. Assessing the clinical effectiveness of preventive maneuvers: analytic principles and systematic methods in reviewing evidence and developing clinical practice recommendations. J Clin Epidemiol 1990;43(9):891–905.
11. Ransohoff DF, Feinstein AR. Problems of spectrum and bias in evaluating the efficacy of diagnostic tests. N Engl J Med 1978;29(9)‹6–929.
12. Ringenberg B.J., et al.: Rational ordering of cervical spine radiographs following trauma. Ann Emerg Med 1988;17:792–796.
13. Macdonald R.L., et al.. Diagnosis of cervical spine injury in motor vehicle crash victims: how many x-rays are enough? J Trauma 1990;(30)4:392–397.
14. Irwig L, et al.: Guidelines for meta-analyses evaluating diagnostic tests. Ann Int Med 120(3):667–676.
15. Hayward RS, Laupacis A. Initiating, conducting and maintaining guidelines development programs. Can Med Assoc J 1993;4:507–512
16. Bullock MR et al. Guidelines for the management of severe head injury. J Neurotrauma 1996;13(11): 639–734.
17. Johnson KB, Hirshfeld EB, Iie ML, et al. Legal implications of practice parameters. Chicago: American Medical Association, 1990.
18. Brockman J: Agent of the third culture. Wired, 1993; 3(8):119.
19. Grimshaw JM, Russell IT: Effect of clinical guidelines

on medical practice: A systematic review of rigorous evaluations. Lancet 1993;342:1317–1322.

SUGGESTED READINGS

American Medical Association. Attributes to guide the development of practice parameters. Chicago: American Medical Association, 1990.

American Medical Association. Directory of Practice Parameters. Chicago: American Medical Association, 1989.

American Medical Association. Directory of Practice Parameters. Chicago: American Medical Association, 1990.

American Medical Association. Directory of Practice Parameters. Chicago: American Medical Association, 1991.

American Medical Association. Directory of Practice Parameters. Chicago: American Medical Association, 1992.

American Medical Association. Directory of Practice Parameters. Chicago: American Medical Association, 1993.

American Medical Association. Directory of Practice Parameters. Chicago: American Medical Association, 1994.

American Medical Association. Directory of Practice Parameters. Chicago: American Medical Association, 1995.

American Medical Association. Directory of Practice Parameters. Chicago: American Medical Association, 1996.

American Medical Association. Implementing Practice Parameters on the Local/State/Regional Level. Chicago, 1993.

American Medical Association. Using practice parameters in quality assessment, quality assurance, and quality improvement programs. Chicago: American Medical Association, 1992.

Anderson FA, Wheeler HB, Goldberg RJ, Hosmer DW, Forcier A, Patwardham NA. Changing clinical practice: Prospective study of the impact of continuing medical education and quality assurance programs on use of prophylaxis for venous thromboembolism. Arch Intern Med 1994; 154:669–677.

Anderson G. Guidelines workshop. Implementing practice guidelines. Can Med Assoc J 1993;148(5):753–755.

Asaph JW, Janoff K, Wayson K, Kilberg L, Graham M. Carotid endarterectomy in a community hospital: A change in physicians' practice patterns. Am J Surgery 1991;161:616–618.

Aucott JN, Taylor AL, Wright JT, et al. Developing guidelines for local use: Algorithms for cost-efficient outpatient management of cardiovascular disorders in a VA medical center. J Qual Improv 1994;20:17–32.

Battista RN, Hodge MJ. Clinical practice guidelines: Between science and art. Can Med Assoc J. 1993;148(3): 385–388.

Bernstein SJ, Hilborne LH, Leape LL, et al. The appropriateness of use of coronary angiography in New York State. JAMA 1993;269:766–769.

Bernstein SJ, McGlynn EA, Siu AL, et al. The appropriateness of hysterectomy: A comparison of care in seven health plans. JAMA 1993;269:2398–2402.

Brennan T. Overview of legal issues. J Qual Improv 1993; 19:319–321.

Burke M. Clinical quality initiatives: The search for meaningful and accurate measures. Hospitals. 1992;March: 26–36.

Burns LR, Denton M, Goldfein S, Warrick L, Morenz B, Sales B. The use of continuous quality improvement methods in the development and dissemination of medical practice guidelines. QRB Qual Rev Bull 1992; 18:434–439.

Canadian Task Force on the Periodic Health Examination. The periodic health examination: 2. 1987 update. Can Med Assoc J 1988;138:618–626.

Carpenter CE, Nash DB, Johnson LE. Evaluating the cost containment potential of clinical outcomes. QRB Qual Rev Bull 1993;19:119–123.

Carter A. Clinical practice guidelines. Can Med Assoc J 1992; 147(11):1649–1650.

Carter A. Guidelines workshop. Background to the ''Guidelines for Guidelines'' series. Can Med Assoc J. 1993; 148(3):383.

Chassin MR, Kosecoff J, Park RE, et al. Does inappropriate use explain geographic variations in the use of health care services? A study of three procedures. JAMA 1987; 258(18):2533–2537.

Committee to Advise the Public Health Service on Clinical Practice Guidelines (Institute of Medicine). Clinical practice guidelines: Directions for a new program. Washington DC: Natl Acad Pr, 1990:38.

Cordero CE, Christensen L. Practice guidelines are adding value to managed care. Business & Health 1992:22–27.

CPG Strategies: Putting guidelines into practice. Chicago: American Hospital Association, 1992.

Cranford CO, Gorton A, Golden WE, et al. Demonstration of dissemination of medical technology using area health education centers. Little Rock, Arkansas: Area Health Education Centers, University of Arkansas for Medical Sciences, 1993.

Deber RB. Translating technology assessment into policy: conceptual issues and tough choices. Int J Tech Assess Health Care 1992;8:131–137.

Department of Health Care and Promotion, Canadian Medical Association. Guidelines workshop. Workshop on clinical practice guidelines: Summary of proceedings. Can Med Assoc J 1993;148(9):1459–1462.

Dolan JG, Bordley DR. Using the analytic hierarchy process (AHP) to develop and disseminate guidelines. QRB Qual Rev Bull 1992;18:440–447.

Eagle KA, Mulley AG, Skates SJ, et al. Length of stay in the intensive care unit: Effects of practice guidelines and feedback. JAMA 1990;264:992–997.

Eddy DM. A Manual for Assessing Health Practices & Designing Practice Policies. Philadelphia: American College of Physicians, 1992.

Eddy DM. Anatomy of a decision. JAMA 1990; 263:441–443.

Eddy DM. Applying cost-effectiveness analysis: the inside story. JAMA 1992;268:2575–2582.

Eddy DM. Broadening the responsibilities of practitioners: the team approach. JAMA 1993;269:1849–1855.

Eddy DM. Clinical decision making: from theory to practice. Cost-effectiveness analysis. Is it up to the task? JAMA 1992;267:3342–3348.

Eddy DM. Comparing benefits and harms: The balance sheet. JAMA 1990;263:2493,2498,2501,2505.

Eddy DM. Connecting value and cost: Whom do we ask, and what do we ask them? JAMA 1990;264:1737–1739.

Eddy DM. Cost-effectiveness analysis: A conversation with my father. JAMA 1992;267:1674–1675.

· Eddy DM. Practice policies: Guidelines for methods. JAMA 1990;263:1839–1841.

Eddy DM. Practice policies: What are they? JAMA 1990; 263:877–880.

Eddy DM. Practice policies: Where do they come from? JAMA 1990;263:1265–1273.

Eddy DM. Principles for making difficult decisions in difficult times. JAMA 1994;271:1792–1798.

Eddy DM. Resolving conflicts in practice policies. JAMA 1990;264:389–391.

Eddy DM. What do we do about costs? JAMA 1990; 264:1161–1170.

Ellrodt AG, Conner L, Riedinger MS, Weingarten S. Implementing practice guidelines through a utilization management strategy: the potential and the challenges. QRB Qual Rev Bull 1992;18:456–460.

Fahs MC, Mandelblatt J, Schechter C, Muller C. Cost effectiveness of cervical cancer screening for the elderly. Ann of Intern Med. 1992;117:520–527.

Favaretti C, Selle V, Marcolongo A, Orsini A. The appropriateness of human albumin use in the hospital of Padova, Italy. Qual Assur Health Care 1993;5:49–55.

Field MJ. Overview: Prospects and options for local and national guidelines in the courts. J Qual Improv 1993; 19:313–318.

Findlay S. Medicine by the book: A gusher of guidelines for doctors can educate patients, too. US News World Rep 1992:68–70.

Flagle CD, Cahn MA. AHCPR-NLM joint initiative for health services research information: 1992 update on OHSRI. QRB Qual Rev Bull 1992;18:410–412.

Gates PE. Clinical quality improvement: getting physicians involved. QRB Qual Rev Bull 1993;19:56–61.

Gilmore A. Clinical practice guidelines: Weapons for patients, or shields for MDs? Can Med Assoc J. 1993; 148(3):429–431.

Ginsburg WH. When does a guideline become a standard? The new American Society of Anesthesiologists guidelines give us a clue. Ann Emerg Med 1993;22:121–126.

Gottlieb LK, Margolis SC, Schoenbaum SC. Clinical practice guidelines at an HMP: development and implementation in a quality improvement model. QRB Qual Rev Bull 1990;16:80–86.

Graboys TB, Biegelsen B, Lampert S, Blatt CM, Lown B. Results of a second-opinion trial among patients recommended for coronary angiography. JAMA 1992; 268:2537–2540.

Greco PJ, Eisenberg JM. Changing physicians' practices. N Eng J Med. 1993;329:1271–1274.

Gronseth GS, Greenberg MK. The utility of the electroencephalogram in the evaluation of patients presenting with headache: A review of literature. Neurology 1995; 45:1263–1267.

Guidelines for Canadian Clinical Practice Guidelines. Canadian Medical Association. 1994.

Guyatt GH, Cairns J, Churchill D, et al. Evidence-based medicine: A new approach to teaching the practice of medicine. JAMA 1992;268:2420–2425.

Guyatt GH, Rennie D. User's Guides to the Medical Literature [Editorial]. JAMA 1993;270:2096–2097

Guyatt GH, Sackett DL, Cook DJ. Users' guides to the medical literature: How to use an article about therapy or prevention. JAMA 1993;270:2598–2601.

Hadorn D, Baker D, Dracup K, Pitt B. Making judgements about treatment effectiveness based on health outcomes: theoretical and practical issues. J Qual Improv 1994; 20:547–554.

Hadorn DC, Brook RH. The health care resource allocation debate: defining our terms. JAMA 1991;266:3328–3331.

Hadorn DC, McCormick K, Diokno A. An annotated algorithm approach to clinical guideline development. JAMA 1992;267:3311–3314.

Handley MR, Stuart ME. An evidence-based approach to evaluating and improving clinical practice: guideline development. HMO Practice 1994;8:10–19.

Harvey K. The clinical practice guideline process: exploring key issues. Ontario Med Rev 1994;(April):25–29.

Harvey K. Evidence-based medicine and the clinical decision-making process. Ontario Med. Rev. 1994; (May): 23–25.

Hastings K. A view from the Agency for Health Care Policy and research: the use of language in clinical practice guidelines. J Qual Improv 1993;19:335–341.

Hayward RS, Wilson MC, Tunis SR, Bass EB, Rubin HR, Haynes B. More informative abstracts of articles describing clinical practice guidelines. Ann Intern Med 1993; 118:731–737.

Headrick LA, Speroff T, Pelecanos HI, Cebul RD. Efforts to improve compliance with the national cholesterol education program guidelines. Arch Intern Med 1992; 152:2490–2496.

Herman R. Harvard HMO improves Pap smear screening. QAR 1989;1:2–3.

Herrmann J. Practice parameters—Hospitals and physicians working together. Health Systems Rev 1992; March/April:24,26,28,73.

Hewitt P, Chalmers TC. Using MEDLINE to peruse the literature. Controlled Clin Trials 1985;6:75–83.

Hilborne LH, Leape LL, Bernstein SJ, et al. The appropriatemess of use of percutaneous transluminal coronary angioplasty in New York state. JAMA 1993;269:761–765.

Hillman AL, Pauly MV, Kerstein JJ. How do financial incentives affect physicians' clinical decisions and the financial performance of health maintenance organizations? N Engl J Med 1989; 321(2):86–92.

Hirshfeld EB. Should practice parameters be the standard of care in malpractice litigation? JAMA 1991; 266:2886–2891.

Hirshfeld EB. Use of practice parameters as standards of care and in health reform: A view from the American Medical Association. J Qual Improv 1993;19:322–329.

Hirshfeld EB, Iie ML. Practice parameters: The legal implications. FOCUS 1992;1.

Hoffmann PA. Critical path method: An important tool for coordinating clinical care. J Qual Improv 1993; 19:235–246.

Hyams AL, Brandenburg JA, Lipsitz SR, Brennan TA. Report to Physician Payment Review Commission: Practice guidelines and malpractice litigation. Boston, MA: Harvard School of Public Health, Department of Health Policy and Management, Harvard University, 1994.

Iezzoni LI, Greenburg LG. Widespread assessment of risk-adjusted outcomes: Lessons from local initiatives. J Qual Improv 1994;20:305–316.

Jaeschke R, Guyatt G, Sackett DL. Users' guides to the medical literature: How to use an article about a diagnostic test. JAMA 1994;271:389–391.

Jencks SF, Wilensky GR. The health care quality improvement initiative: A new approach to quality assurance in Medicare. JAMA 1992;268:900–903.

Johnston ME, Langton KB, Haynes RB, Mathieu A. Effects of computer-based clinical decision support systems on clinician performance and patient outcome: a critical appraisal of research. Ann Intern Med 1994;120:135–142.

Jutras D. Guidelines Workshop: Clinical practice guidelines as legal norms. Can Med Assoc J 1993;148(6):905–908.

Kaegi L. How good are medicine's new recipes? The kitchen debate continues. J Qual Improv 1994;20:465–468.

Kane RL, Lurie N. Appropriate effectiveness: A tale of carts and horses. QRB Qual Rev Bull 1992;18:322–326.

Kapp MB. The legal status of clinical practice parameters: An annotated bibliography. Am J of Med Qual 1993;8:24–27.

Kassierer JP. The quality of care and the quality of measuring it. N Eng J Med 1993;329:1263–1265.

Kellie SE, Kelly JT. Medicare Peer Review Organization preprocedure review criteria: An analysis of criteria for three procedures. JAMA 1991;265:1265–1270.

Kelly JT, Kellie SE. Appropriateness of medical care. Arch Pathol Lab Med 1990;114:1119–1121.

Kelly JT, Swartwout JE. Development of practice parameters by physician organizations. QRB Qual Rev Bull 1990;16:54–57.

Kelly JT, Toepp MC. Development, evaluation, and implementation of medical practice parameters. Med Staff Couns 1992;6:45–49.

Kelly JT, Toepp MC. Practice parameters: Development, evaluation, dissemination, and implementation. QRB Qual Rev Bull 1992;18:405–409.

Kelly JT, Toepp MC. The medical community and evolving strategies for parameter implementation. Internist 1991;32:16–18.

Kibbe DC, Kaluzny AD, McLaughlin CP. Intergrating guidelines with continuous quality improvement: doing the right thing the right way to achieve the right goals. J Qual Improv 1994;20:181–191.

Kinney E. New standards for the Standard of Care. Legal Times 1991(suppl):22–25.

Knaus WA, Wagner D, Zimmerman JE, Draper EA. Variations in mortality and length of stay in intensive care units. Ann Intern Med 1993;118:753–761.

Kosecoff J, Kanouse DE, Rogers WH, McCloskey L, Winslow CM, Brook RH. Effects of the National Institutes of Health Consensus Development Program on Physician Practice. JAMA 1987; 258(19):2708–2713.

L'Abbe KC, Detsky AS, O'Rourke K. Meta-analysis in clinical research. Ann Intern Med 1987; 107:224–233.

Lamas GA, Pfeffer MA, Hamm P, Wertheimer J, Rouleau JL, Braunwald E. Do the results of randomized clinical trials of cardiovascular drugs influence medical practice? N Engl J Med. 1992; 327(4):241–247.

Larsen RA, Evans RS, Burke JP, Pestotnik SL, Gardner RM, Slassen DC. Improved perioperative antibiotic use and reduced surgical wound infection through use of computer decision analysis. Infect Control Hosp Epidemiol 1989;10:316–320.

Leape LL, Hilborne LH, Park RE, et al. The appropriateness of use of coronary artery bypass graft surgery in New York state. JAMA 1993;269:753–760.

Leavenworth G. Case studies: After reviewing past procedures, three hospitals, an HMO, and an employer found compelling reasons to use guidelines. Business & Health. 1994;12(suppl B):13–17.

Leavenworth G. Quality costs less: By helping to eliminate inappropriate care, guidelines are improving quality and outcomes. Business & Health 1994;12(suppl B):6–11.

Leavenworth G. The value of outcomes: One of the most effective ways to develop guidelines is to do so in concert with collecting and analyzing outcomes data. Business & Health. 1994;12 (suppl B):18–22.

Liability premiums reduced for anesthesiologists. QAR 1989;1:6.

Linton AL, Peachey DK. Guidelines for medical practice: 1. The reasons why. Can Med Assoc J. 1990; 143(6):485–490.

Lipowski EE, Becker M. Presentation of drug prescribing guidelines and physician response. QRB Qual Rev Bull 1992;18:461–470.

Litzelman DK, Ditus RS, Miller ME, Tierney WM. Requiring physicians to respond to computerized reminders improves their compliance with preventive care protocols. J Gen Intern Med 1993;8:311–317.

Lohr KN. Guidelines for clinical practice: applications for primary care. Int J Qual Health Care 1994;6:17–25.

Lohr KN, Schyve PM. Reasonable Expectations: From the Institute of Medicine. QRB Qual Rev Bull 1992;18:393–396.

Lomas J, Anderson GM, Domnick-Pierre K, Vayda E, Enkin MW, Hannah WJ. Do practice guidelines guide practice? The effect of a consensus statement on the practice of physicians. N Engl J Med 1989; 321(19):1306–1311.

Lomas J, Enkin M, Anderson GM, Hannah WJ, Vayda E, Singer J. Opinion leaders vs. audit and feedback to implement practice guidelines. JAMA 1991;265:2202–2207.

Lomas J, Haynes RB. A taxonomy and critical review of tested strategies for the application of clinical practice recommendations: from "official" to "individual" clinical policy. Am J Prev Med 1988;4:77–94.

McDonald CJ, Overhage JM. Guidelines You Can Follow and Can Trust. An Ideal and an Example. JAMA 1994;271(11):872–873.

Meeker CI. A consensus-based approach to practice parameters. Obstet Gynecol 1992;79:790–793.

Meeker CI. How practice guidelines aid patient management. Contemp OB/GYN 1993:21–31.

Merz SM. Clinical practice guidelines: Policy issues and legal implications. J Qual Improv 1993;19:306–312.

Mittman BS, Tonesk X, Jacobson PD. Implementing clinical practice guidelines: social influence strategies and practitioner behavior change. QRB Qual Rev Bull 1992:18:413–422.

Moller JH, Borbas C, Hagler DJ, McKay CJ, Stone FM. Pediatric cardiac care consortium: demonstrated value of a physician-directed quality assessment system. Minn Med 1990;73:2632.

Montague J. CME: a school for survival? Hospitals & Health Networks 1994:54–56.

Murrey KO, Gottlieb LK, Schoenbaum SC. Implementing clinical guidelines: A quality management approach to reminder systems. QRB Qual Rev Bull 1992;18:423–433.

Myers SA, Gleicher N. A successful program to lower cesarean-section rates. N Eng J Med 1989;319:1511–1516.

Owens DK, Nease RF. Development of outcome-based practice guidelines: A method for structuring problems and synthesizing evidence. J Qual Improv 1993;19:248–263.

Oxman AD, Cook DJ, Guyatt GH. Users' guides to the medical literature: How to use an overview. JAMA 1994:272:1367–1371.

Oxman AD, et al. Quality Care; Evidence-based care:4. Improving performance: How can we improve the way we manage this problem. Can Med Assoc J 1994;150(11):1771–1772;1793–1796.

Oxman AD, Sackett DL, Guyatt GH. Users' Guides to the Medical Literature 1.How to Get Started. JAMA 1993; 270(17):2093–2095.

Pashos CL, Newhouse JP, McNeil BJ. Temporal changes in the care and outcomes of elderly patients with acute myocardial infarction, 1987 through 1990. JAMA. 1993; 270:1832–1836.

Peachey DK, Linton AL. Guidelines for medical practice: 2. A possible strategy. Can Med Assoc J 1990; 143(7): 629–632.

Phelps CE. The methodologic foundations of studies of the appropriateness of medical care. N Eng J Med 1993; 329:1241–1245.

Pierce EC. The development of anesthesia guidelines and standards. QRB Qual Rev Bull 1990;16:61–64.

Pilote L, Thomas RJ, Dennis C, et al. Return to work after uncomplicated myocardial infarction: a trial of practice guidelines in the community. Ann Intern Med 1992; 117:383–389.

Ramsey SD, Hillman AL, Renshaw LR, Kimberly JR, Paul MV, Schwartz JS. How important is the scientific literature in guiding clinical decisions? The case of magnetic resonance imaging. Int J Tech Assess Health Care 1993; 9:253–262.

Richardson GE, Venzon DJ, Phelps R, et al. Application of an algorithm for staging small-cell lung cancer can save one third of the initial evaluation costs. Arch Intern Med 1993;153:329–337.

Ring JJ. Why Mds believe in practice parameters. J Health Care Benefits 1992;1:4–7.

Rosen AB, Peterson ED. Influence of data sources on outcomes research. J Outcomes Manag 1994:9–14.

Rothschild RD. Practice parameters benefit all: Patient management strategies improve outcomes for patients, lower costs for payers. Health Prog 1993; Sept:24–29.

Sapienza PE, Levine GM, Pomerantz S, Davidson JH, Weinryb J, Glassman J. Impact of a quality assurance program on gastrointestinal endoscopy. Gastroenterology 1992; 102:387–393.

Schriefer J. The synergy of pathways and algorithms: Two tools work better than one. J Qual Improv 1994; 20:485–499.

Smith GH. A case study in progress: Practice guidelines and the affirmative defense in Maine. J Qual Improv 1993; 19:355–360.

Somerville MA. Guidelines Workshop: Ethics and clinical practice guidelines. Can Med Assoc J. 1993;148(7): 1133–1137.

Spernak SM, Budetti PP, Zweig F. Use of language in clinical practice guidelines. Washington, DC: Center for Health Policy Research, The George Washington University for the Agency for Health Care Policy and Research; 1992.

Stiell IG, Greenberg GH, McKnight RD. Decision rules for the use of radiography in acute ankle injuries: refinement and prospective validation. JAMA 1993;269:1127–1132.

Stiell IG, McKnight RD, Greenberg GH, et al. Implementation of the Ottawa Ankle Rules. JAMA 1994; 271(11): 827–832.

Strickland D. The future of guidelines. Business & Health 1994;12(suppl B):27–30.

Tanenbaum SJ. Sounding board: What physicians know. N Eng J Med 1993;329:1268–1270.

Temple PC, DeCola D. Practice guidelines: Do they work? Experience from the Ohio State University College of Medicine on cost savings from guidelines for the routine adult physical examination. Managed Care Med 1994:27–30.

Tingley FW. The use of guidelines to reduce costs and improve quality: A perspective from insurers. J Qual Improv 1993;19:330–334.

Thomasson GO. Participating risk management: promoting physician compliance with practice guidelines. J Qual Improv 1994;20:317–329.

Topol EJ, Califf RM. Scorecard cardiovascular medicine: its impact and future directions. Ann Intern Med 1994; 120:65–70.

VanAmringe M, Shannon TE. Awareness, assimilation, and adoption: The challenge of effective dissemination and the first AHCPR-sponsored guidelines. QRB Qual Rev Bull 1992;18:397–404.

Venable RS. Quality and outcomes management: Facilitating optimal results with caring and technology. Managed Care Med 1994:12–16.

Watanabe M, Noseworthy T. Creating a culture of evidence-based decision-making in Health. Ann RCPSC 1997; 30(3):137–139.

Watchel TJ, O'Sullivan P. Practice guidelines to reduce testing in the hospital. J Gen Intern Med 1990;5:335–341.

Webb LZ, Kuykendall DH, Zeiger RS, et al. The impact of status asthmaticus practice guidelines on patient outcome and physician behavior. QRB Qual Rev Bull 1992; 18:471–476.

Weingarten S, Agocs L, Tankel N, Sheng A, Ellrodt AG. Reducing lengths of stay for patients hospitalized with chest pain using medical practice guidelines and opinion leaders. Am J Cardiol 1993;71:259–262.

Weingarten S, Ellrodt AG. The case for intensive dissemination: adoption of practice guidelines in the coronary care unit. QRB Qual Rev Bull 1992;18:449–455.

Weingarten S, Ermann B, Bolus R, et al. Early "step-down" transfer of low-risk patients with chest pain. Ann Intern Med. 1990;113:283–289.

Wennberg JE, Gittelsohn A. Variations in medical care among small areas. Sci Am 1982;246:120–135.

Wennberg JE. Unwanted Variations in the Rules of Practice. JAMA 1991;265(10):1306–1307.

Winslow CM, Solomon DH, Chassin MR, Kosecoff J, Merrick NJ, Brook RH. The appropriateness of carotid endarterectomy. N Engl JMed 1988;318:721–727.

Woolf SH. Practice guidelines: A new reality in medicine, I: Recent developments. Arch Intern Med 1990; 150:1811–1818.

Woolf SH. Practice guidelines: A new reality in medicine, III: Impact on patient care. Arch Intern Med 1993; 153:2646–2655.

Zweig FM, Witt HA. Assisting judges in screening medical practice guidelines for health care litigation. J Qual Improv 1993;19:342–354.

CHAPTER 7

The Neurosurgical Workforce: Market Effects, Public Policy, and Professional Constraints

A. JOHN POPP, M.D.

INTRODUCTION

The costs associated with medical care in the United States, currently estimated to be in the range of 15% of the gross domestic product, have grown dramatically in recent years. This increase in health-care costs has had a profound and alarming impact on both federal and state budgets, but the implications of unrestrained health-care costs go beyond governmental spending, affecting all segments of our economy. The critical importance of health-care costs for our nation's economy was underscored by President Clinton's resolve to make substantive health care reform a national priority during his first term. The failure of this initiative did not bring an end to efforts to control the cost of health care in the United States, however. Rather, the health-care reform movement provided an impetus for the subsequent growth of managed care, which is now the predominant mode of health-care delivery. Managed care has, as its primary goal, the control of health-care costs. This control is accomplished through capitation, gatekeeping, and limiting hospitalizations. These approaches to cost containment have had the secondary effect of decreasing the demand for physicians, particularly specialists, thereby calling into question the size of the physician workforce. The issue of workforce size has become an increasingly important one for neurosurgery, as it is a specialty that is consistently perceived as having a surplus of practitioners, despite its representing less than 1% of the total physician workforce.

Are there too many neurosurgeons? The answer is complex and depends on one's perspective. From the vantage point of a neurosurgeon, there are too many neurosurgeons if the number and type of operative procedures performed by that neurosurgeon are too few to maintain technical proficiency; or if the neurosurgeon is not sufficiently busy to derive professional satisfaction from his or her practice; or if third-party insurers can bring neurosurgeons to bid against each other, resulting in an unacceptably low level of compensation, considering the neurosurgeon's responsibilities and level of training. Conversely, from the perspective of a patient residing in a sparsely populated state who must travel a long distance or wait an excessively long period of time for treatment, or of a hospital administrator who is unable to arrange neurosurgical emergency room coverage, there may appear to be too few neurosurgeons. Confounding the issue of workforce size are decisions being made by national policy groups, based on an assumption of an abundance of physicians in the specialty workforce, without taking into account such factors as regional needs, specialty differences, and individual choice. Thus, the answer to the question of whether there are too many neurosurgeons in practice or being trained depends on whom you ask.

The term workforce, when applied to an industrial model, is an inclusive term that refers to the total number of individuals, including those with different skills, training, and responsibilities, who are needed to complete a finished product. The term neurosurgical workforce, however, is generally defined more narrowly, referring exclusively to neurosurgeons who perform clinical neurosurgery. Although this distinction may seem unnecessarily pedantic, the difference in the two definitions illustrates several key aspects of the workforce debate currently facing the specialty of neurosurgery. For instance, most workforce analyses of medical specialties consider work to be limited to clinical activities. These analyses fail to take into account for many of the non—income-generating activities in which neurosurgeons engage, such as education, research, and administrative duties, which are best performed by neurosurgeons and which are necessary to preserve the integrity of the specialty. Yet another factor to consider is the role that others in the medical workforce, including physician assistants, nurses, physiatrists, orthopedic surgeons, and vascular surgeons, among others, play in managing the conditions that neurosurgeons include in their ''universe'' of practice activities.

This chapter reviews the methodology of workforce analysis; the history of neurosurgical workforce analysis; the current status of the workforce debate, including some of the forces presently influencing the workforce environment; and some proposed solutions and strategies for addressing workforce concerns as they relate to neurosurgery.

A METHODOLOGY FOR WORKFORCE ANALYSIS

An understanding of the workforce needs in neurosurgery necessarily involves an evaluation of the supply of neurosurgeons and the demand for neurosurgical services. Inherent to the supply of a service or commodity, however, are temporal fluctuations, during which periods of surplus or scarcity can occur. In neurosurgery, this temporal component must be considered in terms of decades, because of the length of the training program. A distinction must also be made between demands or wants, which correlate with a patient's desires or expectations related to medical care, and needs, which are those services that are actually required to maintain or regain health. This distinction is important because the gap between needed services and desired or demanded services can be bridged by educating patients and their families about what

constitutes quality care and what types of services are actually needed to maintain or improve their health. Ideally, the supply of neurosurgeons should exactly match the need for neurosurgical services, resulting in a balanced equation.

The following model of the neurosurgical workforce explores the dynamic between the supply of neurosurgeons and the demand/need for their services. Such a model is helpful in exploring the numerous influences on workforce needs, as well as in validating the complex backdrop against which workforce size must be evaluated to allow meaningful conclusions to be drawn about optimal neurosurgical staffing. The use of mathematical modeling gives workforce analysis the semblance of a science, but although such conceptualizations help to elucidate the various factors involved in workforce assessment, a valid statistical analysis of physician workforce is virtually impossible because of the numerous societal and economic variables involved.

Factors Influencing the Supply Side

The supply side of the equation (Fig. 7.1) appears to be the easiest to quantify accurately, but there are variables that only can be estimated, and, in some instances, those estimates represent only educated guesses. For example, if we use the present number of neurosurgeons in practice to derive estimates of future workforce size, we must, at the outset, recognize that the available data bases on the number and location of practicing neurosurgeons change almost daily. For example, the New York State Neurological Society's 1997 membership roster lists the names, addresses, and approximate number (267) of neurosurgeons in New York State. Ignoring the fact that differing data bases containing lists of New York State neurosurgeons provide somewhat different data, the information compiled will undoubtedly change within a few months, making accurate computation of workforce distribution and size in New York State impossible. Furthermore, this list of neurosurgeons is unlikely to be complete, as it does not account for part-time practitioners, nor does it take into account the services provided to a significant number of patients from outside New York State. Thus, computation of either a clinical full-time equivalent (FTE) or the physician-to-population ratio is difficult and fraught with error.

The goal of most studies of physician supply

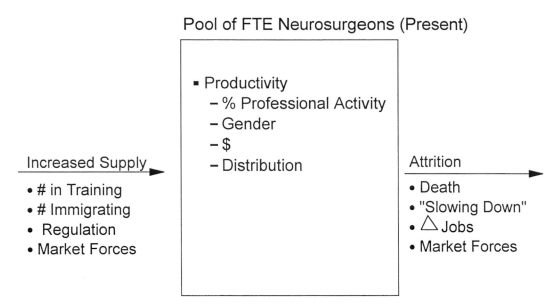

Figure 7.1. A model of the supply of neurosurgeons showing the present pool of FTE neurosurgeons and some of the factors that may modify the present numbers of FTEs in this pool. Also shown are influences on the rate of increase in the size of this pool over time and factors influencing the rate of attrition over time.

is to determine the number of physicians needed to provide clinical services. This calculation involves determining the efforts of a single clinical FTE, the combined efforts of the entire physician pool, and the resultant total number of FTEs delivering service. If we simply consider a static number, representing the present pool of U.S. neurosurgeons, without considering the increase or decrease in the number of practitioners over time, we find a number of variables that influence the number of clinical services (and hence the functional size of the FTE pool) rendered by that pool. Moreover, a component of this computation is based on the productivity of that pool of individuals, and determination of that level of productivity is based partly on the percentage of time the individuals in that pool are engaged in clinical activity. There may be certain members of that pool who are counted as neurosurgeons, despite only 50% of their time being spent performing clinical neurosurgery with the remainder of their professional time being devoted to teaching, research, or administrative activities. Then, too, in some workforce analyses, gender has been found to influence the amount of time spent in clinical activities. For example, it is estimated that female physicians may work only 85% as much as their male counterparts

because of family responsibilities (1–4). Whether a similar percentage applies to women in neurosurgery is unknown. However, if this statistic proves to be valid for the specialty of neurosurgery, as the number of women in neurosurgery increases, gender may increasingly be a factor in determining the clinical productivity of the neurosurgical workforce. Likewise, productivity in the present pool of neurological surgeons is influenced by fiscal considerations. In some instances, surgeons have compensated for falling salaries by increasing surgical volume. Based on these same fiscal pressures, other neurosurgeons have been influenced to decrease their clinical load or retire. A final factor influencing the productivity of neurosurgeons is their distribution. Although the prevailing perception in the United States may be that there are too many neurosurgeons in some areas of the country, there are other areas where the queue for neurosurgical services is long, or where the closest neurosurgical care is hundreds of miles away.

To view the size of the present pool of neurosurgeons as static despite our inability to measure it precisely downplays the dynamics of the situation. Indeed, the size and distribution of the current pool of the neurosurgical workforce is changing on a daily basis because of newly trained neurosurgeons entering and others leaving the workforce. These factors must be taken into account if a reasonable model of the supply side of the neurosurgical workforce is to be developed. Thus, factors that influence the rate of increase or attrition in the workforce must be considered. Factors influencing the rate of increase of the present pool of neurosurgeons include the number of residents in training in the US and the number immigrating from other countries, particularly Canada. In the future, these numbers may be influenced by such forces as government regulation of either the size of training programs or the number of surgeons allowed to immigrate to this country. The numbers involved in training may also be influenced by policies adopted by the specialty of neurosurgery to reduce or increase the number of residency programs. Finally, the number of neurosurgical trainees may be influenced by the market forces, such as the perception of medical students that the value of neurosurgery has declined, because of falling salaries on reduced job opportunities. The size of the present pool of neurosurgeons is also affected by the rate of attrition attributable to death, decreased volume of clinical practice, or job changes. Finances are a factor, as well, as some older neurosurgeons in the managed care environment find that, with

reduction of salaries, it is no longer desirable or economically feasible to continue practicing.

Thus, estimating the supply side of the neurosurgical workforce equation presents significant challenges to workforce pundits. However, these challenges are related solely to defining the actual number of FTE neurosurgeons providing service now and in the future. Even more daunting are the complex economic and societal variables that must be considered when estimating the demand/need for neurosurgical services.

Factors Influencing the Demand Side

The demand/need side of the equation includes the present pool of patients who require neurosurgical services (Fig. 7.2). The size of this pool is determined by the types of disorders for which neurosurgeons presently provide care. Disease prevalence, the range of neurosurgical services offered, market share, physician distribution, and the ability of patients to pay for services are also among the factors that modulate the size of the patient pool. The size of this patient pool may increase or decrease according to fluctuations in disease prevalence or scope of practice variations, as reflected by the percentage of procedures, such as spinal surgery or carotid endarterectomy, performed by neurosurgeons as compared to physicians in other

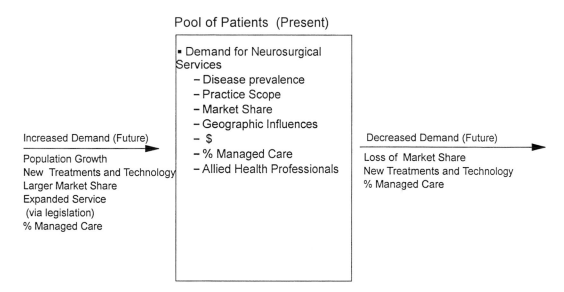

Figure 7.2.   A model of demand for neurosurgical services showing the present size of the patient pool and some factors determining the size of that pool. Included are factors that in time will increase the apparent demand for services and factors that will likely reduce the demand for services.

specialties. Moreover, population growth in the future and a burgeoning elderly population, coupled with a concomitant rise in the incidence of stroke and brain tumors, will increase the demand for neurosurgical services. Whether the neurosurgeon's market share of patients with spinal disease will increase or decrease is dependent partially on the success or failure of orthopedic spine surgeons in maintaining their own market share in spinal surgery. Similarly, neurosurgeons will compete with specialties in other areas. Success in these initiatives will influence the number of neurosurgeons needed to provide service. New technology, procedures, or medications may either enlarge or shrink neurosurgery's practice universe, depending in part on the degree to which neurosurgeons are involved in their development and application.

Another significant influence on demand is the availability of and access to insurance that pays for neurosurgical services. Governmental programs increasing medical coverage will result in a larger patient population pool. However, it has been estimated that if the entire United States population were cared for in a managed care practice, the need for the number of neurosurgeons in this country would be less than half the present number (5). This restricted need is unlikely to occur, however, with managed care market preferences shifting to specialty disease management and specialty direct access and with persistence of fee-for-service coverage and network contracting models requiring a higher number of FTE neurosurgeons. In addition, careful assessment of present managed care patient demographics suggests that an upward adjustment in workforce size will be necessary when the managed care population includes a higher percentage of elderly and uninsured individuals, whose need for medical services is greater, and when the necessary adjustments are made for the decreased physician productivity that may occur in managed care practices (1). Moreover, recent data have indicated that prolonged primary care treatment of some diseases is more expensive in the long term than earlier referral for specialty care; response to these data would thus necessitate another upward adjustment in the need for neurosurgical services (1). Although a number of these factors might increase the need for neurosurgical services over those currently estimated for the managed care setting, other mitigating factors may counterbalance this need, such as the trend to use less costly allied health professionals, such as physician's assistants and nurse practitioners, to deliver some of the outpatient care traditionally provided by neurosurgeons.

In the final analysis of the model, the ideal relationship between supply and demand/need should result in a balanced equation, with just the right number of neurosurgeons to deliver the neurosurgical care needed by society. Under these ideal conditions, neurosurgeons would perform enough neurosurgery to maintain technical competency, would work a reasonable number of hours, and would derive satisfaction from achieving their professional goals. Likewise, patients would have easy access to high-quality neurosurgical care whenever it was needed. Although this ideal balance might be a goal of workforce analysis and policy, it is a difficult goal to achieve, given the numerous variables and changing circumstances involved. Even if precise information concerning these variables were available, it is unlikely that decisions could be made that would result in a consistent balance between supply and demand. On the other hand, as presented later in this chapter, precise analytical data may not be prerequisites for drawing some conclusions about the dynamic between the supply of neurosurgeons and the demand for their services.

HISTORICAL PERSPECTIVE OF THE NEUROSURGICAL WORKFORCE DEBATE

An historical overview of neurosurgery's involvement in workforce analysis serves as a framework for grasping the current issues surrounding the workforce controversy. Although some aspects of this historical overview focus specifically on neurosurgery, many of the factors driving the workforce debate represent general trends in the medical workforce.

At the time of the Flexner report in 1910, which resulted in closure or reorganization of numerous medical schools in the United States, the size of the medical workforce was already a topic of discussion, and it has remained an integral part of every national medical policy analysis since then. During the first quarter of this century, Harvey Cushing addressed the issue of neurosurgical workforce density, recommending a ratio of one neurosurgeon to a population of one million be adopted as the ideal (6). This was an opinion that perhaps originated early in Cushing's career when William Halstead advised Cushing against studying neurosurgery on the grounds that there were only two patients on the ward who would require his services. Similarly, when Eldridge Campbell first came to Albany, New York in 1936, fresh from residency at Johns Hopkins, he was advised by then Chairman of Surgery at Albany Medical Center, Arthur Wells Elting, to continue to perform general surgery, as there was not thought to be sufficient neurosurgical cases in the region to keep even one person busy (7). Presently, there are 10 neurosurgeons practicing in Albany proper and approximately another 10 practicing in the region of Campbell's initial "catchment" area.

Admittedly, a number of factors have changed in the ensuing years. For example, the population has grown and the breadth of the specialty has expanded, not so much in its anatomical scope, which has remained stable over the past 70 years, but rather in the types of operations that have been developed and the efficacy of surgical intervention in the treatment of an increasing number of disorders.

Since the advent of the modern era of neurosurgical workforce debate in the early 1970s, the intensity of the debate has waxed and waned. In 1971, Senator Edward Kennedy was already asking the question, "Why do we have the same number of neurosurgeons in Massachusetts [which has] a population of 5 million people, as they have in England [which has] a population of 40 million people (17)? " Richard Bergland's article, "Neurosurgery May Die," published in 1973, stirred considerable debate among neurosurgeons (10) over its underlying premise that neurosurgery had stopped evolving and that the number of neurosurgeons being trained had increased, a development that was sure to have long-term consequences. Numerous neurosurgical journal articles and editorials of the time focused on issues concerning neurosurgical workforce distribution, size, and other facets of the workforce debate (8, 9, 11–16).

In the early 1970s, the leadership of American neurosurgery was resolute in its desire to investigate the issue of workforce. The American Association of Neurological Surgeons (AANS) appointed a special workforce committee to study the problem for which financial support was obtained through a contract with the National Institute of Neurological and Communicative Disorders and Stroke (18). The ensuing report of the AANS Manpower Commission suggested that there was an overproduction of neurosurgeons and advocated a 20 to 25% reduction in the annual number of neurosurgical trainees. Moreover, the Commission recommended the formation of a Manpower Monitoring Committee to periodically review the implementation process and statistical data so as to determine whether the number of trained neurosurgeons was appropriate or whether further adjustments should be made (19).

In the mid-1970s, The Study on Surgical Services for the United States ("SOSSUS") was conducted jointly by the American College of Surgeons and the American Surgical Association in an attempt to evaluate surgical care in the United States. Concern was expressed about the status of neurosurgery, especially since the number of neurosurgeons being trained had exceeded by 6 to 10% the growth rate for the nation's population. Furthermore, the study data indicated no evidence of an area underserved by neurosurgeons and concluded that neurosurgeons were distributed equally in communities with populations exceeding 75,000. The workload of individual surgeons was also investigated as an area of concern because some of the most common procedures included in the study were diagnostic procedures, such as myelography and angiography, which, in many institutions, are now performed by neuroradiologists. At that time, complex operative procedures were performed relatively rarely; hence, the issue was raised whether the clinical competency of a neurosurgeon could be maintained and whether a resident could be trained thoroughly enough to perform these operative procedures. Ultimately, SOSSUS recommended a reduction of approximately 20% reduction in the size of residency training programs, not only in neurosurgery, but in other surgical specialties as well (20).

In 1976, the Graduate Medical Education National Advisory Committee (GMENAC) was convened to develop workforce strategies to advise the Department of Health, Education, and Welfare (DHEW). The committee developed a needs-based analysis utilizing a modified delphi process to estimate workforce for different subspecialties. It was predicted that, by 1990, there would be a surplus of 70,000 physicians, which surplus would increase to 145,000 in the year

2000 (21). For the neurosurgery workforce, it was estimated that between 2500 and 2800 surgeons would be needed to deliver care in 1990 (22). Although fairly accurate in some of its estimates, GMENAC seriously underestimated the number of international medical graduate (IMG) trainees by approximately 400%. Presently, there are more than 6900 IMGs entering United States medical/surgical residency programs each year—equivalent to the annual output of 44 medical schools having a class size of 125 (23).

Thus, although the size of the physician workforce in general—and that of the neurosurgical workforce specifically—has received a great deal of attention over the past several decades, there has been an inexorable increase in the number of practicing neurosurgeons. Moreover, although the number of noncertified neurosurgeons, as a percentage of the total, has gradually declined, and the number of neurosurgeons certified annually by the American Board of Neurological Surgeons (ABNS) has stabilized at approximately 110, the total number of neurosurgeons delivering clinical care in this country has increased to levels beyond that predicted by GMENAC and warned about by SOS-SUS. A discussion of the current medical environment in this country and the factors influencing appropriate workforce size are reviewed in the next section to give the reader additional insight into the present workforce debate.

TRENDS INFLUENCING THE NEUROSURGICAL WORKFORCE DEBATE

The intensity of the current national debate over the size of the physician workforce is acute. Given the relatively small size of the neurosurgical specialty, it may seem somewhat surprising that this specialty has been a prominent focus of the debate. Its position of prominence is likely attributable to some estimates of workforce need that, in this era of managed care, show neurosurgery at or near the top of the list of overpopulated specialties when classified by specialty. To understand this phenomenon, it may be helpful to examine the current economic and medical trends in the United States that have a bearing on the issue of neurosurgical workforce.

Managed Care

The 1990s have seen managed care emerge as the solution for health-care cost containment in the United States. The decline in the fee-for-service mode of health-care delivery accompanying the rise of health maintenance organizations (HMOs) as the coverage of choice has brought free market and corporate economic incentives to what was once a supplier-dominated cottage industry. Patient choice and physician-to-physician referral have become less significant as cost containment has become the driving force in medical care. As a result, the primary care physician's value has risen, while the specialist has been devalued—viewed as an expense to be avoided by managed care organizations. This trend is especially evident in southern California, where the managed care penetration is approximately 90%. This has resulted in a decline in hospital use, hospital occupancy rates, and specialist's incomes, and a surplus of hospital beds (24). Furthermore, by the year 2000, it is projected that 50% of hospitals and 60% of acute inpatient beds will be closed (25). Thus, although managed care organizations have demonstrated an ability to control costs, this has generally been accomplished by decreasing the use of specialty services. Thus, the prevailing perception is that the number of primary care physicians appears to be adequate but that the number of specialty physicians, such as neurosurgeons, appears to be too high given the need for services.

The initial report by GMENAC (21) suggested a 92% surplus in neurosurgery for the year 1990. However, as early as 1986, Tarlov (26), Chairman of GEMNAC, speculated that the estimated surplus of neurosurgeons needed to be adjusted further upward to take into account the unprecedented growth of HMOs. Concerns over the surplus were heightened when other reports were published, such as that of Wennberg et al. (27), which described the specialty of neurosurgery as having 2.5 times the workforce needed if the entire country were converted to an HMO delivery system (Fig. 7.3). These authors, furthermore, asserted that, even with immediate closure of all residency training programs in neurosurgery, it would take until the year 2018 before the supply of neurosurgeons approached a level that was in balance with the needs for neurosurgical services (Fig. 7.4). Weiner, et al. (5) studied the same issue, assuming that by the year 2000, 40 to 65% of Americans would be receiving care from integrated managed care networks. They forecast that there would be a surplus of 165,000 physicians, mostly in the area of specialty care, where the supply of specialty physicians exceeded need by 61 to 67%. Using this model, the present ratio of 1.4:100,000 neurosurgeon to population substantially exceeded the ratio (.04/100,000) needed by an aggressively managed staff-model HMO.

Although alarming, the results of these reports must be considered in light of the methodological problems inherent in extrapolating data from existing HMOs and applying them to an entire nation's health-care needs. For example, when elderly and indigent patients are added to an HMOs patient base, the intensity of care increases, and, hence, so does the number of specialists needed for the delivery of care. A recent study of physician staffing ratios in a staff-model HMO reevaluated the ratio of physicians used in the HMO setting (28). Earlier computational analyses of HMO physician staffing density had excluded medical care provided by non-HMO physicians, whose services were arranged on a contractual basis. When the services provided by these physicians were included in the computation for two HMOs in the Puget Sound area, the specialist to population ratios were significantly raised. For example, the newly computed neurosurgeon-to-population ratio, which reflected the newly computed HMO use of neurosurgical services, was 1 FTE neurosurgeon: 100,000 population, as compared to the initial computation of 0.4:100,000. Clearly, the more recent computation more closely approximates the present United States rate of 1.4:100,000. These findings suggest that previous projections of the magnitude of physician oversupply could be based on flawed methodology; thus, care should be exercised in implementing any signifi-

Current FTE/ 450,000 Population	Under Capitation FTE/ 450,000 Population	Current Number of Practicing Physicians	Number Required in a Capitated System	Number in Surplus	Percent Surplus
8.1	3	4,501	1,658	2,843	63.2%

Figure 7.3. The neurosurgical workforce in the era of capitation showing the current number of physicians per 450,000 population, the number needed under capitation, the current number of practicing neurosurgeons, and those required in a capitated system. (Adapted from Kronick R, Goodman DC, Wennberg J, Wagner E. The marketplace in healthcare reform: The demographic limitations of managed competition. N Engl J Med 1993;328:148–152.)

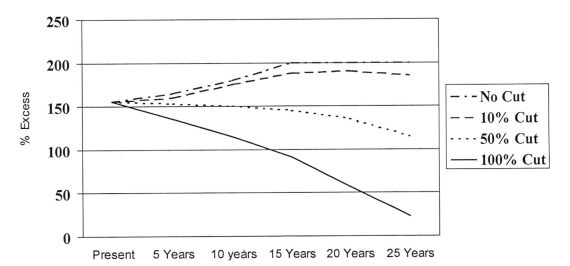

Figure 7.4. The percentage of neurosurgical workforce in excess of the size required in the classic HMO setting based on the percentage of reduction in the number of residents trained per year. (Adapted from Wennberg JE, Goodman DC, Nease RF, Keller RD. Finding equilibrium in U.S. physician supply. Health Aff 1993;12:90–103.)

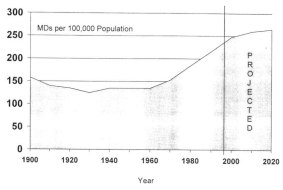

Figure 7.5. Physician workforce of active physicians per 100,000 population demonstrating the growth in physician workforce since 1900 and projected into the future. (Adapted from Academic medicine: Institutions, programs and issues. 7th ed. Washington DC: Association American Medical Colleges, 1997.)

cant corrective actions designed to reduce the supply of specialists.

Growth of the Physician Workforce

The perceived excess of physicians in the current managed care setting would have been far less likely to have arisen if the number of physicians being trained had remained at the level produced in the early 1960s (Fig. 7.5). However, in the mid-1960s, believing that there was a shortage of 50,000 physicians in the United States, Congress relaxed immigration laws for physicians in training and allocated increased funding for a number of medical schools, as well as increase in class sizes. At that time, the physician to population ratio was 156:100,000. By 1980, this ratio had increased to 196:100,000; in 1990 to 237/100,000; and by the year 2000, it is predicted that the ratio of active physicians to population will increase to 261:100,000 (29).

Although the growth in physician-to-population ratio signifies a possible surplus in the workforce, there is also evidence of maldistribution of that workforce. For example, the East Coast population center, which extends from Boston to Washington, D.C., comprises 21% of the nation's population, but has 28% of the physicians, reflecting an average physician-to-population ratio of 270:100,000. At the other extreme is the state of Mississippi, which has a physician-to-population ratio of 118:100,000 (30).

Growth in the Number of Neurosurgical Residency Positions and Practicing Neurosurgeons

The number of neurosurgeons has steadily increased over the past several decades owing to several factors. What's more, not only has the number of neurosurgeons trained exceeded the attrition rate, but the overall number of neurosurgeons being trained has increased. In 1952, there were 94 approved institutions for neurosurgical training, with a total of 241 trainees total in all years of training (31). By 1977, there were 91 approved neurosurgical residency training programs, a total number of 480 residents, and a net output of 100 residents per year. Today, there are approximately the same number of training programs (97), but the number of residents completing their training each year has risen to approximately 140, with 650 residents at other levels of training (32). From 1983 to 1995, the number of residency training programs grew from 94 to 97. Although this represents only a 3% increase in the number of programs, during the same time, the total number of graduating residents increased 44% from 98 to 141 each year, and the total number of residents grew by 23% from 664 to 817 for all years (ML Sanderson, personal communication, 1997).

Despite this growth in the number and size of training programs over the past 40 years, the ABNS has continued to certify an average of only 111 new neurosurgeons annually (1975–1995) (Fig. 7.6). Over the past 4 years, the total number of Board-certified neurosur-

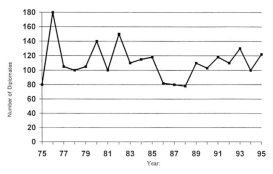

Figure 7.6. Number of Diplomats certified by the American Board of Neurological Surgery from 1975 to the present (Adapted from American Board of Neurological Surgery, 121st Office Meeting Agenda Book, 1996).

geons who are in active practice in this country appears to have stabilized at about 3200.

In the past, data on the output of Canadian training programs in neurological surgery were included in estimates of the U.S. workforce, because the number of neurosurgeons immigrating to the United States was substantial. However, recent limitations on cross-certification between the ABNS and the Royal College of Surgeons (Canada) are expected to reduce and, ultimately, to eliminate this trend.

Density of Neurosurgeons in Other Countries

Using the neurosurgeon-to-population ratio in other countries as an indicator of the need for neurosurgical services in the United States (as is suggested by some in the public sector) is a comparison fraught with serious difficulties. Currently, there is 1 neurosurgeon per 66,000 population nationwide. In other industrialized nations, such as Great Britain and Austria, the ratio of neurosurgeons to population is 1:500,000 (33) and 1:132,000 (W Koos, personal communication, 1995), respectively. In India, the ratio is 1:2,000,000 (PN Tandon, personal communication, 1995), and some countries have one or no neurosurgeons.

Any comparison of neurosurgical workforce size in the United States with that in other countries must take into account the differing focus of neurosurgery in different countries. For example, British neurosurgical practice focuses predominantly on intracranial procedures, whereas spinal and head injuries, which represent a large portion of any U.S. neurosurgeon's practice, are managed by other specialties. Thus, although studying the international neurosurgeon-to-population ratio is interesting and may hold clues to the future of American neurosurgery, any extrapolation about need or supply in the United States based on international practice should be done with considerable caution (34).

International Medical Graduates

The training of international medical graduates (IMGs) is frequently cited as a cause of physician surplus. Indeed, the growth in the total number of IMGs has been dramatic. Presently, IMGs constitute 20% of all the residents in the United States. By contrast, during the past decade in neurosurgery, the number of IMGs concluding a successful match has changed very lit-

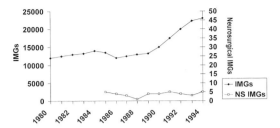

Figure 7.7. Total number of international medical school graduates in residency training programs since 1980, including growth and overall numbers and comparison with the number of IMGs in neurosurgical residency training programs since 1986 (Adapted from Pevehouse BC, Colenbrander A. Education Issues of the Journal of the American Medical Association and from the United States neurological surgery residency matching program. Neurosurgery 1994; 35:1172–1182.)

tle, averaging approximately 4 annually (Fig. 7.7). Considering the small number of IMGs in neurosurgical training programs, their impact on workforce strategy is likely to be minimal.

However, there are philosophical issues concerning IMGs that should be addressed by the neurosurgical community. Such issues have been debated more vociferously in other areas of medicine, where the percentage of IMGs in the workforce and in residency training is higher. Those who advocate allowing IMGs to train in the United States assert that competition for training slots should be based on merit, regardless of the applicant's country of origin. In addition, these supporters point out that, in the past, when there has been a need to increase the number of trainees in American residency training programs, IMGs have been the ones who have filled the vacancies, often taking assignments in inner-city facilities.

One of the opposing arguments cites the concern about "brain drain." If the brightest and best medical students come to the United States for training and ultimately stay in America, then their countries of origin, many of which have a greater need for highly qualified medical practitioners than does the United States, never benefit from their expertise. A second point of opposition lies in the fact that American taxpayers subsidize residency training slots. "Why," the opposition asks, "should this subsidization allow preferential training of a foreign national, even if that trainee ultimately becomes a citizen of this country?''

Late in 1996, President Clinton signed new immigration legislation into law, a portion of which affects IMGs who are in the United States on a J-1 exchange visitor visa. Previously, the J-1 visa required the holder to return to his or her country of origin for at least 2 years prior to immigrating to the United States. In the past, a waiver for the residency requirement could be granted if the physician agreed to practice in an area that was medically underserved. The newly enacted law makes it more difficult for IMGs to obtain their green card and is more consistent with the original intent of allowing foreign physicians to train in the United States and then return to their country of origin. However, despite the labyrinthine nature of this new process, it is anticipated that IMGs will continue to constitute a percentage of the residents in training, even in a small specialty like neurosurgery.

Scope of Neurosurgical Practice

The scope of neurosurgical practice is defined by the breadth of training provided, the development of new treatments and technologies, the degree to which neurosurgeons are successful in competing for patients whose care could be managed by physicians from other specialties, and even the definition the specialty has established for itself.

The AANS bylaws define neurosurgery as:

> . . . a medical discipline that provides the operative and nonoperative management (i.e., prevention, diagnosis, evaluation, treatment, critical care, and rehabilitation) of disorders that affect the central, peripheral, and autonomic nervous systems, including their supportive structures and vascular supply, and the operative and nonoperative management of pain. As such, neurological surgery encompasses disorders of the brain, meninges, skull, and their blood supply, including the extracranial carotid and vertebral arteries; disorders of the pituitary gland; spinal cord, meninges, and spine, including those that may require treatment by spinal fusion or instrumentation; disorders of the cranial and spinal nerves throughout their distributions; and disorders of the autonomic nervous system (35).

Although the definition of neurosurgery as a specialty appears to differ slightly depending on the organization of origin (AANS versus ABNS versus ACGME, the Accreditation Council on Graduate Medical Education), all of the definitions delineate firm and exclusionary boundaries that define the domain of neurosurgery. However, an examination of the definitions of such specialties as orthopedic surgery, vascular surgery, and otorhinolaryngology reveals some areas of overlap with neurosurgery, underscoring the complexity of delineating scope of practice. Indeed, each of these specialties has claimed some area of neurosurgery—spinal surgery, carotid artery surgery, and skull base surgery, respectively—as lying within their purview of care.

Beyond the definitions that neurosurgeons and others use to define their specialties, the scope of neurosurgical practice is also influenced by neurosurgery's ability to compete with other specialties. In this regard, carotid endarterectomy, spinal surgery, and peripheral nerve surgery represent either areas of opportunity or lost market share for the specialty of neurosurgery. Presently, neurosurgeons do less than 10% of all carotid endartertectomies. Furthermore, according to the Comprehensive Neurosurgical Practice Survey (CNPS) (36) of 1995, 67% of the neurosurgeons who responded believe that there is more competition today between neurosurgeons and orthopedic surgeons than there was 5 years ago (CNPS 1995). The same insights concerning competition surely have occurred to those in specialties that compete directly with neurosurgery, and all involved undoubtedly view successful competition as both critical to their specialty and a means for ameliorating workforce concerns.

The scope of neurosurgical practice can be further defined by examining the breadth of training that residents receive during their neurosurgical programs. This scope is not static. Continual developments in the management of neurosurgical disorders mandate that residency training programs be consistently updated and revised so that they incorporate new science, technology, and techniques. Program directors are responsible for overseeing the orderly incorporation of these changes into the training programs to ensure that residents are thoroughly prepared to offer a full range of neurosurgical care and treatment when they enter the job market.

Finally, just as certain new developments in medicine and technology (e.g., endovascular therapy) threaten to reduce the need for neurosurgical procedures, the development of new interventions that are effective in treating neurologic disorders will ensure the future of our specialty. A case in point is coronary artery bypass surgery. The increased use of coronary bypass procedures to treat occlusive coronary artery disease increased dramatically the number of procedures performed by cardiac surgeons. As a result, the cardiothoracic surgery workforce, which previously appeared to be sufficient to manage the relatively small number of patients with congenital heart disease and those needing other types of open heart procedures, proved inadequate to meet the new needs. Although perhaps not as dramatic, similar examples abound in neurosurgery. For example, the development of skull-base surgery and stereotactic radiosurgery are but two examples of new technology or procedures that have broadened the horizons of the specialty of neurosurgery.

Results of Recent Economic Surveys of the Neurosurgical Community

Several recent economic surveys have been conducted by various neurosurgical organizations in an attempt to elucidate some of the issues that have a bearing on the neurosurgical workforce. The first, sponsored by the AANS/CNS, is the 1995 CNPS (36). This survey continues the inquiry begun by the practice surveys of 1987 and 1992. Some pertinent information relating to the topic of neurosurgical workforce has been extracted.

Of the 1008 respondents, only 8.6% cited an oversupply of neurosurgeons to be one of the major challenges facing the neurosurgical specialty in the next 2 to 3 years. Of more pressing concern were the development of managed care and the increasing competition with orthopedic surgeons, selected as the major challenges by 21% and 10.3% of the respondents, respectively. Approximately half of the respondents (49.7%) thought that the number of neurosurgeons currently in practice was the right number to meet patients' needs. However, 45% of the respondents believed that there were too many neurosurgeons in practice; only 5% thought that there were not enough. Of the respondents in prepaid health plan/HMOs, 61% believed that there were too many neurosurgeons, as compared with 43% of those in private neurosurgical practice and 54% of those in medical school or university practice. A majority (59%) of physicians practicing in the Pacific census region believed that there were too many neurosurgeons in their region; by comparison, only 37% of those practic-

ing in New England shared that perception. Only 29% of the neurosurgeons located in cities with populations of 50,000 to 99,000 were of the opinion that there were too many neurosurgeons. At the other end of the spectrum were those neurosurgeons practicing in cities with populations exceeding 2,000,000, 64% of whom thought there were too many neurosurgeons. Between the time that the 1992 and 1995 surveys were administered, the percentage of neurosurgeons who believed that too many neurosurgeons were being trained increased from 34 to 45%. Forty-nine percent of the respondents indicated that they were in favor of the federal government setting limits on the number of surgical residency positions, and 47% favored reducing the number of neurosurgery resident positions.

Other factors influencing workforce size were also explored, including stability of professional revenues, age at retirement, practice productivity, and the influence of managed care on practice. Some interesting results of the CNPS regarding these topics, not all of which signify excessive workforce in all areas of the country, are presented in the following section.

Of greatest interest was the finding that the gross professional revenues from patient care services had increased between 1992 and 1995 for all respondents, except those from the New England, West North Central, and Pacific census regions. In these areas, there had been a small decline in gross professional revenues.

The average age at retirement was found to have decreased over the period covered by the three surveys, decreasing from 63.0 years in 1987 to 62.4 years in 1992 to 61.9 years to in 1995. A significant change in the 1995 survey was a doubling of the percentage of individuals that retired between 56 and 60 years of age, increasing from 14.3% to 27% of those retiring in 1992 and 1995 respectively.

Sixty-six percent of the respondents performed between 3 and 6 operations per week. The mean number of operations performed was 5. Thirty-five percent of the respondents indicated that they would like to perform an additional 1 to 2 operations per week. However, 53% of the respondents did not wish to increase their office caseload during the course of the work week.

The pervasiveness of managed care in neurosurgical practice was indicated by 83% of respondents who reported accepting an increased number of managed care contracts during the 3 years prior to the survey. A particularly significant development was the increase in the mean size of multispecialty groups from 34 physicians in 1992 to 149 in 1995. This percentage signifies the ongoing appeal of multispecialty group practices to neurosurgeons attempting to cope with the changes in the health-care environment.

Several surveys concerning workforce issues have been conducted as a result of the efforts of the Joint Council of State Neurosurgical Societies (JCSNS). The first was a survey conducted among residency training program directors, which sought to determine the effect of the present environment on the perception of residency training program directors relative to workforce (38). More than 55% of the responding training directors indicated that too many neurosurgeons were currently being trained. Factors contributing to this perception included concerns about managed care, present job availability, and changes in workload and/or income. In addition, 53% of the training directors believed that there were too many neurosurgeons currently practicing within their geographic area. Despite these concerns, some training directors indicated a desire to increase the number of residency positions within their program positions; in the instance of medical schools approved by the LCME (Liaison Committee on Medical Education) without neurosurgical residency training programs, several heads of neurosurgery indicated a desire to develop a new residency training program. Thus, although residency program size is only one aspect of workforce dynamics, it is an important factor as the residency training pool continues to fuel the growth in the neurosurgical workforce.

The second survey developed by the JCSNS (37) sought to determine, among other things, the current status of the neurosurgical workforce and the effect of managed care on the clinical practice of neurosurgery. This study asked a number of questions similar to those included in the CNPS of 1995. The results indicated that managed care had penetrated all areas of the country to a significant extent, including communities with populations of less than 500,000. Furthermore, managed care systems appeared to have increased office workload by 10 to 30%, and to have decreased surgical workloads by 10 to 20%. In addition, the survey revealed that managed care was thought to have decreased neurosurgical incomes significantly—by as much as 50% in some areas of California.

The Role of Allied Health Professionals

The increased role of allied health professionals in managing patient care traditionally provided by physicians appears to be attributable partly to economic factors and partly to the willingness of physicians and patients to allow care to be rendered by allied health professionals. This competition for patient care services that has arisen between physicians and allied health professionals seems unlikely to diminish in the future. Although this trend is particularly prevalent in primary care medicine, it may also influence the size of the neurosurgical workforce. The use of allied health professionals can increase the efficiency of a neurosurgeon in addition to decreasing costs, but their use in the outpatient setting or in a managed care environment could, in theory, also decrease the need for trained neurosurgeons.

The Government's Role in Workforce Policy

The federal and state governments have had a long-term interest in the size of the physician workforce. In the 1960s, a perceived shortage of physicians led to governmental programs that resulted in the enlargement of existing medical schools and an increase in the overall number of medical schools. The resultant expansion in the physician workforce has led to the current concern about an oversupply of physicians, particularly among those engaged in specialty practice. Nevertheless, the government seems poised to take steps to modulate workforce size. One might ask whether the results of any such governmental intervention to reduce the size of the workforce will result in another overcorrection in the future, perhaps radically depleting the supply of physicians and resulting in a concomitant decline in the quality of graduates. One also may be prompted to ask why, of all the existing professions, the government feels it has the right to influence the size of the physician workforce, rather than letting market dynamics dictate trends.

Although the economics of the marketplace appear to work in many professions and many industries, market forces do not seem to work as well in health care. In the fee-for-service environment that dominated medicine in the past, an increasing supply of physicians, each working to maximize income, resulted in an increased utilization of the health-care system. This dynamic runs contrary to the usual forces of supply and demand, whereby increased competition, because of oversupply of labor, results in a decrease in the cost of services. Furthermore, because of enormous sums of money being spent on health care in the United States and the perception that the health of the citizens in this country is of prime importance, there seems to be a societal perception of a governmental responsibility to ensure smooth functioning of the health-care system.

These philosophical perceptions, among others, fueled President Clinton's proposed 1994 Health Security Act, which set forth a series of regulations limiting the number of trained physicians in the United States. Although this legislation was unsuccessful, other economic incentives are being used by the federal government to encourage physicians to enter primary care medicine. An example of these is Medicare's resource-based relative value scale (RBRVS), which was designed, in part, to shift payment from procedure-based specialties to evaluation-based office practices. Although these inducements plus market forces, appear to be having the desired effect of shifting new physicians from specialties to primary care, other governmental initiatives designed to influence the workforce, such as declining reimbursements for graduate medical education, will likely follow.

National Policy Groups

Concern about the physician workforce has led to recommendations by several national policy groups, including the Institute of Medicine (IOM), the Council on Graduate Medical Education (COGME), the PEW Commission, and, most recently, a consensus statement from six United States medical associations. The statements appear to arise from differing motivations, including legislated responsibilities, self-interest, and concern for public welfare.

Created in 1970 by the National Academy of Science to examine health policy matters, the IOM recently presented the recommendations of their committee, established to examine physician workforce issues (39). Major recommendations included the following: (*a*) no new medical school should be opened, and existing class size should not increase; (*b*) the number of first-year

residency positions should reflect the number of U.S. medical school graduates; (*c*) a mechanism for replacement funding of IMG-dependent hospitals should be devised; and (*d*) the Department of Health and Human Services should collect information and fund investigations concerning physician workforce, including career opportunities, and make this information available to all interested parties.

The COGME was created by Congress in 1988 because of concerns about workforce size and the cost of graduate medical education. In their first report, COGME concluded that no steps should be taken by the government to decrease the size of the physician workforce, as projections of workforce needs were based on numerous uncertainties that limited the validity of the projections (40). More recently, COGME has indicated support for reducing the available number of residency positions from the current 144% of U.S. medical school graduates to 110% (a decrease from 24,170 to 18,490 residency positions). This would be accomplished gradually, rather than abruptly, in order to minimize the impact on hospitals for which the effect would be significant, such as those located in inner cities and rural areas.

The PEW Commission set forth recommendations relating to the health-care profession in the 21st century (25). These recommendations targeted not only medicine, but also nursing and other allied health fields. The PEW Commission's recommendations for the physician workforce included the following: (*a*) create a payment pool funded by health insurance premiums for support of health-care professionals' education; (*b*) reduce the number of first-year residency training positions to 110% of the present number of U.S. medical school graduates; (*c*)achieve the goal of 50% of residents in primary care and 50% in specialty care by the year 2004; and (*d*) reduce the size of medical school classes by 20% over a period of 10 years by closing medical schools, not by reducing class size.

A recent consensus statement (41) on physician workforce, developed by six of the nation's medical associations, including the American Association of Colleges of Osteopathic Medicine, the American Medical Association, the American Osteopathic Association, the Association of Academic Health Centers, the Association of American Medical Colleges, and the National Medical Association advocated some of the same steps. They issued the following recommendations: (*a*) the number of first-year resident positions in the Graduate Medical Education system should be more closely aligned with the number of graduates of accredited United States medical schools, and this alignment should be achieved by eliminating federal funding of GME positions; (*b*) the United States should continue to provide Graduate Medical Education opportunities to foreign-born physicians under the J-1 exchange visitor program, recognizing the importance of these physicians returning to their country after completing their GME; (*c*)a National All Payers Fund should be established to provide a stable source of funding for the direct costs of GME; (*d*) transitional funds should be made available to aid teaching hospitals that lose resident physicians; (*e*) a National Physician Workforce Advisory body should be established to monitor and periodically reassess the physician workforce.

Thus, most of the reports by national policy groups seem to focus on reducing the number of resident positions available, while maintaining funds for graduate medical education programs and monitoring physician workforce. Transition funding that eases the impact on IMG-dependent hospitals recognizes the plight of the inner city and underserved populations and makes this approach more palatable to those states that rely heavily on IMG trainee services. Although these recommendations by highly visible and respected groups serve to draw attention to this topic and may influence future governmental policy, changes occurring in the workforce seem to be most easily influenced by more local initiatives. Even if the recommendations of the national policy group were formalized by legislation, none would appear to have a direct bearing on the specialty of neurosurgery at this time.

Local Initiatives

Other health-care initiatives are occurring at the state level. For example, a demonstration project, recently announced by the Health Care Financing Administration (HCFA), would pay New York hospitals $400,000,000 over a period of 6 years not to train physicians. This plan, conceived as a solution to physician excess, would allow time for teaching hospitals to redesign their graduate medical education programs. Forty-one hospitals volunteered to reduce their residency training positions by between 20 and 25% over 6 years, thereby reducing by 2000 the number of positions offered (42).

Traditionally, it has been a lucrative undertaking for hospitals to train residents, especially in light of Medicare reimbursement for direct medical education (Part A) and the indirect medical education funding intended to offset the higher inpatient operating costs resulting from a patient mix that includes indigent and more severely ill patients (Part B). This demonstration project funding will not only serve to reduce the number of residents in training, but will also help provide transition funding for the substitution of allied health-care professionals for residents and/or the maximization of efficiency in caring for patients in these hospitals. It is expected that teaching hospitals can more easily be weaned from GME funding if the plan includes a transition period. This approach addresses some of the problems inherent in inner city hospitals where residents provide low-cost care for an underserved population. This program is especially important for New York State, which contains approximately 15% of the resident population of the country, but such tactics might not be successful in other regions of the country.

Programs such as these recognize the regional influences in health care and allow residency training institutions to make decisions concerning right-sizing by providing a vehicle for funding during a period of transition. Whether such programs will affect neurosurgical residency programs and, hence, the size of the neurosurgical workforce, is being studied. In programs with one resident per year, a reduction might render residency training unfeasible. Larger neurosurgical training programs whose size is, in part, determined by greater patient volume, may be more affected by such programs since a greater emphasis on education, rather than delivery of service, might allow these training programs to constrict in size.

Initiatives of Neurosurgical Organizations

Many practitioners in neurosurgery believe that the various neurosurgical organizations have been unresponsive to their concerns about the number of neurosurgeons in practice. Some have urged the ABNS or the Residency Review Committee (RRC) or the AANS or the Congress of Neurological Surgeons (CNS) or the JCSNS to ''do something about the number of neurosurgeons being trained.'' While the goals of these neurosurgical groups are to enhance neurosurgical practice by various techniques, such as ensuring residency training quality, improving neurosurgical marketplace position, and implementing other strategies that affect the workforce issue, regulations imposed by the Federal Trade Commission (FTC) and the Department of Justice (DOJ) prohibit these groups from taking any action that would directly regulate the size of the workforce. Such activity would be considered restraint of trade under the Sherman Anti-Trust Act (43).

How, then, can ''organized'' neurosurgery affect the workforce in a positive way? The current policies of the ABNS and RRC are directed towards enhancing and preserving the quality of residency training programs, a fundamental underpinning of neurosurgical residency training since its inception. Indeed, their continuing efforts to develop and maintain policies that improve educational quality, perhaps more than any other strategy, have advanced and improved the environment of the neurosurgical workforce. By working to ensure that the graduates of neurosurgical training programs have the best education available and access to training that develops clinically competent, independent practitioners with good common sense, the organizations have helped to give neurosurgery a competitive advantage in the market.

One component of ensuring quality is to prevent quality from decreasing as the number of years in practice increases. From this point of view, the AANS and CNS provide a service for all of neurosurgery by their ongoing commitment to education and professional development. Neurosurgical residents learn early that they must make a commitment to a lifetime of learning, not only the facts of neurosurgery, but also the techniques. By building on this early indoctrination in the importance of continued learning, the AANS and CNS provide a means by which this commitment can be honored.

In addition, the AANS and CNS work jointly to ensure that the small group of neurosurgeons practicing in this country has a voice and maintains a presence at the federal level. The Washington Committee, previously chaired by Russell Travis and currently chaired by Arthur Day, together with Katie Orrico, Director of the Washington Office, has been effective in advancing the aims of neurosurgery at the fed-

eral level and in keeping the neurosurgical community apprised of trends in the government concerning workforce and other issues affecting the specialty.

Similar initiatives are being carried out at both state and local levels. The Key Person program of the AANS and CNS recognizes the importance of developing useful personal relationships with political representatives at all levels. Such programs have also led to an improved understanding among neurosurgeons of the important issues affecting the specialty, as well as appropriate strategies for addressing them.

POSSIBLE STRATEGIES AND SOLUTIONS

The previous sections in this chapter have discussed the details of workforce analysis, the history of such efforts, and the factors currently influencing the neurosurgical workforce. Given the complexity of workforce issues, it is unlikely that any one solution can be found that would resolve the problems identified thus far. However, the following section explores some possible strategies and identifies the use that may be beneficial to the specialty.

Strategy 1: Ignore the Problem, Do Nothing, or Let the Marketplace Provide a Solution

Given the imprecision of workforce analysis and recalibration, some would argue with policy-driven workforce change, but watchful waiting or complacency is not a good strategy for the field of neurosurgery either. Unregulated market forces tend to create an oversupply, followed by a period of undersupply. Both extremes result in problems: an undersupply of physicians causes poor access to health care, whereas an oversupply results in an increase in health-care costs and dissatisfaction among physicians.

There are compelling reasons to conclude that there are too many neurosurgeons. First, managed care organizations can, in many instances, access all of the neurosurgical services they need without contracting with all the neurosurgeons in the region. Second, in many areas, market conditions suggest a glut of neurosurgeons, as evidenced by declining reimbursement for neurosurgical procedures. Unlike the previously unrestrained growth of health-care costs in the fee-for-service environment, this stepwise decline in payment for neurological services follows the economic law of supply and demand. In the past, many neurosurgeons compensated for reduced reimbursement by increasing practice volume. This strategy, however, is unsuccessful in a capitated reimbursement system.

New graduates of residency training programs have reported fewer opportunities in the job market. This decline in employment opportunities has affected different specialties differently—e.g., urology, in which every graduate found employment and pathology, in which 10.8% of graduates were unsuccessful in securing employment. Anesthesiology recently estimated a 6.6% unemployment rate (44), but a later survey of graduates and training directors indicated that this figure was too high (45). These conflicting data underscore the need for development of a data base to study workforce longitudinally for each specialty.

Strategy 2: Develop Workforce Policy Based on Analysis

Using a longitudinal study of surgical residents (46), specialties such as pediatric surgery have carefully followed the number of trainees for a 20-year period. This has validated not only the number, but the geographic location, of all active pediatric surgeons in the United States (47). Although the workforce of pediatric surgery is smaller than that of neurosurgery, it seems that this type of data collection and ongoing analysis could be beneficial to the specialty of neurosurgery, especially when discussions of the size of the neurosurgical workforce arise with national policy groups. This course seems preferable to allowing the vagaries of the marketplace to dictate how many neurosurgeons should be trained. Some information is presently available from the ABNS, the AANS, the ACS, the AMA, and the Neurological Surgery Residency Matching Program, but there are inconsistencies from data set to data set, and none of these databases is considered to be comprehensive.

Some specialties, such as gastroenterology, have formalized the data collection process by setting up a manpower study committee comprised of representatives from various gastroenterology societies (48). This group has recommended that gastroenterology training numbers be reduced by 50% over the next 5 years, and, in many instances, reduction has already been done voluntarily. Whether such an approach would work in neurosurgery is uncertain, but the concept requires further consideration. Perhaps and initial focus on supply, rather than need, would be easiest to accomplish, both theoretically and practically. Such an analysis would not only determine the actual numbers of neurosurgeons, but also the distribution of these specialists throughout the country. As mentioned earlier, any action taken in response to these data would have to be voluntary, as active downsizing would come under the scrutiny of federal enforcement agencies for restraint of trade. Increasing residency training programs by another year would be only a temporary solution, and would be difficult in neurosurgery, because of the current length of the residency training program and the lack of funding for or advantage of an additional year of neurosurgical training.

Strategy 3: Support the Efforts of "Organized" Neurosurgery

Residency training directors know only too well the conflicts created by trying to balance the perception that there are too many neurosurgeons with the desire to maintain high-quality residency training programs. Some training directors believe that, at least in their region, there is a need for more neurosurgeons, and that their training program should remain unchanged. Others believe that they are training their competition. As individual training program directors, they have the ability to downsize, if appropriate in their individual programs, without fear of retribution from the Federal Trade Commission.

All neurosurgeons should strive to participate in the AANS and CNS. These organizations have developed strategies for improving the quality and efficiency of neurosurgical care in this country. These initiatives range from programs that seek to influence governmental policy, to continuing education, professional development, and quality initiatives. Recently, a political action committee unrelated to these societies was created to enhance neurosurgery's voice in the political arena. These efforts are all laudable, but their success will be directly related to the support they receive from the neurosurgical community.

Strategy 4: Educate Medical Students and Residents About Workforce Trends

Individuals who pursue a career in neurosurgery generally do so because they are attracted to the content and challenges of the specialty. Program directors and others in neurosurgery must be frank with students about the present economic climate and the potential oversupply of neurosurgeons, so that those entering the field will make informed decisions and will be less inclined to feel disillusioned when confronting the challenges of a potentially overcrowded specialty.

Although many medical students continue to believe that any investment of time and energy will result in a satisfying professional career, there is evidence that they select a specialty area to meet their personal future goals. In the past, it was widely assumed that medical students who completed an accredited residency program were assured future employment. Recent evidence would suggest that there is cause for diminished optimism. One needs only to consider the increase (to 73%) since 1990 in the number of students matching in primary care residency training programs or the decrease (of 72 and 33%, respectively) in the number of applicants for anesthesiology and radiology training programs, to recognize that students are responding to availability of employment opportunities (49). In some specialties, even if a graduate is able to find a position, the financial package is often not as lucrative as anticipated (50).

Because income potential appears to have considerable influence on the fields chosen by medical students (51, 52), how will neurosurgery as a specialty fare in the future if there are excessive numbers of practitioners in the field? At the present time, no decrement in the number of students applying for neurosurgical residency training programs has been observed, despite the concern about incomes and job availability. Thus far, students entering this specialty seem to be motivated more by their interest in the field than by the economics of the discipline.

Furthermore, despite the concerns noted elsewhere, there continue to be opportunities for talented practitioners in all branches of medicine. Hence, neurosurgery likely will remain an attractive specialty for medical students.

It is important that the "brightest and best" continue to be attracted to neurosurgery and that training programs continue to provide a quality education in order to maintain the quality for which neurosurgery is known. Medical students should be introduced to the neurosciences and should be assigned specialty rotations in neuro-

surgery. The standards of education should be raised, and the RRC should continue their focus on quality resident education.

The educational experience should be elevated. There should to be an uncoupling of the education component of residency training from the clinical service needs of the teaching institution. This separation may require that some patient care be provided by health-care professionals other than residents (e.g., by attending neurosurgeons or allied health professionals). Moreover, this must all be accomplished in a setting of diminished federal funding for graduate medical education. Thus, we will need to identify alternative strategies for funding resident education.

Strategy 5: Develop a Viable Approach to IMG Education

In the author's estimation, United States neurosurgical training has attained a level that is unequaled in the world. This preeminence stems from the neurosurgical tradition, the educational efforts of residency training programs, and the diligence and oversight of the ABNS and the Neurosurgical RRC. An area of opportunity for IMGs may exist in residency training provided by U.S. neurosurgical residency training programs. It is possible that federal legislation could be enacted that would allow U.S. programs to continue to train foreign nationals, with the aim of improving the quality of neurosurgery in their home country. This would allow United States programs to export education to areas of the world that have a dirth of qualified neurosurgeons, thereby reversing the "brain drain" associated with the immigration of these individuals. When one considers that the United States has approximately 20% of the world's neurosurgeons and less than 10% of the world's population, it becomes clear that there is ample educational capacity for training outstanding individuals from other countries who would then return to their own countries to offer the quality of neurosurgery that U.S. patients have come to expect. This would reduce the number of trained neurosurgeons in the United States, yet would maintain residency training programs, particularly in those inner city institutions that rely on them for the staffing.

A similar proposal was made more than 20 years ago, when it was suggested that foreign medical graduates could be trained in a foreign fellowship in neurosurgery; this would ensure that sufficient training was received to provide adequate care in the trainee's country of origin, but the duration of training would be insufficient for ABNS certification (53). This coupled with more stringent immigration requirements, might close the loophole that has long allowed IMG trainees to remain in this country.

Strategy 6: Increase Neurosurgery's Competitiveness

It is in the interest of neurosurgery to create new markets by strengthening the research initiative in the neurosciences. This will result in new treatments for known diseases and the identification of new diseases that can be managed by neurosurgical intervention. Other means of enhancing neurosurgery's competitiveness include professional development and training in the use of new technology, as well as documentation of quality care. Outcome analyses are excellent tools by which consumers (patients) can evaluate the difference in quality between one provider (physician) and another. It is important for neurosurgery to conduct outcome studies so as to document the quality of care provided. In so doing, our specialty will be able to maintain a competitive edge in attracting patients whose care could be managed by other specialties. Indeed, the Joint Committee for Assessment of Quality of the AANS and CNS has assigned this initiative top priority. Given the results of outcome studies, it is reasonable to assume that patients would wish their care to be rendered by physicians providing better outcomes. If neurosurgeons could document their worth in terms of quality and outcome of care, the problem of excess workforce in neurosurgery could rapidly diminish.

By applying these strategies, neurosurgeons can remain competitive in areas in which there is overlap with other specialties. Although neurosurgeons have been labeled, by themselves and others as ''brain'' surgeons, they also treat other systems and other disorders. Indeed, if the distribution of the type of patients treated by neurosurgeons is examined, they would more accurately be labeled ''spine'' surgeons rather than ''brain'' surgeons.

Consideration should also be given to training different types of neurosurgeons to fill different niches in our specialty, thereby becoming more competitive with other specialties. This differential training might be accomplished by offering 3 years of core neurosurgical training followed by 2 additional years of specialization, such as in spine or head injury, or, for a few, advanced training in cerebrovascular surgery, brain tumors, epilepsy, and the like. In this regard, it makes sense for neurosurgeons to participate on disease-based teams, (e.g., a stroke team or an integrated spine team). In general, the neurosurgeon's training and leadership skills will ensure that neurosurgeons remain central to patient care in these areas. In such an environment, neurosurgeons should not willingly give up responsibility for treating disorders, such as head injuries, despite the often onerous responsibilities associated with the care of these patients (e.g., coverage, night call, reimbursement, and liability).

SUMMARY

The dynamics of the neurosurgical workforce affect virtually all aspects of neurosurgery, including economics, clinical practice, education, and research. In the past, unrestrained growth in the number of neurosurgical practitioners has not resulted in a significant adverse impact on the specialty. However, the current perception is that there are too many specialty physicians, including neurosurgeons, to meet the medical needs of our country, and that steps should be taken to right-size the workforce. Right-sizing can occur either passively—if allowed to be driven by market forces—or actively, by the development of policy based on analysis. As a small specialty, neurosurgery must be active in this analysis or risk having those outside the specialty determine workforce policy for neurosurgery. What the future holds in this regard is uncertain. However, because a strong (healthy) workforce is fundamental to the evolution and survival of neurosurgery, actively developing a strategy for guiding work force decisions, rather than passively allowing a nonneurosurgical policymaker or the marketplace to hold sway, appears to be a rational approach.

Acknowledgments

The author gratefully acknowledges the support of the H. Schaffer Foundation, the expert secretarial assistance of Jo Anne Olender, and the editorial assistance of Elizabeth Cole, Adele O'Connell, and Ann-Lorraine Edwards.

REFERENCES

1. Cooper RA. Seeking a balanced physician workforce for the 21st century. JAMA 1994;272(9):680–686.
2. Kletke PR, Marder WD, Silberger AB. The growing proportion of female physicians: Implications for U.S. physician supply. Am J Pub Health 1990;80: 300–304.
3. Schroeder SA. The health manpower challenge to internal medicine. Ann Intern Med 1987;106:768–770.
4. Schwartz WB, Sloan FA, Mendelson DN. Why there will be little or no physician surplus between now and the year 2000. N Engl J Med 1988;318:892–897.
5. Weiner J. Forecasting the effects of health reform on U.S. physician workforce requirement. JAMA 1994; 272:222–230.
6. Mayfield FH. Should the number and quality of neurosurgeons be determined by control or by the market? In: Morley TP, ed. Current controversies in neurosurgery. Philadelphia: WB Saunders, 1976:5–14.
7. Popp AJ. Eldridge Houston Campbell, Jr. Surg Neurol 1988;29:347–349.
8. Ablin G. Are there too many, too few, or just the right number of neurological surgeons? Clin Neurosurg 1974;22:516–520.
9. Alexander E. Perspective on neurosurgery: Presidential address. J Neurosurg 27:189–206, 1967.
10. Bergland RM, Neurosurgery may die. N Engl J Med 2973;288:1043–1046.
11. Bucy PC. How many neurosurgeons? Surg Neurol 1975; 3:201–206.
12. Bucy PC. The distribution of neurological surgeons in the United States and Canada. Surg Neurol 1976;6: 201–203.
13. Bucy PC. Whoa! (Editorial) Surg Neurol 1977;7: 161–162.
14. Clark KW. Manpower surveys and other myths. Clin Neurosurg 1970;22:566–572.
15. Drake CG. Neurosurgery: Considerations for strength and quality. The 1978 AANS Presidential Address. J Neurosurg 1978;49:485–501.
16. Ginzberg E. Manpower of neurosurgery: Seeing ourselves as others see us. The 1977 Harvey Cushing oration. J Neurosurg 1977;47:803–809.
17. Kennedy E. Nation health security. Tufts Health Sci Rev 1971;2:8–11.
18. Odom GL. Neurological surgery in our changing times. The 1972 AANS presidential address. J Neurosurg 1972;37:255–268.
19. Schneider R. The ''future trends'' in neurosurgery are here. The 1975 AANS Presidential Address. J Neurosurg 1975;3:651–660.
20. Zuidema GD. The SOSSUS report and its impact on neurosurgery. J Neurosurg 1977;46:135–44.
21. Report of the Graduate Medical Education National Advisory Committee, US Department of Health and Human Services, Health Resources Administration. 1980;1(77): 2:273–274.
22. Watts C. Neurosurgical manpower requirements for 1990: An estimate of the Graduate Medical Education National Advisory Committee. Neurosurgery 1981; 8:277–279.
23. Schroeder SA. How can we tell if there are too many or too few physicians? JAMA, 1996;276(22): 1841–1843.
24. Cochran JD. Scenes from Aspen Integrated Health Care Report, September 1996, 1–9.
25. Critical Challenges: Revitalizing the health professions for the 21st century (15). San Francisco: PEW Health Commission, 1996.
26. Tarlov R. HMO growth of physicians: The third compartment. Health Aff 1986; 314:217–222.
27. Wennberg JE, Goodman DC, Nease RF, Keller RD. Finding equilibrium in U.S. physician supply. Health Aff 1993;Summer: 89–102.
28. Hart LG, Wagner E, Sarmad P, Nelson AS, Rosenblatt RA. Physician staffing ratios in staff-model HMO's: A cautionary tale. Health Aff 1997;16:(l)55–70.
29. Rivo ML, Kindig DA. A report card on physician workforce in the United States. N Eng J Med 1996;334 (14):892–896.
30. Cooper RA. Perspectives on physician workforce to the year 2020. JAMA 1995;274(19):1534–1543.
31. German, WJ. Neurological surgery. Its past, present and future. J Neurosurg 1952;10:526–537.
32. Pevehouse BC, Colenbrander A. The United States neurological surgery residency matching program. Neurosurgery 1994;35:1172–1182.
33. Maurice-Williams RS. Enough British neurosurgeons? Br J Neurosurg 1987;1:301–304.
34. Mosberg W. Medical manpower needs at home and abroad. Neurosurgery 1992;30:639–648.
35. 1997 Guide to The American Association of Neurological Surgeons. Park Ridge IL: AANS,1997.
36. Pevehouse BC, the Gary Siegel Organization. Comprehensive Neurosurgery Practice Survey. Park Ridge IL: American Association of Neurological Surgeons and the Congress of Neurological Surgeons, 1995.
37. Harrington T. Neurosurgical manpower needs-achieving balance. Surg Neurol 1997;47:316–325.
38. Popp AJ. Neurosurgical residency training programs and the work force debate. AANS Bulletin, Spring 1996;22–27.
39. Lohr, KN, Vanselow NA, Detmer DE, eds. The nation's physician workforce: Options for balancing supply and requirements. Institute of Medicine. Washington, DC: National Academy Press, 1996
40. Council on Graduate Medical Education. Improving access to health care through physician workforce reform: Directions for the 21st century. Washington, DC: Public Health Service, Health Resources and Services Administration, US Dept. of Health and Human Services, 1992.
41. American Association of Colleges of Osteopathic Medicine, American Medical Association, American Osteopathic Association, Association of Academic Health Centers, Association of American Medical Colleges, National Medical Association. Consensus Statement on Physician Workforce 1997.
42. Mitka, Mike. States jump on, and off, GME reform bandwagon. AMA News June 16, 1997, 5.
43. Popp AJ, Toselli R. Work force requirements for neurosurgery. Surg Neurol 1996;46:181–185.
44. Miller RS, Jonas HS, Witcomb ME. The initial employment status of physicians completing training in 1994. JAMA 1996;275 (9):708–712.

45. Vaughn RW, Vaughan MS. Using anesthesiology as a model for change. Physic Ex 1997; (February): 4–12.

46. Kwakwa, F, Jonasson O. The longitudinal study of surgical residents, 1993 to 1994. J Am Coll Surg 1996; 183(5):425–433.

47. O'Neil JA. Workforce issues in pediatric surgery. Bull Am Coll Surg 1981;(4): 34–37.

48. Meyer GS, Jacoby I, Krakauer H, Powell DW, Aurand J, Mcardle P. Gastroenterology workforce modeling. JAMA 1996;276(9):689–694.

49. National Resident Matching Program, NRMP Data,1991–1995. Washington, DC: Association of American Medical Colleges, 1996.

50. Anders G. Once hot specialty, anesthesiology cools as insures scale back. Washington DC: Wall Street Journal, March 17, 1995, 1.

51. Ebel MH. Choice of specialty: It's money that matters in the USA. JAMA 1989;262:1630.

52. Shulkin DJ. Choice of specialty: It's money that matters in the USA. JAMA 1989, 262:1630.

53. Selby R. Neurosurgical training. (Letter to the editor) J Neurosurg 1974;40:136.

CHAPTER 8

Health-care Reform and Neurosurgery Training

JULIAN T. HOFF, M.D., MICHAEL N. POLINSKY, M.D., JAMES R. BEAN, M.D.

INTRODUCTION

Neurosurgical training is organized and conducted under a standard residency program design, which evolved over decades from the standard Halstead hospital-based apprentice model (1). Academic neurosurgical training programs grew in parallel with expanding academic medical centers, sharing in the responsibilities and rewards conferred on academic centers by federal and state tax support, private endowment, and, not least, health insurance funding over the past 40 years. The triadic academic mission of service, teaching, and research is the guiding aim within academic programs, expressing an ideal, but expensive, time-consuming, and often conflicting menu of responsibilities.

The academic mission can be accomplished only through a generous balance of financial resources and time available to both instructor and trainee in the academic program. Time spent in patient care often takes precedence, and, although obviously of vital individual and social importance, the demands of patient care may obscure the need for, and rob the time available for, instruction, study, and clinical or basic research. Protecting that time and funding has been important to academic program success.

Financing of the academic mission creates special needs that have been accommodated over time from several income sources (2). Research money comes from National Institutes of Health (NIH) and other public and private research grant funding sources. Medicare direct and indirect medical education funding to academic (3) centers for graduate training has grown to $7 billion over the past 30 years. The disproportionate share of hospital (DSH) payments for indigent and uncompensated care ex-

panded dramatically in the early 1990s from $0.4 billion to $17 billion from 1988 to 1992, with academic medical centers receiving a substantial proportion. Clinical revenues accounted for 37 to 57% of medical schools' revenues in 1995, depending on the type of school (4). Cross-subsidization of academic training programs and basic science draws funds from clinical practice income and redistributes high earning specialty revenue through academic center discretionary funds, the so-called "dean's tax." Each source has been important in supporting growth, balance, and differentiation within the academic agenda.

However, that financial support basis is fragile and it is traditionally dependent on a generous revenue margin from clinical services charged on a cost-plus fee-for-service basis to both private insurers and public payers. Costs and budgets have been expansionary throughout the century, and insurance-based financing to support that unrestricted expansion has been a vital ingredient. Despite periodic declarations of a health-care cost "crisis," dating back to the Nixon administration, soon after implementation of the Medicare program, health-care cost continued to rise at a rate of 10 to 12% per year until 1994, far exceeding the growth rate in any other economic sector. The cost of care in the United States reached 14% of the gross domestic product (GDP), about 30% higher than the next most expensive nation, Canada, whose cost hovers at just under 10% of its GDP (5).

Health-care reform, for all its quality, preventive, and cost-effectiveness language, is a euphemism for any change to this expansionary trend in health care in the United States, and the phrase translates to reduced growth in funding for health care and indirectly for specialty care training. For academic programs, the change has far-reaching consequences. Not only is clinical income threatened, but the very design of the residency training program, if not the existence of the training program itself, is at risk.

In this chapter, the specific effects that health-care "reform" (in the form of private managed care and federal funding and regulatory change) has had on neurosurgery training programs is examined.

SOCIETAL PRESSURE STIMULATING HEALTH-CARE REFORM

The health-care reform debate that preceded the proposed and failed Clinton Health Security Act in 1994 expressed the aims of reform in three categories: access, quality, and cost. Of these three goals, cost was the only truly driving motive in sparking any serious consideration of legislative action. To be sure, 35 million, or 15% of the American public were without health insurance in 1991, a number that has only grown to an estimated 40 million by 1995. But Congressional debate made it clear that public sentiment for reform did not include support for increased tax payment for premium subsidies or expanded Medicaid eligibility for the uninsured. Quality was never debated as a serious issue, despite the observation that the United States ranks below most other Western industrialized nations in virtually all standard population health indicators, such as infant mortality, maternal mortality, and life expectancy. The single driving issue was cost, both to public programs (Medicare, Medicaid) and to private payers (primarily employers, with rising employee health benefit costs).

The source of rising costs in the United States health-care market is traceable to the traditionally dominant form of payment for health-care services. With few exceptions (as outlined in Dr. Kusske's chapter), fee-for-service payment characterized medical reimbursement throughout the 20th century, until the emergence of bundled case rates and capitation in the 1980s. Health insurance benefits, which expanded rapidly after WW II, covered virtually all large personal health-care costs and hid the cost from immediate view. Economic theory suggests that indemnity insurance coverage for routine health services is as responsible for much of the unrestrained rise in total medical costs. Indemnity coverage characterized employer health benefit plans, which grew rapidly in numbers following exemption of employer health benefits from federal personal income taxation in the 1950s. Indemnity coverage, that is, paying billed charges, was also adopted by the Medicare and Medicaid programs in 1966, a political compromise allowing the federal programs to mirror private health coverage without appearing to intervene in medical decision-making.

Public expectations, at least for those covered by insurance, rose in tandem with technical improvements in and available access to health services. Unrestricted physician choice and unlimited resource availability based on need became widely accepted social principles. Even the uninsured gained new access to health care, funded either by public charity programs or by cost-shifting uncompensated care costs to indemnity covered patients through higher charges. Medical decision-making and determination of need remained a physician and patient choice, without today's familiar preadmission authorizations, length of stay restrictions, and emphasis on out-patient care.

Complicating the open access and unrestricted payment method was rapid development and widespread deployment of sophisticated and expensive diagnostic and therapeutic tools, such as computed tomography (CT), joint prostheses, magnetic resonance imaging (MRI), and organ transplantation. In addition, medical school enrollment doubled from 8000 to 16,000 per year from 1960 to 1985 through federal support, thus expanding the available workforce, programs to train them, and expenditures generated by their availability.

The stage was set for a reaction to health-care costs when employer health benefit costs rose from under 15% to over 60% of pretax profits from 1965 to 1985, and Medicare program costs showed a similar 11% or more annual increases, with a cost-doubling time of 5 to 7 years (6).

RESPONSE TO RISING HEALTH-CARE COSTS

The national cost of health care reached 12% of GDP in the early 1990s, and it was projected to rise to 20% by 2000, in the absence of substantial change in health-care structure and financing. The sense of alarm caused by such projections set the stage for both another attempt at federal health-care reform by legislation and for private insurer business and management strategies to rein in costs.

A decade earlier, Medicare had attacked the growing budget problem by controlling first hospital reimbursement and then physician fees. In 1983, Medicare instituted case-rate reimbursement for hospitals, based on average costs for 460 Diagnostic Related Groups (DRGs). Hospitals began receiving payment by a lump sum per admission, regardless of length of stay or volume of services. In 1992, Medicare implemented the first year of a 4-year transition from usual, customary, and reasonable (UCR) fee reimbursement for physicians, to a Medicare Fee Schedule based on a Resource-Based Relative Value Scale (RBRVS) methodology. The RBRVS, with its separate work, practice expense, and malpractice expense components, sought to control cost rise by controlling physician service price increases. Annual price (fee) increases are determined by a dollar conversion factor ($40 for surgical services in 1997), which is multiplied by each CPT code's relative value units (RVUs) to arrive at the actual fee.

The RBRVS basis of the Medicare Fee Schedule was designed for adoption by private insurers as well (7). This strategy has gained growing acceptance, as more and more private payers convert to Medicare's RBRVS, using their own conversion factor. Thus the Health Care Finance Administration (HCFA) has achieved the de facto role of reimbursement structure designer for fee-for-service medical reimbursement. The effects of the RBRVS have included substantial reduction in reimbursement for procedural CPT codes, with corresponding increase in payment for cognitive (nonprocedural) Evaluation and Management (E&M) CPT codes. Surgical specialty reimbursement will further decline with proposed unification of the three part Medicare conversion factor (surgical, primary care, and "other"), and with conversion of the practice expense relative value units to a "resource base," rather than the original historical cost base. With growing competition in the health-care market and the growing size and negotiating strength of HMOs, reimbursement in the private market, which is using the Medicare Fee Schedule and conversion factor as a benchmark toward which the rest of the market aims, is shrinking.

The private response to rising costs has been in the form of various managed care strategies. Managed care refers to any form of contractual agreement between an insurer and provider in which price limits, financial incentives or penalties, and/or medical decision-making limitations are accepted. Managed care involves several strategies of increasing complexity and control.

The federal HMO act of 1973 created the opportunity to offer an alternative form of health care: prepaid services. Although group model, salaried staff model, and network model HMO structures vary somewhat in their methods, several features are consistent across different HMO health plans. Primary care is emphasized, often with primary care gatekeeper roles, while specialty care is de-emphasized, or frankly discouraged. Primary care physicians are frequently paid on a capitated basis, eliminating the incentive to increase the number of their own services to augment income. At the same time, primary care bonus incentives for reduced specialty referral and hospital use effectively reduce specialty use and workforce requirement. Physician provider panels, particularly specialty panels, are limited by selective contracting. Specialty income is reduced by negotiated steep fee discounts or, more recently, by paying on a specialty risk-bearing capitation basis. Hospital margins are reduced by similarly negotiated discounts, generally on a per-diem rate basis. The overall effect is reduced hospital and specialty revenue, particularly the padded revenue margins of earlier years, by which practice revenue could cross-subsidize treatment of uninsured patients or other research or teaching activities.

The entity most at risk under these conditions is the academic medical center. Costs of care in academic centers are on an average 25% higher when compared to community hospitals (8). The number of uninsured, nonpaying patients is often higher in teaching hospitals, increasing their uncompensated, internal costs. The burden of high cost, high technical complexity cases tends to be higher in academic centers, making them financially vulnerable, if adequate direct or cross-subsidized funding is not available (9). In a market in which contracting is based on price and degree of discount, academic centers may have difficulty competing with nonteaching hospitals for patients, based on their higher overhead costs. In short, managed care confronts academic centers with exclusion from contracts for care or reimbursement below the cost of care.

Penetration of managed care has proceeded at different rates in different geographic markets. Academic centers in the most heavily penetrated markets have been most seriously affected. The highly managed health-care market in Minneapolis has had profound effects on the University of Minnesota Medical Center stemming from exclusions and income reductions, and the university hospital has merged with a local community hospital system. Exclusion of Tufts University New England Medical Center from the Harvard Pilgrim Health Care HMO has threatened economic survival of the hospital and its academic programs. Several academic hospitals, including Tulane, UC Irvine, George Washington University, Presbyterian in New York (Columbia University), and South Carolina Medical College, are negotiating or have completed acquisition deals with for-profit hospital corporations, such as Columbia-HCA (10).

THE EFFECT OF HEALTH-CARE REFORM ON NEUROSURGERY TRAINING

In February, 1997, the authors asked 95 residency training program directors to assess the effect of health-care reform on their neurosurgery training programs. Questions addressed four areas: teaching, research, patient care, and administration. Seventy-seven (81%) responded The questions addressed six specific issues. First, how has health-care reform affected resident supervision by faculty and how do residents and faculty view this change? Second, has reform changed the quality of patient care? Third, do patients have less access to the university hospital and has this affected the case mix of the program? Fourth, have administrative duties changed? Fifth, has research funding availability changed? Sixth, is academic neurosurgery losing its appeal as a career choice for residents in training? The responses are summarized in three tables below.

The questions dealt with issues common to all training programs. Perceptions of both faculty and house staff were sought. The survey was intended to sample the atmosphere created for training programs by health-care reform over the past five years.

Teaching

Teaching is an inherently inefficient process, but nevertheless essential for the development of safe and competent neurosurgeons. Teaching and learning take time. Teaching institutions are, by their nature, more expensive, because they are inefficient compared to nonteaching hospitals. The presence and involvement of a trainee influences the entire hospitalization process, from the admitting physical examination, to the use of important monitoring devices, to the induction of anesthesia, to the performance of surgery, and to early postoperative care in the recovery room, an intensive care unit, or both. In particular, the operating room, per unit of time, is the most costly place in a hospital. Operating room hospital charges and anesthesiology billing are proportional to time; both are substantially increased by resident involvement. In-hospital teaching, therefore, becomes an added expense that must be compensated by either professional fees, hospital charges, or both. In recent months, the length of stay for hospitalized patients has shortened noticeably, because of the need to control cost. Less in-hospital teaching is a direct result of the shorter hospital stay, because trainees have less access and exposure to patients during the stay. Teaching has necessarily shifted to the outpatient setting, before and after hospitalization.

Methods to control cost have become important priorities of training. Reducing laboratory and radiological testing, days in the hospital, and dependence on consultation with other specialties has intensified the responsibility of faculty and house staff within the discipline. Less use of high-cost units, such as intensive care and recovery rooms, has occurred. Admissions to the hospital before surgery and for preoperative evaluations have practically been eliminated. Measures necessary to control costs, including staff reductions and bed closures, have become realities.

Scrutiny of reimbursement by federal agencies has increased substantially in recent months. Federal investigations of academic medical centers for improper, or allegedly fraudulent, billing has intensified since the initiation of the ''PATH'' (Physicians At Teaching Hospitals) initiative by the Office of Inspector General (OIG) of the Department of Health and Human Services (DHHS) in 1996. In December 1995, HCFA revised regulations regarding teaching physician presence and documentation of service to be eligible for Medicare billing. No longer will a countersignature suffice. The regu-

TABLE 8.1
Resident Supervision*

	More	Same	Less
Amount of supervision	56	40	4

	Positive	No Change	Negative
Resident assessment	58	4	38
Faculty assessment	50	2	48

* Values reflect percentage of responses.

TABLE 8.2
Quality of Care*

	Better	Same	Worse
Patient care	44	5	51
Patient access	43	26	31

	More	Same	Less
Case complexity	68	29	3
Administration time	95	5	0

* Values reflect percentage of responses.

lations require the teaching physician's presence during all procedures and documentation in the physician's own hand for Evaluation & Management (E&M) services (11). For surgical procedures, this means that the teaching physician must be personally present during the "key" portion of the procedure, and "immediately available" during the entire procedure. The regulations limit alternative activities teaching physicians may conduct while a resident is performing a procedure for which the responsible teaching physician will bill. Using the federal Civil Monetary Penalties Act and the Civil War-period False Claims Act, the OIG has applied the regulation retroactively for care rendered and billed during 1990 to 1995 and has initiated investigations at several academic centers. Following "PATH" investigations, the University of Pennsylvania (Philadelphia) settled for $30 million, and Thomas Jefferson University (Philadelphia) settled for $11 million to avoid larger penalties for billing violations found during audits for that period (12).

The revised HCFA regulations and the PATH initiative have resulted in increased supervision of residents and increased documentation of all activities related to patients. Many program directors view these changes positively, and even more detect a positive response from their residents (Table 8.1).

Patient Care

Increased faculty involvement in patient care could theoretically improve the overall quality of care. However, more than half of program directors believe the quality of care has fallen during the last 5 years. This may reflect the increasing administrative responsibilities required of academic faculty, which detract from the delivery of quality health care (Table 8.2).

Teaching hospitals continue to absorb patients without insurance and accept and treat patients that have already been treated at other hospitals to the limits of their insurance. At the same time, complex and high-cost cases continue to be referred to teaching hospitals for their "teaching value" in an evolving health-care system that only marginally supports the cost of complex care (Table 8.2).Because patient care depends heavily upon cost-effective delivery, there is an increasing need for paraprofessionals, such as nurse practitioners, physician assistants, and social workers to expedite the process of health care. Students and house officers in such an environment slow the process by their inexperience.

Certain problems inherent to a training curriculum remain unsolved, such as continuity of patient care in programs that include service rotation for trainees and resident training using the basic principle of "progressive responsibility."

Research

Training programs face new problems because of health-care reform. Faculty protected time, which allows the academician to probe new frontiers of research and conduct other scholarly activities, has been curtailed substantially by patient care requirements and administrative responsibilities. At the same time, protected time remains vital for the academic growth of faculty members. Because of the reduction in protected time, resulting from increased patient service demands, research productivity of faculty members is more and more threatened. Academic faculty members must focus increasingly on patient care and clinical revenue-generating activities, with correspondingly less commitment to teaching and research. Involvement in any activity that consumes time without reimbursement, such as service to the community or to regional or national profes-

TABLE 8.3
Academic Appeal*

Appeal to Residents	more—25	same—34	less—41
Resident Placement	harder—61	same—33	easier—6
Access to Funding	harder—90	same—10	easier—0
Extramural Funding	yes—94	no—6	
Intramural Funding	<10K—9	10K—100K—60	>100K—31
NIH Funding	yes—72	no—28	
Change in NIH Funding	increased—29	same—38	decreased—23

* Values reflect percentage of responses.

sional organizations, must be limited and budgeted. Thus, due to financial factors, the traditional academic mission is changing for faculty members, although their responsibility to train neurosurgeons remains undiminished. Faculty members, as well as those planning a future in academics, must contend with this paradox.

Time is money, costs are high, and efficient time management is vital for neurosurgeons in training programs. Time for research has become an unaffordable luxury for faculty members without extramural funding sources and for residents in training as well, if facilities, mentors, and money are not available. The research obligation for academic neurosurgeons continues, but, because extramural funding is so essential for research by faculty, those without it find their academic careers imperiled, because they simply cannot afford the time or money for unfunded research. The dilemma lacks solution and threatens to worsen.

Fifteen percent of training programs receive under $10,000 per year of extramural funding annually (Table 8.3). Tighter budgets and prioritization of research dollars have become universal problems for all academic programs. The majority of program directors find access to funding more limited now compared to 5 years ago, even though 72% currently have NIH funds for research. Consequently, research has become vulnerable as a cornerstone of training programs. In order to improve their financial position and establish long-term research funding, programs have become increasingly dependent upon philanthropy and industry for resources.

Administrative

The administrative burden on an academic faculty has increased from several sources. Personal documentation of patient care and heightened patient-record detail needed to satisfy private payers and Medicare guidelines increase the time commitment to patient care without adding to patient benefit or time efficiency. Practice management to increase efficiency and decrease expenses requires time and understanding of business management principles that were foreign to neurosurgeons only a few years ago. These new requirements come on top of traditional academic administrative duties, such as faculty committee assignments and academic departmental oversight.

PRESERVING THE ACADEMIC MISSION OF NEUROSURGERY TRAINING PROGRAMS DURING HEALTH-CARE REFORM AND BEYOND
Teaching

The academic mission of residency programs in the United States includes training safe and competent neurosurgeons. In order to accomplish that mission, training programs must maintain an abundant volume of patients with a broad spectrum of illnesses or disorders within the domain of neurosurgery. The faculties of training programs must compete successfully with others who provide similar care, but are unburdened by trainee teaching or research responsibilities. Marketing, networking, and contracting thus become important, even for academic centers. Providers in training programs, from the most junior to the most senior, must endorse such a focused approach to clinical care in order for the program to survive and thrive.

Residents and students should be incorporated into every outpatient encounter. Most patients who undergo neurological surgery today are admitted on the same day, precluding in-hospital preoperative examinations by trainees. Follow-up visits in an outpatient setting provide continuity of care that is essential for good training.

Teaching efficiency and cost control are now emphasized in training programs. Clinical faculty members in practice can teach the socioeconomics of health care. Lectures and seminars focused on the business of practice, database accumulation and management, and outcomes research methodology are other avenues that can improve the productivity of the training program and educate its trainees in the practicalities of life beyond residency.

Patient Care

Faculty clinical competency and ability to generate referrals are essential to a successful academic practice and will remain so. A substantial volume of patients with a variety of disorders is vitally important for the resident learning experience. The inclusion of clinical faculty who have clinical expertise and are willing to teach is one method to assure access of residents to a sufficient volume and variety of patients. Creating a regional network for neurosurgical care with a training program at the hub can have a positive effect on all those involved, both academic and private practices. Consultations by telecommunication, educational experiences, and academic stimulation are benefits of a collaborative arrangement developed among those in private practice and those in academic centers.

Research

Protected time for an academic faculty is essential. Interdisciplinary collaborations can be highly productive and may help compensate for the loss of protected time by sharing the burden; such collaborations should be included in every research activity. Funding for basic research is and will continue to be a problem for clinical neurosurgeons. Again, collaboration can provide a solution. The recent emphasis by research funding agencies on clinical relevance is a welcome change for clinicians who want to pursue investigations. Clinical research with protocols based on clear-cut hypotheses is emphasized now more than ever before. An interdisciplinary approach is key; e.g., the establishment of a stroke center utilizing a variety of specialists working as a team with a common goal. Programmatic efforts such as spine centers and brain tumor centers are other examples.

The goals of training programs may need to be adjusted to keep research and clinical care in perspective. All residents may not need an extensive research exposure during their training. While many programs today offer a substantial research experience, some have reduced their research training in order to cope with tighter budgets and less time for research. Research may seem less important than clinical care, because of the emphasis of health-care reform on efficient patient care and cost reduction, but research will emerge again in the future as a high priority, and it is the only means to assure progress in the specialty.

Administration

Academic realities remain the same, despite the effects of health-care reform. An academic faculty member continues to be held to the ''publish or perish'' principle and to promotion expectations. The cost of health care has had a direct effect on reimbursement for providers, reducing salaries for many faculty members in training programs. Pressures on faculty to provide more care for less pay and, at the same time, engage in research and teaching, have clearly affected the atmosphere in training programs. As a result, many program directors have noted declining interest in academic neurosurgery among their residents (Table 8.3). Adapting to changing priorities in academics, i.e., clinical activity versus research, has continued to be a major problem for many.

SUMMARY

Academic priorities have changed for neurosurgeons in training programs because of health-care reform. Pressures to provide more patient care because of the reimbursement it provides have caused a reduction in resources for research and time for teaching. The alignment of priorities in academic neurosurgery has threatened the creativity that comes from protected time for the academic who yearns for a research opportunity and for the fulfillment that comes from teaching trainees. Health-care reform tests, and will continue to test, the flexibility, and possibly the viability, of neurosurgery training in the United States.

REFERENCES

1. Long D. Assurance of competency in residency training: Neurosurgical education in the twenty-first century. In: Bean JR. Neurosurgery in transition: The transformation of neurosurgical practice. Baltimore: Williams & Wilkins, 1997.

2. Pardes H. The future of medical schools and teaching hospitals in the era of managed care. Acad Med 1997; 72:97–102.

3. Financing graduate medical education and teaching hospitals from a trust fund. Physician Payment Review Commission Annual Report 1997:381–395.

4. The financing of medical schools—A report of the AAMC Task Force on Medical School Financing. Washington DC: AAMC, 1996

5. Evans R. Going for the gold. J Health Polit Pol Law 1997;22:427–465.

6. Context: The rising cost of medical care. Physician Payment Review Commission Annual Report 1993: 1–11.

7. Assuring equitable payment under the Medicare Fee Schedule. Physician Payment Review Commission Annual Report 1992:23–86.

8. Thorpe K. Health system in transition. J Health Polit Pol Law 1997;22:339–361.

9. Mechanic R., Dobson A. The impact of managed care on clinical research: A preliminary investigation. Health Aff 1996;15:72–89.

10. 42 CFR § 415.170 et seq. In: 60 Federal Register 63123. December 8, 1995.

11. Bureau of National Affairs. New York representatives ask Shalala to ensure fairness of PATH audits. Washington DC: Bureau of National Affairs Medicare Report. May 2, 1997:8:403–404.

CHAPTER 9

Academic Neurosurgical Practice: The Role, Challenges, and Changes of the Academic Mission in the Age of Accountability

LYAL G. LEIBROCK, M.D., F.A.C.S., LESLIE C. HELLBUSCH, M.D.

BRIDGING THE ACADEMIC/PRIVATE PRACTICE DIVIDE: BACKGROUND

Neurosurgical postgraduate training has traversed a multiplicity of changes since the beginning of the century. In the early 1900s, physicians with an interest in surgery of the brain and spinal column learned by practice after obtaining training in surgical principles and techniques. Subsequently, a system like an apprenticeship evolved in which more proficient individuals offered their services as teachers to physicians with an interest in the field of neurosurgery. There was no fixed time period in which the training was accomplished. The relationship continued until the student was deemed skilled in his mentor's art. In the 1920s, 1930s, and 1940s, neurosurgery training developed along with the system of graduate medical education, with identifiable training originating at private and university institutions. The American Board of Neurological Surgeons began certifying in 1940. Through the 1940s and early 1950s, American medicine began to organize, certify, and evaluate the teaching and educational components of training through graduate medical education committees set up by the Accreditation Council for Graduate Medical Education from its five parents organizations: the American Board of Medical Specialties, American Hospital Association, American Association of Medical Colleges, Council of Medical Specialty Societies, and the American Medical Association.

The next step was formalized residency training, which began in the mid-1940s with private practitioners providing most clinical instruction at affiliated hospitals. Substantial government funding and control was added to the mix in the mid-1960s. This separated academic and private practitioners in graduate medical education. The mid-1980s ushered in an era of growing perceptions of excess numbers of physicians, particularly in the specialties, and with this perception, attempts to control the cost of medical care. This led governmental, social, business, and philosophical organizations in the country to review how graduate medical education is obtained and what mix and number of physicians are required at what cost. The revolution in graduate medical education resulting from this review continues today.

One issue being addressed is how to merge the divergent worlds of academic training centers with the private practice of neurosurgery to obtain better quality and variety of service, education, research, and value in resident education. To achieve education with good value to the individual, to private practice, the academic university center, patients, and the body politic in general, one must produce individuals trained to perform evaluations, diagnostics, and surgical or medical care of good quality at reasonable cost. This review arises because of three precipitating factors causing major disruptions in postgraduate medical education. These factors are proceeding concurrently with the continuing evolution of medical care delivery, which is increasingly complex and technically sophisticated. The factors are: (*a*) the continuing aging of the population, which requires more medical care; (*b*) the presumed oversupply of medical specialists; and (*c*) economic and political constraints, which are face to face with the demand for increasingly complex technical care. These three issues in their relationship to medical care delivery and a demand for value in education by the payers for medical care (business, the populace, insurance companies, and government) have forced reevaluation of graduate medical education. Federal and state governments have given large sums of money to postgraduate medical education and now perceive that the investment has produced an excess of medical specialists, a costly result, not only in terms of training, but also throughout the practice life of the trained specialists. The competitive environment which was expected to generate lower costs as a consequence of large physician numbers did not materialize as anticipated after government-subsidized graduate medical education was initiated.

In determining how good quality neurosurgical education, research, and service can be provided at a good value, one must bridge the academic and private practice divide generated when the government adopted a policy of providing enormous sums of money to hospitals and universities to train physicians. This resulted in a large increase of specialists through the 1960s, 1970s, and early 1980s, with the majority entering private practice. Government funding is now being reduced, making it imperative that educators who direct graduate training programs seek the association of community neurosurgeons, neurologists, neuroscientists in general, and the public as a way to provide quality and variety in education, research, and service opportunities to residents in training. This will assure that neurosurgery residency training programs survive with quality and good value.

PHILOSOPHY

Inclusiveness of All Neurosurgeons and Neuroscientists in a Clinical Cachement Region Should Be a Mission of Neurosurgery Training Programs

Beyond the directly affiliated group or groups, the academic center needs to ensure that other private practitioners, partnerships, or groups in its clinical cachement area are included in training efforts. This creates a responsibility for the training medical center to address continuing educational, clinical, and economic requirements, and the psychological support of neurosurgeons who find themselves in increasingly difficult times.

How does the training center achieve inclusiveness in the increasingly competitive medical environment? To accomplish this goal, the academic center and its partners in the academic consortium must provide several services and opportunities that will involve private practitioners for the mutual benefit of both academic and private practice communities. Methods of achieving inclusiveness include: accepting referred patients, providing support with difficult cases or complications, encouraging participation in the educational process, fostering involvement with visiting faculty, and offering continuing education opportunities.

Referrals

If the academic group has specialists in neurosurgical skills not possessed by private neurosurgeons in the clinical cachement area, the center will accept referred patients. Other patients may be referred to give residents the opportunity to see an unusual or complicated case or to have a case discussed at a conference. The referred patients are cared for at the center, but without any deprecation by consortium faculty, residents, or students of the neurosurgical skills of referring individuals. Rather, the emphasis of any explanation of the referral can and should reasonably stress outstanding facilities at the academic center.

Providing Support

A second way to be inclusive is to enable neurosurgeons in the cachement area to access the training consortium for support with a difficult case or complex complication. If a neurosurgeon requests transfer, the patient is always accepted, regardless of economic remuneration or social distress. The training center establishes the principle of accepting all patients with any disease or complication from any source at any time and of providing the best care according to the center's ability. This principle makes an effective working relationship between the training center and neurosurgeons in the region.

Participation in Education

A third way of achieving inclusiveness is making practitioners an active part of the neurosurgery resident, allied health, nurse and medical student education process. Practitioners can be used extensively in teaching. Regional neurosurgeons can provide education in the laboratory year for residents who are not interested in bench research and want to perform clinical work. Residents can be assigned to one of the private practice groups for a month or more and thus gain additional clinical experience. The neurosurgeons are on the clinical faculty. This role helps them maintain contact with the consortium training center. While the resident's service is lost to the center for a month or more, the relationship with the practitioners means many of these individuals will refer unusual cases or teaching lesions, such as an intraventricular tumor or a difficult aneurysm to the consortium training center. This increases the educational variety at the center and enhances resident experience. Because regional neurosurgeons know the residents, they will call residents personally. Practitioners in the region who are included in teaching and training are also more willing to contribute to the economic viability of the training program through donations of money for resident or medical student education.

There usually are several excellent private practice groups in a region, and if a second- or third-year medical student requests a neurosurgical experience to explore a career in neurosurgery, that student is assigned to one of the private practice groups to work for a month. When the students return after a month of living and working with individuals in the group, most know if they wish to pursue a career in neurosurgery.

Visiting Faculty

The fourth way to accomplish inclusion is by inviting the clinical faculty to participate actively whenever a visiting professor is teaching. The clinical faculty may have dinner collectively and also have individual time for discussion with the visitor. Not only do the residents and academic faculty benefit from such visitors, but the clinical faculty in the region also gain.

Continuing Education

An essential effort of the academic training consortium is to provide for the continuing education of neurosurgeons in the community, state, and region. If regional neurosurgeons wish faculty to help with surgery, a faculty member will help. Recently at our medical center, one of the private partnerships requested help organizing instrumentation of the spine in a patient. The academic center's spine surgeon went out to help them organize this effort. If regional neurosurgeons want help with stereotaxic, seizure, or skull base surgery, or other specialties, the same principle applies. The academic program faculty will travel to the requesting location and help provide the service. If the clinical faculty wish, they can spend time learning at the consortium training center. This cooperation and assistance makes community neurosurgeons willing to help in the teaching and education of neurosurgery residents, medical students, and allied health professionals.

MODEL SYSTEM

The University of Nebraska Medical Center Neurosurgery Residency Program has thrived in the hybrid environment of both academic and private-practice-based mentoring; using this system as a model demonstrates the practical and philosophical underpinnings of the consortium arrangement and model system.

Administration

The chief administrative officer must be the academic chairman. The academic training center needs governance input into the group or groups with which it affiliates in the community. At each private sector site, there should be a training director responsible for economics, technical and intellectual education, research, conferences, and clinical service. The program director at the academic institution must have the authority to direct, replace, or counsel the training director at the private practice site if the individual is not performing adequately. This might happen, for example, if the surgeon is focused not on education, but primarily on the delivery of service. In a practice of three or more individuals, a chairman should be able to identify one member of the group to be responsible for the success of resident training at that site. If a training director has to be replaced, the program director can negotiate the change diplomatically with the private practice group and change training directors without disrupting the affiliation arrangement or the training director's practice.

A critical factor in making this system work at the University of Nebraska is having little in writing. Written agreements can lead to difficulties, particularly with academic institutions. Universities have a tendency to be administratively heavy-handed. Administrators find value in their jobs by performing and enforcing administrative policies. If policies are specified, administrators will try continually to nudge things to gain control, which is the administrative (product) goal. Academic administrative personnel can ruin agreements established with the private sector community. Workable academic-private practice affiliations cannot have fixed, written documents that give the academic center the opportunity for total control. Control is clearly the goal of administrators; whether in private practice or in the academic medical center. Neurosurgeons in private practice abhor external control. The agreements therefore have to be conceived out of mutual respect between the chief at the academic center and the training director or directors at the private facilities. The fraternity of neurosurgeons in the community, state, or region must have mutual respect and trust. Verbal agreements require more personal meetings than written contracts, but provide the safety factor of remaining outside the province of the administrative tigers in the various entities in which neurosurgical service is provided, i.e., the academic center, managed care organizations, insurance companies, hospital, and the private sector. The administrative goal should be a fraternity of neurosurgeons involved in education, research, and service, and economic viability to support these efforts. This is accomplished with mutual respect and trust, based on verbal agreements without contractual arrangements.

Numbers

To bridge the divide between academic and private practice involves identifying one or two private neurosurgery practices with which to partner in the community. It is optimum to incorporate groups of neurosurgeons, rather than an individual or a partnership. Groups of three or more neurosurgeons providing a variety of services offer a better opportunity. Even more attractive is a group with not only neurosurgeons, but neurologists, neuroradiologists, neuropathologists, and/or electrophysiologists. The types of groups depend upon the community and how private practice is organized, whether in small, medium-sized, or large practice groups.

The second numbers issue is determining at how many locations residents can effectively be educated besides the academic center. Experience at the University of Nebraska demonstrates that travel, education, and conference restrictions make it difficult for residents to work in more than three locations, particularly if the hospitals are any distance apart.

In special circumstances, a resident can, for a specific educational purpose, be directed to a facility for training not available at an affiliated private training consortium. For example, in pediatric neurosurgery, there may not be enough cases even with the private practice group affiliations. Arranging for residents to go for several months to another location to receive this education is an acceptable way of completing their training.

Economics

It is difficult for private practice groups to incorporate significantly into the economic system of academic centers. The academic center imposes "taxes" of large sums on the clinical enterprise of its neurosurgical section, division, or department. The private group requires that money earned be contributed to maintain the economic viability of the practice. The major affiliation between the two entities, therefore, has to be in the areas of education, service, and clinical research. One means of economic support that can come from the private groups is to have the clinical faculty provide service at the academic center, with the individuals allowing a portion of the income generated to be retained by the academic center. Such service takes away from the private practice because it takes time from the practice, so good service agreements will ensure that the independent practice is able to remain economically viable. Private practice affiliates can obtain support for the training program from the hospital or hospitals with which they are affiliated, for residents' salaries, visiting professorships, clinical research, space, and training grants. The private practice can donate money from their practice to the residency training program, via a university foundation account for example, an arrangement which allows the money to be tax-deductible. Such money can be used to enhance resident travel, education, and training.

When bridging the academic/private practice divide, the academic center must take care not to hurt the affiliated independent practice group or groups economically. Instead, the arrangement should enhance the practice with resident workforce and reduced need for physician assistants or nurse practitioners. The affiliated practices will be more integrally incorporated in the training if the residents rotate through facilities at which the groups practice. If there is one hospital with two groups practicing there, or two groups at two hospitals that are fairly close together geographically, residents can rotate through these sites without spending all of their time in cars, rather than in service and education. It is important to make sure the practice affiliates' hospitals pay the resident salaries when the residents rotate, providing service at the affiliate hospital. The affiliates' hospitals should also help economically with the education of the residents. Forms of such support, which can be negotiated with the help of the private practice group, are conference facilities, on-call sleep rooms, educational space, and eating facilities.

Conferences

Conference responsibilities are shared with the group practice sites. At the University of Nebraska, about 60 to 70% of conferences occur at the academic center, with the remainder at the private practice site. Academic conferences are held at the university center, because educators in the support sciences are available there. Conferences at the private affiliations sites are clinical and morbidity and mortality conferences.

Clinical conferences at the private center include Grand Rounds, brain tumor, spine, and a monthly morbidity & mortality conference on cases performed at the private practice center. The off-site facility provides one visiting professorship per year, funded through the resources of the hospitals and practice group. The academic center provides one visiting professorship per year, so the residents have an experience at both locations with visiting professors. The academic conferences at the University are on neuroanatomy, neurophysiology, neuropharmacology, neuroradiology, neuropathology, and neurology. A monthly Journal Club is divided evenly between academic and private sites.

Facilities

The private group guides the offsite hospital in providing facilities support. The practice site must provide an office for the residents, including computer facilities, a desk, a telephone, and supplies for paperwork and dictation. The practice must also provide an examination room to evaluate patients, which can be the same room used by the clinical faculty. This will make it convenient for residents to see patients, dictate office notes, and work with the faculty at the practice site. If the group is unable or unwilling to provide such facilities to support the training of neurosurgery residents, the program cannot have the residents rotate at this site.

CONCLUSION

Cooperative agreements contribute to value in educating a neurosurgeon, but the academic and private practice relationship must be beneficial to every person involved. Residents gain experience by performing surgery under the direct supervision of a larger, more diverse faculty, and when residents make rounds, the faculty is supportive and present. With private practice affiliations, a neurosurgery resident can be technically and clinically educated at approximately half the cost and with improved quality, as contrasted with the academic medical center serving as the sole source of training. Medical students also receive quality education at less financial cost to the medical college. Using part-time and clinical faculty reduces requirements for full-time university faculty. The merged faculties provide greater opportunity for education, clinical variety, specialization, clinical, and basic science research. As an illustration, the academic center may provide salaries for only three full-time positions, making it impossible to have seven or eight subspecialies represented at the center, but, if the funds are divided over six to nine part-time faculty members, the department can have pediatric, functional, spine, skull-base, tumor, trauma, and cerebrovascular neurosurgeons. The same amount of money can thus increase educational and research potential.

The agreement benefits the clinical faculty because of services provided by residents, and the teaching and mentoring provides intellectual stimulus to clinical faculty participants, so that most neurosurgeons are delighted to participate. The consortium must not hurt the community neurosurgeons economically: the academic center is working with them, not taking patients from the practice. A patient in a managed care environment may be told, ''You can't go to the community hospital. We've resigned from the contract and we've signed a new one with the university hospital.'' With an affiliation at the academic center, the cerebrovascular neurosurgeon who performs aneurysms at the community hospital can perform them at the center. If the stereotaxic physician is at the academic center and the managed care plan signs a contract moving stereotaxis to the community center, the physician can perform the stereotaxis procedure at the community hospital. If agreements incorporate two groups in two different hospitals and two different managed care systems or organizations, a point can be reached where a provider is obliged to work with the consortium neurosurgery group no matter how contracts are constructed by the managed care organizations, insurance carriers, physician-hospital organizations, or academic centers. These contractural entities then have to work out affiliation agreements with the consortium practice. This leads to an increased number of patients available for resident training and an increased number of patients for medical students to examine, review, and learn from. In summary, the academic/private practice relationship provides good quality education for neurosurgery residents at probably half the cost involved if the academic medical center had to bear the entire cost—thus, good quality at reasonable cost and, therefore, good value for all concerned.

CHAPTER 10

Assurance of Competency in Residency Training: Neurosurgical Education in the Twenty-First Century

DON M. LONG, M.D., PH.D.

INTRODUCTION

Assurance of competency is the goal of all of the regulation of residency training. The requirements and regulations are designed to verify that the trainees have an adequate fund of knowledge and at least have experienced the management of a representative group of neurosurgical patients. Yet nothing in the current system truly assesses an individual's competence to manage complex neurosurgical patients or actually perform the needed surgeries (14). Verification of competence is left to the discretion of individual program directors. The Bosk Report, commissioned by and presented to the Society of Neurological Surgeons, reported that approximately 10% of residents change their mind about neurosurgery as a specialty at some phase of training and leave the field. Another 10% were dismissed, usually for apparent psychological mismatch with the specialty. Neither group has a significant impact on the practice of neurosurgery in the United States. However, a third category of residents identified are of concern. Program directors questioned the overall competence of a small, but real percentage of chief residents completing their programs. A small percentage of chief residents also were concerned that their experience during training was not sufficient.

While these concerns about competence of a small percentage of individuals completing neurosurgical training are important to examine and correct, they are less important than the concept that the competence of all trainees can be im-

proved by increased emphasis on a few fundamentals within neurosurgical training programs (8).

There are a complex of other issues brought about by the current or impending socioeconomic changes in biomedicine that will impact on trainees and training programs as well.

How many neurosurgeons are needed to care for our population's health needs and what should they do? *Length of training* is important because of cost. How many years does it really take to train a competent clinician? What about *research*? Why is research training required? The *spectrum of experience* is also an important issue. Does every trainee and every program really have enough of all procedures so that competence is assured? What should be done if they do not? Should trainees be certified only in those areas where they do have enough demonstrated experience? *Verification of outcomes* as a measure of competence is likely to become important. Health maintenance organizations currently compete on cost. Should they not compete by outcomes?

All of these questions must be answered as training programs evolve to meet the needs of a new century (Table 10.1).

The Halsted Residency

It is always worthwhile to remember the steps by which neurosurgical training reached its current situation. The training plan introduced by William Halsted 100 years ago radically

TABLE 10.1
Ideal Neurosurgical Training

1. Produces the needed number of practice and academic surgeons and no more
2. Does so in the shortest time commensurate with competence
3. Provides research training for those who will engage in a research career
4. Provides the full spectrum of all neurosurgical procedures to the trainee
5. Provides for active participation in all to assure competence
6. Allows enfolding of additional subspecialty experience in the residency context
7. Engenders the habit of lifelong critical learning to continuously improve practice.

changed surgical training and remains the foundation of all the residency system today (7).

Even before Halsted made his revolutionary changes in the education of young surgeons, there were other changes in medical education that were fundamental and necessary to allow the concept of the defined residency to develop. Welch had implemented controversial and even more revolutionary changes for the selection and education of medical students. For the new Johns Hopkins School of Medicine, of which Welch was the dean, a college degree was required; a limited number of students were chosen by competition; women were allowed to compete for positions equally with men; a student's progress was assessed by regular examination; and competence to practice medicine was verified at the time of graduation. All these requirements were rejected initially by most medical educators of the day. Osler implemented a suggestion made by Sydenham 100 years earlier to take teaching to the bedside and require practical experience with patients as a part of the medical school curriculum. Surgical training at this time was ill-defined. It might be a short period of observation or it might be indentured servitude at the whim of the professor. There was no specified content, and surgical experience was not necessary. The great professors of surgery often operated in amphitheaters with hundreds of observers. There was no certainty that a young surgeon completing training had ever done an operation of any kind. The public was understandably apprehensive about contacts with young physicians.

The Halsted principles for surgical training began with a fixed period of time during which

that training would occur. A small number of residents were chosen competitively to be trained, and the content of what they would be expected to learn was defined. The training was directly with patients, and patient care was based on an escalating schedule of responsibilities. Surgical skills were taught rigorously. At the end of formal training, a year of supervised independent practice was required.

It is of interest to note that Halsted believed that students and surgical residents should obtain all the fundamental skills of tissue handling, instrument control, and knot tying in the laboratory before they were allowed to come to the operating room, even as assistants. An extensive operative experience was a required part of the training.

In 1901, the final component of the Halsted residency was put in place with the foundation of The Hunterian Laboratory. The first director of the laboratory was Harvey Cushing, and it appears probable that Cushing's decision to return to Johns Hopkins after his year with Kocher in Bern was predicated on the directorship of this laboratory. Cushing and Halsted developed the current concept of the clinician/scientist. Cushing himself was the prototype, and Walter Dandy was one of the earliest products of this system of required research experience in the course of medical school and residency. Learning to do research is now a part of nearly every residency training program in the world.

The fundamentals of the Halsted residency were adopted widely and postgraduate medical education changed from preceptorship to a highly regulated system. Determination of competence of trainees was still the purview of the training chief and solely a matter of that chief's opinion. Concerns over competence led next to the board certification movement. The various specialties developed combinations of oral and written examinations, frequently coupled with practice review. Successful completion of the examinations was one assurance to patients that the individual was competent in the opinion of a peer group. In parallel with the board movement, the residency review concept developed through the sponsorship of several national organizations. The board examination was designed to determine the abilities of an individual. The residency review established minimum criteria for training and examined training programs and their ability to meet the minimum criteria. While these two adjuncts to training are extremely important, there has been no change in the fundamental structure of residency training introduced by Halsted 100 years ago (7).

THE PHILOSOPHY OF EDUCATION AND LEARNING

Acquisition of Skills and Knowledge

The residency as the fundamental process for postgraduate medical education in clinical areas was introduced at a time of enormous change in American education (5). The *progressive education* theory, introduced by Hall and popularized by Dewey, minimized the value of learning a corpus of material and emphasized the forms of thinking (4). Since we are all a product of progressive education, it is not surprising that we generally believe (without evidence) that exposure alone produces a framework by which to think about and analyze problems. This is most evident in resident training in the ongoing belief that one learns to think through exposure to research and science. This is contrary to data that indicates that scientists think no more rationally on subjects outside their specific research interests than does the general population (2).

The lecture has been the fundamental tool of postgraduate medical education in the clinical areas for many years. Most residents equate the didactic program with lecture. By contrast the seminar has been the fundamental tool in postgraduate scientific training. There is good evidence that learning is retarded by formal lectures and that adherence to a defined *pedagogical* learning form produces information that will be outdated within 5 years. Adult education, which is also correctly termed *androgological*, holds that student and teacher learn together in open forum and that the habit of lifelong learning is instilled in the student. In such a system, the student is the teacher and requires only guidance and explanation from the professors (1, 9, 10).

Much has been learned in the past century about the ways people acquire and use knowledge. An important issue is learning style. The population is divided into two equal groups with a small minority constituting the third general group of learning styles. Some are *topic learners*. That is, they acquire knowledge best by examining a topic from beginning to end and then going on to another topic. They synthesize the separate topics independently. Another large group learns best in *random* fashion. That is, they may study some part of any topic, then move to another topic, and later synthesize the topics themselves independently. A small group of people have what is termed an *omnivorous* style. These individuals usually try to learn everything without weighing importance or regard for relevance. No one of these techniques has proven to be better than another and opportunities for all should be included in the didactic portions of all training programs (3).

The application of knowledge is another issue which has been studied extensively (6). The formulations of Rasmussen are particularly germane to neurosurgery, though they have been applied most extensively to military decision making (12, 13). The parallels are obvious. Rasmussen has theorized that there are three basic phases of knowledge acquisition and application. The first he terms the *skills* phase; the second, the *rules* phase; and the third, the *knowledge-based* phase. The *skills* phase occurs when the neophyte first acquires technical knowledge and manual skills, while the appropriate application of the knowledge and techniques often are well beyond their understanding. Clearly, this is true for the young surgeon who often can do surgical manipulations under supervision without fully understanding when and why they are applied. Acquisition of these skills is critical, for without them it is not possible to progress in the field. The second phase is termed *rules-based*. In this stage, the trainee has enough information and experience to follow algorithms of rules that will lead to the desired result most of the time. Generally, these rules will be applied to all situations and there is no individualization on a case by case basis. The individual may not understand the situation fully, but comprehends the principles well enough to recognize what rules are to be applied. At some undefined point some people move from the *rules* phase to *knowledge-based* practice. No all do. In this phase, each individual situation is recognized, analyzed, and correct decisions are made without following a sequence of rules. There is strong evidence that most great clinicians practice in this mode (6). They are a minority, and, unfortunately, no one knows how the transition is made from following the rules to independent judgments. It is not surprising that there is no certainty how one can be taught to make knowledge-based judgments. It is clear that the transition requires a broad base of knowledge and experience.

There are a number of other theoretical formulations of how people acquire and use knowledge. The important issue is not that one or another is correct or best for neurosurgery. What is important is that this kind of educational information be incorporated into training programs in a rational way and that the impact of utilizing information theory be examined in the training process.

Changes in Training in the Twenty First Century

Three issues stand out as the most important which confront those responsible for neurosurgery training in the next century. These issues, which are manpower needs, parsimonious use of time in training, and verification of competence, are key training questions. The question of *manpower* can be reduced to: How many neurosurgeons do we need and for what purposes? Other important questions for training design must also be answered. What is the most *efficient training* for neurosurgeons? What do neurosurgeons need to know and how long should it take them to learn it? How is competence related to knowledge and how is each verified? The next logical issue is how to ensure the *lifelong acquisition of knowledge* and improvement of practice. Finally, the issue of *verification of outcome* as a measure of competence must be confronted.

There is an assumption implicit in these questions and their answers, which may not be obvious, but must be understood. That is, the training process is not limited to the formal requirements of residency, but rather is a lifelong process that never ends for the duration of practice. And the responsibilities of the training program should not end either.

Manpower Requirements

One of the important issues facing neursourgery as a whole and all program directors is: How many neurosurgeons are needed to serve the health needs of the nation and the academic requirements that go with those needs? None of the manpower requirement schema currently available is likely to be correct. All have flaws, even as regards the provision of health care, and none takes into account the manpower needs for education and the generation of new knowledge. There is an urgent need for manpower assessments in neurosurgery that take these needs into account.

There are three categories of practitioners of neurosurgery, whose programs of training have to be significantly different. One reason that manpower needs must be considered in the assessment of changes in our training programs is that the cost of training will become an important issue. We cannot afford to spend the amount of money required to train a significant surplus of neurosurgeons. An individual who plans on a research career in an academic institution needs substantially more training than is required to be a competent practitioner of neurosurgery. The committed academician needs to learn how to teach, how to administer, and how to conduct and report research. It is unnecessarily expensive to give residents extensive training in areas that will never again be a part of their practice. A fundamental change in training philosophy, which should be incorporated into training programs, is to individualize the training according to the aspirations and needs of the individual trainee.

Clinical Practice of Neurosurgery

Evidence from board examinations indicates there is a reasonable understanding of what is required to practice competent neurosurgery. The quality of neurosurgical care in the United States is very high. Even though the Bosk report figures on competency are disturbing, the percentages of questionable trainees and programs are low. As a profession, no deviation from a competency standard should be accepted, but the magnitude of the problem currently is not great. Current training generally produces competent clinicians. However, there are training issues that go well beyond minimum competency. The first is length of time in training. The current requirements were chosen arbitrarily and have never been validated as necessary. It is probable, if not certain, that residents can gain all the fundamentals of clinical neurosurgery in a substantially shorter time than current training programs require. This theme will be developed in the discussions of the competency-based training program.

Another important issue is research training for clinical neurosurgeons. It is an article of quasi-religious faith among academic neurosurgeons that research training is good for residents and teaches them how to think. This is a relic of our progressive education. There is no evidence that individuals learn to read and think critically or apply the scientific method through experience in research. Most objective data indicate they do not. If teaching critical reading, assessment of data, and critical thinking is the aim, then that should be done directly—not indirectly through expensive research experiences, which will never be applied again in the individual's career. Basic research training should be restricted to those who will apply these techniques in a research-oriented career. Practicing clinicians need to understand principles of clinical research and how new procedures are correctly introduced into medicine in order to assess new information and use it properly in patient care. Exposure to the details of good clinical research may be helpful, though there is no objective data which says it is.

Clinical neurosurgeons should be trained to do clinical neurosurgery, and this training can probably be accomplished in a substantially shorter period of time than is currently required.

Academic Neurosurgery

Training needs for those committed to an academic career are significantly different. Clinical skills must be equivalent, but the academic surgeon needs research and teaching qualifications that are not required for the general practice of neurosurgery. A very small group of individuals will apply basic research techniques to neurosurgical problems. An M.D./Ph.D. program or its equivalent is important if these few are to be competitive researchers. They are an extremely valuable group, for they can do things that no other basic researchers can do. Traditionally, the number of such individuals in neurosurgery has been very small. Emphasis should be placed on the importance of those who can study neurosurgical disease with basic science tools, and the number should be increased.

The majority of academicians are more likely to be involved in clinical research. In addition to clinical training they will need biostatistics, epidemiology, and study design. A Masters Program in Public Health or its equivalent seems an excellent way for them to become competitive researchers. All academic neurosurgeons need to learn to teach, to think and read critically, and to write effectively.

Critical analysis of data and the techniques for incorporating new data into practice are extremely important issues for all practicing neurosurgeons. There is little or no evidence that these

qualities are learned through a brief unstructured research experience. It is, therefore, important that they be added to the didactic portion of the clinical years for all trainees.

The ideal training program of the future will begin with an intensive clinical education in which the trainee learns to care for patients and do surgery. A core curriculum of applied basic science and an understanding of the principles of clinical research must be integrated. Research experience of 2 or more years at the level of Master's degree will be important for those who will do clinical research in an academic atmosphere, and a basic research experience at the level of Ph.D. will be necessary for those who wish to be competitive researchers with basic techniques. We cannot afford the luxury of adding several years of training to our programs in research disciplines that will not have relevance to the practice and career of the individuals in training. Research training should be limited to those who will use it throughout their careers.

The Competency-Based Residency Training Program

Competency-based training is founded on the theory of continuous improvement in quality in which it is assumed even the best can be made better (1). By quantifying and guaranteeing competence (insofar as it is possible to do so), both students and teachers are reinforced in their opinion of their own abilities or the abilities of their students (8). Verification begins with written record that details experience. By focusing on competency rather than length of training, we can determine how long it actually takes bright young people to gain the skills needed in the practice of neurosurgery. While incompetency is not a major issue in neurosurgery, and elimination of incompetents/incompetence not the goal of the competency-based residency, the cumulative effects of such training will be to reduce that small group in whom competency was questioned to zero.

In order to improve on current residency training, the experience required before one can practice neurosurgery efficiently and well must be considered. Data is not available to allow an answer now for any individual procedure. The periods of training chosen by the various boards are arbitrary and based only on expert opinion. Individuals may vary in the speed with which they acquire skills. There are enormous differences between training programs, both in numbers of patients and procedures which are done, and in the rapidity with which residents are allowed to do them. Few programs retain the year of supervised practice advocated by Halsted. While variation is a good thing, and any attempt to completely standardize our training programs should certainly be resisted, it is probable that current variations in both opportunity and experience within specific programs should be addressed. The standards, which are the minimum experience required, should be determined, and then mastery of the skills within those standards defined. Current board certification assumes that, if a training program has any specific experience available, the trainee has experienced it. The issue of competency is left to the program director. Further, it is assumed that if the board examination is passed, then that individual is capable of carrying out all current neurosurgical procedures and learning all new ones without further concern from the training program or the Board. In practice these contentions are probably largely true, but no data exist to prove them. As the regulation of medicine increases and competition between physicians escalates, it will be necessary to prove the competency of training and reasonable standards of outcome. Establishing the criteria for both is a valid goal of neurosurgical education now.

Competency-Based Training at Johns Hopkins

Undoubtedly there are many ways to verify competency during training. After several years of discussion, the residents and staff at Johns Hopkins together have devised a program that we consider a beginning in competency-based training. The goals are straightforward: (a) to verify the skills needed to perform a specific intervention have been learned, (b) to be certain the resident has experienced all of the subspecialty areas available to them, (c) to assure the resident has acquired the knowledge essential to the skills, (d) to enfold within the residency program subspecialized interests individual to each resident, (e) to provide a variable research experience tailored to the aspirations of each resident.

Implicit in the design is the assumption that residents will gain these skills at different rates and will proceed through levels of responsibility and independence as allowed by their skills

rather than according to a predetermined time table. Since the Board requirements currently are fixed, any time saved is used for the enfolding of additional subspecialization experience.

Verification of Experience and Competence

In order to verify that necessary skills were being acquired, we first created lists of knowledge and skills needed during training in its current time format of rotations. Thus, lists of the information and techniques that should be learned during internship, junior residency, senior residency, and chief residency were created and collated. We asked interns and residents at each stage to list the skills they thought they needed and the sequence during the year in which they should be acquired. We did the same for the clinical information needed to diagnose, understand, and manage typical neurosurgical problems. Once the lists were collated, we decided on a final order and defined the content of the composite lists. We then developed a final list that outlined for the trainees what specific information they are expected to learn in sequence, the skills they are expected to acquire, and the loose order that their peers have thought best for that acquisition. It is then the responsibility of the trainee to be certain that the necessary reading is done and that he or she participates in enough of the requisite procedures to become experienced. It is the responsibility of the staff to be certain the trainees have the opportunities to participate.

Some of the skills are straightforward; lumbar puncture, central line placement, ventriculostomy are examples. In the operating room, procedures may be broken into more complex component parts for the purposes of record keeping. For instance, our sequence in laminectomy and related procedures is: (a) closing the incision, (b) opening the incision, and (c) completing the laminectomy. All other operations are divided into similar components. The residents are expected to keep a list of these composite procedures that they have accomplished. When the resident feels satisfied that the skills to do the component part of the operation have been achieved, at least two staff members are asked to verify this by signing the list of procedures. Then the resident is assumed competent to do the procedure independently within the supervisory framework of the training program. Of course, no truly independent practice is allowed until the final year of supervised practice.

The verification process has several values. Since the residents know that they must become competent in all of the areas we have decided are important in neurosurgical training, their participation in all procedures is guaranteed. They cannot participate exclusively in those things they prefer to do. At least two staff members and the chief must agree that the resident is competent in a given portion of a procedure in order for them to proceed to the next part. There are no time requirements. A trainee can be certified as proficient as rapidly as competency is demonstrated. Residents can progress at very different rates. In the recent past, we have had one first-year resident opening and exposing posterior fossa tumors at a time when another was still working on closure of craniotomy.

We have completed a trial year in which the concept was introduced into residency training. The most obvious immediate effect has been escalation of the acquisition of skills to independence in the operating room. Residents in the program estimate that operating room responsibilities have escalated by one full year. The expansion of experience is also obvious. We are now assured that the trainees experience everything potentially available in the program.

Competency in Research Training in the Neurosciences

The days of 1 year in the laboratory to learn to do research are over. The current board recommendation of a single year may provide rest and recreation with some study time, but has little else to recommend it. There is no valid evidence that one learns to think because of an exposure to science or that the thought processes used in the laboratory transfer to clinical practice (6). This is a myth of progressive education, which has never been validated. The neurosurgeon who wishes to pursue a career in basic or clinical research must compete with those who devote near full time to a research career and have spent years training for that career; a neurosurgeon cannot successfully compete without comparable research training experience. The cost of adding a year or more of training in neurosurgery residency is considerable. It is probable that training programs will not have the luxury of spending time on laboratory efforts that

will not be central to the eventual career of the individuals being trained, even if they wish to do so.

A small number of individuals who seem likely to pursue a research career will have to be identified by competition. This concept is similar to current M.D./Ph.D. programs in medical school. These individuals should be trained in laboratories with track records that makes it likely that their trainees will be successful and will continue in academic practice. Criteria for laboratory training should be defined as stringently as clinical training is defined, and the 10% of neurosurgeons who will pursue thematic basic research should be directed to those institutions. Clinical research requires equally rigorous training. There are probably even fewer places where outstanding training programs in clinical research exist. They certainly can be identified, since most are with schools of public health, and the larger number of trainees who are likely to carry out high quality clinical research can be directed to them.

If an obligatory year of research is to continue as a part of neurosurgical training, it probably should be a focused experience in clinical research, which also teaches critical reading, data analysis, and how to judge the validity of published claims. An obligatory year might also serve as a catalyst for some to seek serious research training. It is unlikely that a year of laboratory research can be justified for all in order to discover the small number who will continue in a thematic research career. Discovering those individuals and optimizing their training is a serious challenge to neurosurgical educators.

Implications of Regionalization of Tertiary Care

The current reorganization of health care delivery emphasizes diffusion of primary care, reduction in specialty consultation, and emphasis on outpatient and satellite services for things that have traditionally been done in major hospitals. Evidence is accumulating that the response for neurosurgery should be regionalization of services and subspecialization. There are a number of reasons for this, which are well beyond the scope of this presentation. They include the enormous cost of doing neurosurgery today. Immediate access to magnetic resonance imaging, CT, portable CT, and the latest in angiographic techniques are all required. Specialized anesthesia, intensive care, and operating rooms are important for virtually all kinds of intracranial surgery. Equipment in operating rooms, including operating microscope, navigational system, ultrasound, and ultrasonic dissectors and lasers may cost millions of dollars. It is unlikely that duplication of this equipment in multiple institutions can be continued in any region, when utilization is partial in all.

Solomon has demonstrated that experience and volume are major determinants of outcome in aneurysm surgery and management of subarachnoid hemorrhage (14). Sung and collaborating vascular surgeons have made the same findings at Johns Hopkins (In preparation) (Sung). Comparing results of the most experienced vascular surgeons in the state operating at one institution with all other hospitals in the state, they demonstrate reductions in mortality and substantially lower cost for aneurysm surgery. The improvement and cost reduction was most striking in the best grade patients. Long and Brem have examined craniotomy for tumors in the same way (In preparation) Long & Brem. They studied outcome for benign and malignant intrinsic tumors, brain metastases, pituitary and related tumors, and all other benign tumors in Maryland. Approximately $\frac{1}{3}$ of all craniotomies were done in a single institution. Mortality of craniotomy was $\frac{1}{2}$ to $\frac{1}{4}$ of the state average and costs were 15 to 20% less.

These data strongly suggest that higher volumes and greater expertise have accompanying improvements in outcome and cost for patients undergoing craniotomy. In the Johns Hopkins model, the hospital facilities are used by a number of neurosurgeons whose primary practice is in other hospitals in the region. Even though severity index studies indicate that these surgeons bring their most complicated procedures to Johns Hopkins, their outcomes are still better than those they achieve in smaller primary- and secondary-care hospitals. These data lead to the conclusion that outcomes could be improved by regionalization.

The implications for residency training are very important. Surgeons, hospitals, and institutions may be in direct competition based on outcome. If outcome data are rigorously applied by those responsible for health care costs, it may mean substantial redistribution of patients, which could have significant influence on training. Concentration of patients in a few regional-

TABLE 10.2
The Residency Training Program of the Future

1. Core institution
   plus
2. Shared regional facilities
3. Affiliated secondary hospitals
4. Office practices
5. Consortia of hospitals for subspecialty experience
6. Affiliates for research training:
   Basic
   Clinical

ized centers could mean reduced experience in some programs and excessive exposure to complex problems in others. One way to approach this problem is to regionalize training with consortia of institutions rather than the current independent training programs.

Conversely, there is no need for the highly specialized facilities required for craniotomy, management of trauma, and management of subarachnoid hemorrhage for many patients in the every day practice of neurosurgery. Improvements in anesthesia mean that simple discectomy, which is the most common neurosurgical operation, can be carried out on an outpatient basis or with minimal hospitalization. Most cervical surgery requires only a little more hospital observation postoperatively and that only until the patient's well being is assured. Even cervical and lumbar laminectomy patients rarely need intensive care. The requirements for the major spinal reconstructive operations are different, but still not as complex as required for craniotomy. Cost considerations may force such patients out of neurological regional centers into their own centers of specialization. Either the centers must develop several cost classes of patient facilities or some operations will have to be done in less expensive hospitals. This means that for trainees to be adequately exposed to the most common operations in neurosurgery, they may have to leave a parent institution and obtain this experience in smaller surrounding hospitals. This will require a major paradigm change for current requirements of the American Board of Neurological Surgery and the Residency Review Committee. The traditional town-gown dichotomy may become very blurred. (Table 10.2).

SUMMARY AND RECOMMENDATIONS

Much of what has been said in this chapter will be opposed by many neurosurgical educators. Nevertheless, these are issues that all in academic neurosurgery must address. The core points of the argument are these.

Manpower studies are needed, which are related to the health needs of the nation for patients with neurological disease, to determine in a rational, intelligent fashion, how many neurosurgeons are required to serve these needs. Training programs must then be tailored to create this number of trainees, with some margin for error.

An equally rigorous examination of the needs for academic neurosurgeons is needed, and assurance must be made that an appropriate number are available to continue required research and teaching.

The educational fundamentals of neurosurgical training must be examined and academicians taught to teach more effectively.

The time requirements of neurosurgical training programs should be examined and programs should move from the century-old concept of specific rotations and exposures to proof of competency through education. This concept is true both for individual trainees and for training programs.

In doing so, the length of time required for training must be examined and programs arranged so that they lead to competency, rather than completion of required times. It is probable that the clinical education of a neurosurgeon can be reduced; and, if time is not reduced, experience can be expanded. (Tables 10.3, 10.4).

The research training in residency programs must be reexamined, tailoring the research experience to national needs and the aspiration of individuals. The costs of indiscriminate research training are too great to allow the luxury of years of never-to-be-utilized research experience.

It is probable that complex neurosurgical procedures will be regionalized into a much smaller number of tertiary centers than now exist. This implies, either or both, increased cooperation be-

tween programs and regionalization of training. Rather than focusing training in a single institution, it is probable that several training programs may need to use a single regional facility for complex intracranial disease and that residents will have to go to office practices and primary or secondary hospitals to experience patients with less complex diseases. Traditional differences between private and academic facilities are likely to be blurred.

The goal of any educational process is first to impart a required body of knowledge and, then, to inculcate the principle of lifelong learning. Educators must be responsible for the quality of care delivered by trainees throughout the entire course of their practice. Training programs must assure that competency in all aspects of neurosurgery is achieved during training and that this competency is maintained for the practice life of the individual. Proof of outcome is going to be required for comparison of institutions and individuals. If well done, determination and comparison of outcomes should lead to cooperation and education. If poorly managed, use of outcomes may lead to destructive competition.

The goal of neurosurgical educators has to be lifelong continuous improvement in the competency of trainees in all phases of practice. This alone is a huge evolutionary step in medical education.

The concept that outcomes will be continuously reviewed throughout practice by any mechanism is revolutionary also. Training will not end with the residency. Nor will the responsibility of the training program. Steps should be taken now to create the ideal training program for the future, rather than to allow uncontrolled events to shape and misshape neurosurgical education in the next century (11).

TABLE 10.4
Training for Academic Neurosurgery Practice

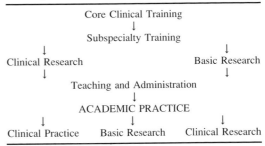

| Core Clinical Training |
| ↓ |
| Subspecialty Training |

| Clinical Research | | Basic Research |
| ↓ | | ↓ |
| Teaching and Administration |
| ↓ |
| ACADEMIC PRACTICE |
| Clinical Practice | Basic Research | Clinical Research |

TABLE 10.3
Clinical Training for Neurosurgery Practice

Core Clinical Training
↓
Specialty Training
↓
Critical Readings and Data Review
Practice Management
↓
PRACTICE

All of these socioeconomic factors, such as regionalization and subspecialization, competition based on outcomes, restriction of specialty trainees, and verification of specific experience for certification, will not develop simultaneously. It may take 5 to 10 years of unequal expression to see them all. There is time to improve neurosurgical education to meet these many challenges. The most important tenet of the next evolutionary phase of neurosurgical training must be assurance of competence in the care of neurosurgical patients.

REFERENCES

1. Adapting Clinical Medical Education to the Needs of Today and Tomorrow. New York: Josiah H. Macy, Jr. Foundation, 1988.
2. Anderson JR, ed. Cognitive Skills and Their Acquisition. Erlbaum, New Jersey: 1981.
3. Blum BI, Sigilliot VG. An expert system for designing information systems. Johns Hopkins APL Technical Digest 1986;7(1):23-31.
4. Dewey J, Dewey E. The schools of tomorrow. New York: Dutton, 1915.
5. Eliot CW. Report of the Committee of Ten on secondary school studies, Washington, DC: Government Printing Office, 1893.
6. Hamill BW and Stewart RI. Modeling the acquisition and representation of knowledge for distributed tactical decision making. Johns Hopkins APL Technical Digest 1986;17(1):31-38.
7. Long DM: Educating neurosurgeons for the 21st century. Neurosurg Q 1996;6(2), 78-88.
8. Hart I, Harden RM, eds. Further developments in assessing clinical competence. Montreal: Can-Heal, 1987.
9. Muller SM, ed. Physicians for the twenty-first century: Report of the Project Panel on the general professional education of the physician and college preparation for medicine. Part 2. J Med Educ 1984;59.
10. Muller S. Wilhelm von Humboldt and the university in the United States. Johns Hopkins APL Technical Digest 1985;6(3):253-256.
11. National Commission on Excellence in Education. A nation at risk: The imperative for educational reform. Washington DC: Government Printing Office, 1983.
12. Rasmussen J. Skills, rules, knowledge: Signals, signs and symbols and other distinctions in human performance models. IEEE Trans Systems, Man and Cybernetics 1983;123:257-66.
13. Rasmussen J, Lind M. A model of human decision making in complex systems and its use for design of system control strategies. Riso-M-2349. Roskilde, Denmark: Riso National Laboratory Report, April, 1982.
14. Solomon RA, Mayer SA, Tarmey JJ. Relationship between the volume of craniotomies for cerebral aneurysm performed at the New York state hospitals and in-hospital mortality. Stroke 1996;27:13–17.
15. Williams RG, et al. Direct, standardized assessment of clinical competence. Med Educ 1987;21:482-489.

CHAPTER 11

The Reformation of Biomedical Research: Influence of the Market and Society

WILLIAM H. BROOKS, M.D., THOMAS L. ROSZMAN, Ph.D.

INTRODUCTION

Generalization of rights in a democratic society, the obligation of the state to assure these rights and the recognition that these entitlements place a fiduciary and fiscal demand on all its citizenry provides the stage on which reform of health care is enacted. According to a former under secretary of the Department of Health, Education and Welfare (HEW), ''In the past, decisions on health-care delivery were largely professional ones. Now the decisions will be largely political'' (1). Polemics concerning an obligation to reform health-care services emerged from two poles of societal concerns: social-democratic and cost. As the expenditures associated with health-care services increased, the initial, coequal concerns of health-care politics and reform tilted away from redistribution (to achieve equity of access) to market concerns about efficiency and cost containment. The discussions of health-care delivery generally have shifted toward who will pay how much rather than who will receive how much.

Science as a socially constructed endeavor is not immune to the consequences of policies designed to reform health-care and health-related services (2, 3). Application of market principles to health-related research demands a definition of cost-effectiveness and value in the context of scientific observation and discovery. Scientific investigation, set in a politicized, market-determined, and economically discursive field, is not easily recoverable in the modern discourse of biomedical research where patients become clients or consumers, therapeutic advances are commodities, and the ideas and conditions for research are evaluated as cost-effective. Accordingly, scientific knowledge, as defined by clinical research, is translated to value; expertise becomes commodity, and eligibility is reconstructed as consumer oriented. Reform of health-related research forces a shift in the collective scientist-physician by redefining this individual as a producer of a commodity about which the market will determine value, set cost and expenditures, and develop as ''needed.'' Thus, the trajectory for cost containment in health-care services undoubtedly will influence funding for basic science and clinical research in accordance with the concerns of the health-market.

Science and the potential of scientific knowledge always has effected greater changes in the imagination of the public than it has on the processes of the diseases that afflict them. Nevertheless, science, scientifically acquired knowledge, and scientifically based theories have been used as paradigms to provide a rationale for the founding of ''reality'' as well as for establishing the infrastructure of medically related research and health care. Concurrent with contributing to the elucidation of disease processes and translation to therapeutics, medically related science engenders complexity and specialization that tend to place knowledge remote from free access by a nonscientific laity. ''The less one could believe 'one's own eyes'—and the new world of science continually prompted that feeling—the more receptive one became to seeing the world through the eyes of those who claimed specialized, technical knowledge, validated by communities of their peers'' (4). These claims that the unaided and uneducated senses of the ''public'' are inadequate to understand the world of medicine and health-related issues provided the basis for the growth of an industry of health-related research directed and controlled solely by medical scientists and physicians.

At the end of the 20th century, scientific formulations of Entropy, Chaos, Organism, and the ''Uncertainty Principle'' have tended to lessen coherence to a linear scientific principle by which a hypothesis perceived may be established as universally and eternally valid (5). Whereas in ''earlier contexts . . . coherence . . . was construed either as a sign of an invisible hand at work, a spontaneous harmony of numerous individual acts, or as a sign of the operation of a nonarbitrary rational agency'' (6), at the close of this century, coherence is replaced by irreducible uncertainties, contingency and nonlinearity of scientific and social inquiry (5). The loss of adherence to a positivist approach to science and the acquisition of scientific knowledge is reflected also in the political and social trajectory toward a ''decline of coherence as a norm or an ideal of public action'' (6). Thus, according to Ezrahi, ''In a society . . . affected by . . . cognitive skepticism, coherence tends to stand for pretense, untenable claims of knowledge and authority, and the unacceptable exercise of power. Incoherence, by contrast, . . . indicates humility, a refusal to suppress subjectivity and diversity, the toleration of numerous notions of purpose, causation and reality'' (7). This rebuff to ''foundationalism,'' i.e., '' a faith in the human capacity to gain access to a permanent, timeless foundation for objective, context-free, certain knowledge'' (8), poses a challenge to the process of validation and valuation of biomedical research.

The insertion of perspectivism into the debates regarding reform policies makes the issues of societal needs and demands problematic. Saltman suggests that a participatory process in health care will require that citizens be empowered with ''real influence in budgetary and resource-allocation decisions'' (9) Inclusion of the public in decisions regarding the possible goals of scientific research calls into question the possibilities for the existence of a ''common'' direc-

tion of medically related research and supports a move to shift the discourse on nonmaterial issues such as science, technology, and the exercise of expert authority ''to closer critical, ethical, and political scrutiny'' (10). Such a societal trajectory threatens to extend beyond the advancements and distribution of health and health-care services to encompass the linguistics and relatedness of ''scientific fact making'' and ''societal importance'' itself (11, 12).

The fulfillment of the Enlightenment, founded on equal access to knowledge and truth, has been eclipsed by a social-democratization and pragmatic interpretation of how scientific knowledge is acquired, formulated and used. It is this interplay of how knowledge is constructed with the nonlinear principles of the ''new'' science exemplified by Uncertainty and/or Chaos Theory and restricted access to scientific ''facts'' by all educated, informed citizens that challenges the authority and autonomy of those involved in biomedical research (5). Too frequently, those involved in clinical research engage individuals as ''patient groups,'' signifying their subjects as ''the other,'' and design therapeutic protocols to support a presupposed conclusion of effectiveness. Preliminary observations are reported as demonstrations that, in turn, are held as scientific-fact by treating physicians. It is the loss of confidence in those who ''make'' rather than behold scientific-knowledge and the applicability of science-knowledge itself to health issues that a diversified society believes important that must be considered in the evolving definition of health-care research elicited by general reforms of health care.

The conjoined participation of knowledge-empowered communities (groups of individuals) and capital-empowered communities (federal and private) in the construction of medical research threatens the credibility of, and the trust in, those actually involved in basic and/or clinical experimentation. These contingencies provide for the possibility of a multiplication of pathways to establish credibility and a diversification of personnel involved in the acquisition and validation of scientific-knowledge beyond the highly credentialed. Thus, biomedical research is being drawn into industrial bureaucratic organizations and simultaneously reconstructed by prevailing social and political trajectories. These inextricable forces shaping reform of health care result in the abdication of authority and autonomy by scientist-physicians to the power of the state, institutions, pharmaceuticals, and the polity.

Social reforms manifestly are heterogeneous and dynamic; never decisive or wholly irreversible, they are redefined continually as a society evolves linguistically, structurally and scientifically. Reform of health care is no exception. It is not our intent to provide a definitive discussion of the effects that reform may have on the mode in which research will be conducted and/or interpreted. Rather our object is to review the genealogy of those conditions that have allowed for and/or demand a restructuring of basic and clinical biomedical research, to investigate the social influences that are becoming integral to health care and health-related research, and, lastly, to formulate questions that will require solution as the purpose of research is redefined and reconstructed by reforms in health care that are initiated by monetary limits and perspectivism. Answers to these questions should provide a framework for reconstructing the goals of research and should suggest strategies as to how they may be achieved in light of democratization and constraints of the market. These abridged questions include:

- What are the dynamics of the acquisition of scientific knowledge when science is scrutinized closely by funding agencies (federal and private) and special interest groups?
- What will be the impact of the "democratization of research" on the assessment of credibility and construction of belief about the specific aims of research and treatments?
- Should the social priority of science be the elucidation of a "scientific" basis for treatment design or access to rapidly developed treatments ?
- Who decides what treatment strategies to pursue or how to develop and evaluate treatment protocols?
- Does current, peer-reviewed "established science" produce the best results for society in the end?
- Precisely what does it mean that a treatment "works"?

ACADEMIC MEDICAL CENTERS IN THE MARKET PLACE

As academic medical centers (AMCs), driven primarily by concern for cost containment, move steadily into the era of managed care, it proves useful to reflect on the propelling forces. Such self reflection is useful if only to avoid the old adage that "those who ignore history are bound to repeat it." The genesis of the modern AMC can be traced to the Johns Hopkins model established in the early 1890s under the leadership of the medical dean, William Welch. Rather than implementing a British model of medical education where medical (basic) science was taught at universities (e.g., Oxford) and clinical training was obtained at urban hospitals located in such places as London, Welch decided on the Berlin model that joined the medical school and the teaching hospital. This remains the predominant structure of AMCs in this country, albeit with some important alterations. In addition to conjoining the medical school and the teaching hospital, the Berlin model was the harbinger of things to come in medical education. Prior to this, medical education, in the main, was chaotic, shoddy, unregulated, and unstructured—with differing views on human physiology and disease theory. This was beginning to change as the nation moved into the 20th century. Not only were advances rapidly occurring in medical sciences, particularly in bacteriology and immunology; the nation also was moving from the coal century to the oil century. Both of these events would have a profound influence on the development of American medicine and medical education.

The culmination of these events occurred in 1910 with the publication of the Flexner report. This report recommended curriculum reform in medical education that essentially remains unchanged today (13). Thus, medical education consists of preclinical or basic sciences followed by the clinical sciences. As hard as some medical school and well-meaning organizations have tried, a "better way" to educate medical students remains to be found. This, of course, is not meant to infer that AMCs have not changed since the Flexner report; obviously, they have changed dramatically. During the 1920s and 1930s, medical schools continued to be staffed by part-time clinical faculty where, except at a few schools, research was a modest endeavor. The AMC as we know it today is a post-World War II phenomenon. This growth and development of AMC was aided greatly by two events that occurred immediately after the war. The first was a report by Vannevar Bush entitled

"Science—The Endless Frontier" that originally was prepared for President Roosevelt but submitted to President Truman in 1945 (14). Bush outlined how the nation should support scientific research in the postwar years. From this came the founding of the National Science Foundation (1950) and the subsequent unparalleled growth of the National Institute of Health (NIH). The second major event was the passage by Congress of the Hill-Burton Act of 1946, which provided federal aid for hospital and medical school construction. These two events provided the infrastructure of the modern AMC. Growth of the AMC industry was enhanced significantly following the launching of Sputnik in 1957; the launch, which caught the nation unaware, led to an outcry for increases in federal funding for science. Less than a decade later, as part of the Great Society, the Johnson administration supported legislation creating Medicare and Medicaid (1965). President Nixon declared "war on cancer" in 1971. Collectively, these events resulted in profound changes in the composition and financing of AMCs. The number of clinical faculty increased dramatically as did the magnitude of the income generated by practice plans. The emphasis of the AMCs became diverted from academic pursuits of primary teaching and research to the generation of large individual incomes derived from clinical practice. During this period until the present, the NIH budget continually has increased in terms of constant dollars. It may well be that we can very soon look back on the last 50 years as the golden age of AMCs.

Managed care carries with it the threat of seriously impacting clinical and basic research in AMCs. These threats to medical research come from many quarters and are being taken seriously by faculty in AMC as well as by Congress. Fortunately, there remains strong support in Congress for generous increases in the NIH budget. When this is taken together with the fact that 50% of all NIH extramural research awards went to medical schools, which represented about 31% of total medical school revenues in the 1995 fiscal year, the importance of NIH support cannot go unappreciated (15). The question remains: How long will Congress continue to grant 6 to 7% increases in the NIH Budget? In addition to this support AMC receive significant monies from such agencies as the Agency for Health Care Policy and Research (AHCPR),

Medicare Direct Graduate Medical Education and Indirect Medical Education adjustments that totaled over $6 billion in 1996. When these monies are factored in with practice plan (approximately $8 billion in 1993) and hospital income as well as state support where applicable, AMCs become economic giants (16). There is little doubt that these monies have contributed to producing the greatest health-care and biomedical research systems in the world. Why then do we want to change it? The answer is simple—it costs too much! The way to fix the health-care industry equally is obvious. We need to offer quality care at affordable prices. To achieve this goal, it is probably not inappropriate to look at how the American automobile industry met the challenge of the Japanese automotive industry in the 1980s. The keys to overhauling the American automobile industry were to reduce labor costs, automate, improve efficiency, close plants, and at the same time, increase the quality of the product. This overhaul was carried out, but a high price was paid by the automobile workers and their unions. The same process will no doubt occur when managed care has fully penetrated the health-care market. But will the public be satisfied with the product and will those of us associated with AMCs like it?

As AMCs move into the next century, managed care has the potential to alter the character of these institutions to the same extent that the Flexner report did for medical education and the Bush report accomplished for medical research. Thus, many concerns are being voiced, and they include reduction in the time clinicians have to do research, the impact of various cost containment measures including reductions in Medicare and Medicaid, increased use of ambulatory care centers, decrease in practice plan income with a reduced ability to cross-subsidize other endeavors, and a decline in NIH research grant support garnered by clinical faculty. The latter is of particular concern because a panel of scientists appointed by the director of NIH to assess the status of clinical research in AMCs estimates that only 30% of the extramural NIH funding is devoted to this type of research (17). In 1996, a bill (H.R. 3587) was introduced in Congress "to amend the Public Service Act to provide additional support for and to expand clinical research." This "Clinical Research Enhancement Act" proposed to provide over $0.5 billion for support for General Clinical Research Centers

(GCRC), Clinical Career Enhancement Awards and Innovative Medical Science Awards. This bill will be reintroduced in the 105th Congress this year. Whether or not this registration is enacted, it confirms that Congress is well aware of the problems facing clinical research by AMCs and presently is willing to help rectify them. If this legislation is passed, these funds would be particularly welcome because the cross-subsidization of clinical research from practice plan income decreases and ultimately disappears.

SOCIETY AND THE RECONSTRUCTION OF BIOMEDICAL RESEARCH

Credibility and trust are the underpinnings of any scientific endeavor (18). However, recent concepts about how science-based knowledge accumulates in conjunction with a reinterpretation of the role of the polity in health-related issues have challenged these precepts as they might apply to biomedical research. Since the 1970s, the sociology of science has argued that "no scientific claim 'shines on its own light'–carries its credibility with it . . ." (19). Credibility becomes a relationship of power rather than neutral, dependent on objective reality and/or devoid of personal interpretations. That investigator whose rhetoric is most persuasive, who is "able to summon up the most compelling citations, and who is able to enlist more allies, patrons and supporters by 'translating' their interest.. [to] correspond with [her/his] own is the one who constructs credible knowledge and gains access to further resources as a result" (20). Therefore, health-related scientists and physicians seemingly "barter their credibility" by securing "external markers," e.g., publications, credentials, and "successfully" translating basic observations for use at the bedside. These investigators and physicians are rewarded by being cast in the venerable role of society's designated gatherers and constructionists of scientific knowledge to the extent that basic and clinical biomedical research is considered of value in improving health and health care. As the technological advances required for this function became increasingly opaque and obscure to the society-at-large, biomedical scientists became cloistered, enhancing their authority without corollary accountability. Thus, Pippen writes, "the growing sophistication of

science and technology, and the difficulties encountered by a lay public in understanding evidence, demonstrations, and the ambiguities and risks inherent in the pursuit of scientific research permit those involved in medical research to grow less accountable in traditional ways shielded by their claim to a greater technological knowledge" (21). This elitism is masked further by the perception that biomedical scientists are "neutral agents of instrumental public actions" (22) and by pronouncements of the public benefits of the ends to which technology can be employed.

Yet as discussed by Epstein, "The failure of experts to solve the problems of AIDS quickly, as they were 'supposed to,' has heightened popular resentment and sparked a 'credibility crisis'" (23). The failure of clinical science to fulfill its "Covenant with Society" also has been emphasized by Ahrens (24). The societal shift in trust seemingly is reinforced as technologies become increasingly sophisticated, influence and mediate more control over individuals, and themselves determine codes of behavior and action (25). It is not surprising that the multiplicity of advanced surgical techniques have resulted in the loss of conviction and unanimity among physicians as to what/which treatment is necessary or sufficient and what results are to be expected. Thus, society challenges an "executive approach" previously endorsed by biomedical researchers to protect their scientific authority and autonomy by seeking only peer-approval (26). Credibility and trust are suspect in a system in which individuals are signified as belonging to groups selected only by technologically driven solutions. This shift in the relations of power, trust, and technology, has produced further alienation of the citizenry from biomedical scientists and practitioners. Discourse is shifted now from questions of who has authority to act to questioning what actions can or should be authorized. To address this query, patients have organized into self-help and special-interest groups. These groups collect and exchange scientific, clinical, and narrative information and hence are well informed about particular illnesses, the validity of current treatments, and the directions and particular achievements of basic and clinical research. These educated citizens demand to be heard, to be listened to and to become instrumental in directing basic biomedical research and rapid translation into clinical practice. Current examples of this trajectory include AIDS, breast and prostate cancer-related research. These "activist" groups have had great success, according to Epstein, "in extending ... [their] ... critique of medical practice into an engagement with the methodologies of biomedical research" (27). This newly rediscovered power of healthy citizens and those with infirmity in collaboration with the power of the market poses a substantial political challenge to the biomedical community in regards to the substantiation of what treatments and scientific endeavors are valuable, appropriate and affordable. It is presupposed that the spontaneous interactions among these diverse groups, nonmedical with medical, can generate a system whose aggregate results will be socially beneficial to all citizens. Biomedical science thus becomes a socially constructed product as demonstrated by the proliferation of "new" institutes at the NIH, the "War on Cancer," and AIDS.

According to Sclove, "If citizens ought to be empowered to participate in determining their society's basic structure, and technologies are an important species of social structure, it follows that technological design and practice should be democratized" (28). It is precisely this movement, in conjunction with the radical transformation in theories and models of the "scientific method" and the demands of an informed, knowledgeable citizenry, that presupposes relevancy of the polity and democratization of health-related science in any discussion of a reformation of health care. This movement is not "anti-science." Confidence in scientifically acquired knowledge remains high (29). It is rather "pro-knowledge" and calls for equity in generation of health-related "facticity." It is a movement "to re-value forms of knowledge that professional science has excluded, rather than devalue scientific knowledge itself" (30). It is a notice served to those in biomedical research that the reliance on an authoritative, "depoliticized" scientific endeavor has resulted in certain social costs and created difficult ethical problems; therefore, the general framework within which health-related research takes place must be altered (31). It is a challenge to avert "The danger that public policy could ... become the captive of a scientific technological elite" (32).

Another socially constructed concept that engages movements of reform is the recent trend toward "the democratization of uniqueness" (33). This is perhaps the most instrumental concept in restructuring medical research. According to this view, each individual is a singular, autonomous, self-created entity, distinct from all others and is without social or political responsibility. This concept of "radical individualism" breaks from the traditional view of "liberal individualism" by rejecting the necessity or usefulness of coordinating "behavior voluntarily in the pursuit of shared social and political goals" (34). This may be summarized as not having one's way rather having a way that is one's own (35). Thus, radical individualism invites those individuals and groups marginalized by uncommon, incurable, and/or costly illnesses to demand immediate input to refocus health-related research toward their particular interests. These requests are not based on the "claim that they are 'like' all others [with commonly shared health-care concerns and needs] but rather they are 'different'" (36). Accordingly, health "is not a socially informed, fixed value, but something that can have a multitude of uniquely distinct meanings and therefore must be negotiated anew in each particular case" (37). Thus, a "trilemma" as to what circumstances constitute "fact," "validity," and "value" is created among socially constructed needs, radical individualist demands, and traditional scientific-medical authority. The result of this confrontation of a democratization of uniqueness with socially responsible democratization of science and market-derived principles is a fragmentation of public goals and of the demands made on scientific inquiry. Fragmentation within basic biomedical scientific research at the level of the larger polity reflects a direction most compatible with an equilibrium or mediocrity in scientific progress rather than with a direction toward amelioration of disease and improvements in health and health care. This tendency is further accentuated as the constraints of costs are applied to social and political goals accompanying reform considerations. Thus, the major focus of biomedical research may become micrological (individualistic) rather than macrological (societal)—the urgency of biomedical research becomes "valuable" as dictated by a democratization of uniqueness with its limited focus rather than conjointly determined by social democracy in science, and, ultimately, facts become relative and "for sale." If society puts money into a particular feeder, the scientists will flock to it!

Democratization of science frequently encourages short-term success at the expense of a wider and long-term view of the global importance of medical and scientific research. Increasingly, pressures are placed on the scientific and medical communities to make basic science readily and rapidly applicable to treatment, "to disengage the goal of advancing medical knowledge for the contest of treatment . . ." (38). Such a trend toward "contemporarization" of health-related research gives "rhetorical advantages to the instantly communicable over that which is communicated only in the course of a longer life span" (39). Long-term accountability of success, value, and the generation of scientific knowledge is sacrificed for the immediate applicability of technological possibilities. Thus, an extraordinary new role for medical technology has emerged in which health and health care are being modified to meet the needs of technological efficiency. As such, health and illnesses are depersonalized concurrent with the evolution of a "neo-technic" approach to medical care. This is exemplified by the increased prevalence of degenerative disc "disease" parallel to the development and availability of magnetic resonance imaging of the spine. Similarly, the frequent use of spinal instrumentation and other technologically driven modalities, e.g., percutaneous "laser-disectomy" for treatment of low back pain, without considerations of unsubstantiated effectiveness to alleviate pain, increase function, and positively influence the over all "quality of life" provides further strong evidence as to the immediate power of technology in determining "fact," "validity," and "value" in health care and health-care services. These technocratic tendencies, the trajectory toward a democratization of science and the continued redefinition of authority and autonomy of its practitioners, will call on scientists and physicians to reexamine their role in shaping medical services and to share with lay persons the processes of defining health-related issues, of shaping decisions regarding what strategies to use in achieving a solution and of deciding to what end these solutions may be implemented in the society. Redefining the orientation of medical research toward discovery of treatment modes rather than primarily toward generation of scientific knowledge aims to protect the integrity of the former from the long-term objects of the latter.

In this discourse, the narrative of the forces of market principles and democratic liberation that cross previously institutionalized boundaries restructures the various forms of power and authority and creates new freedoms and opportunities. However, in response to this discourse, a counternarrative may be evoked in which these new territories within the biomedical scientific community become themselves "reterritoralized" and institutionalized, thereby demanding a shift of policy in which more freedom is less, where research is encouraged and supported, yet focused by limited federal funding or by private companies. Thus, democratizing may promote equity, yet possess a dispiriting effect, i.e., "re-legitimation" rather than reform. Accordingly, new fields of authority are created and encounter limited resources of funding, thereby recasting biomedical research as a socially constructed, approved, and legitimate commodity. It is on this political map that the biomedical investigator must negotiate her/his way. The problem is not so much defining a political "position" (which means choosing from a preexisting set of possibilities no longer available in reform movements) but to imagine and to bring new schema of "politicization," thus to continue to advance medical science and health-care research simultaneously as a socially sensitive and scientific endeavor.

STRATEGIES, BIOMEDICAL RESEARCH, AND REFORM

The constraints placed on the acquisition of scientific knowledge by the marketplace and by the demands of an informed polity invite a reconstructionist view of biomedical research, of its components, of its goals, and those individuals and groups actively engaged. Elucidation of these features provide a framework for strategies that provide the conditions by which biomedical research can be reinvented in the context of monetary constraints and societal demands.

The Territorial Reconstruction of Biomedical Investigation

Biomedical science, according to Ahrens, is of very recent origin (24). This term linking biological and medical initially was coined in the post-World War II era as investigations of the biological effects of radiation from atomic bomb test sites were undertaken. However, in the context of a socially democratized science, a redefinition of health and health-care services is required. As conceptualized during the Enlightenment and Scientific Revolution of the 16th and 17th century, biomedical research might be considered as "pure." Accordingly, scientific-knowledge is believed to be "grounded in impersonal non-private reproducible procedures through which it can be certified by anyone who cares to do so, provided he has the competence and the patience" (40). The "purity" of science is guaranteed by its insulation from external pressures. However, as described above, the inclusion of alternative and multiple components as instrumental to the construction of scientific "fact" necessarily redefines biomedical science as "impure" (20, 41). As an informed polity representing a 'nonscientific' segment of society becomes more involved in influencing the goals, directions, and implementation of biomedically generated discoveries; the more "impure" research will become. More specifically, health-related research becomes increasingly "impure," as it is socially and linguistically reinterpreted by nonexpert laity and recast into a market-driven commodity in which exciting discoveries are valued as being cost-effective. Therefore, in redefining the function of biomedical science in the context of reforming health care in a society, one must consider the nexus of movements toward a democratization of science, the perspective of uniqueness, and cost constraints. Acceptance of the premise that health-related research will be altered by the instrumental interplay of scientific and nonscientific fields with market-oriented principles provides the basis for restructuring a geography of biomedical research. It is the redrawing of traditional territories of science that will determine where the specific modes of clinical research will be performed, that will dictate the educational requirements of those involved in biomedical research, and that will influence the allocation of monetary support.

The mission of the AMC is to perform teaching, patient care, and research. Although all these functions will be altered by managed care, biomedical research has the potential to be redefined the most because it is less amenable to cost analyses. There are three differing but overlapping types of research that AMCs perform—basic, translational, and clinical (patient-oriented clinical research). The majority of basic biomedical research that garners primary support from the NIH and/or the National Science Foundation is performed in preclinical departments. Traditionally, the trends in basic health-related research have been toward elucidation of the cellular and molecular basis of disease. Translational research, representing the confluence of basic research and patient-oriented research, results in direct utilization of knowledge gained from cellular and molecular studies in clinical paradigms. One example of translation research is tissues transplantation. Advances in major histocompatibility antigen typing and immunosuppressive modalities has made transplantation of a variety of different organs possible. Patient-driven research is more diversified, both in its approaches and its funding. However, the trend appears to be more toward "outcome studies" with funding coming from a variety of sources, including NIH, biotechnology and pharmaceutical companies, and managed care systems. At many AMCs, the amount of funded clinical research has decreased. This trend certainly will continue as managed care becomes more prevalent. Basic research will continue to the extent that sufficient funds, primarily from the NIH, are available. The outlook on continued increases in the NIH budget depends on a number of factors, not the least of which is a balanced budget. Currently, Congress considers NIH to be a "sacred cow" and is considering a 6.9% increase for the financial year 1997. There is even some discussion among members of Congress about doubling the NIH budget by the year 2002! This certainly would have a dramatic effect on the current success rate of new investigator generated research proposals, which presently is between 20 to 24%. Such increases in the NIH budget also could have a dramatic effect on translational and clinical research, particularly as more emphasis is diverted to funding these research efforts. Nevertheless, the evolving question to be resolved is whether there will be physicians involved in biomedical research at all, given the observation that only 45% of clinicians devote 20% or more of their time to scientific endeavors (42). An even more relevant number is the number of clinicians who devote 50% or more time to research—a number which is more consistent with active participation in biomedical research.

Patient-Oriented Clinical Research

The common ground for all patient-oriented clinical research (POCR) is the community-at large. It is within the community-based environment, as judged by an informed citizenry and purchasers, where basic biomedical research achieves value as therapeutically relevant to the modulation of disease, contributing to health in general, and contained within the constraints of cost. Health-related research in this milieu, according to C. R. Gaus, should be designed "to determine what works best in clinical practice; [to] encourage the cost-effective use of health-care resources; [to] help *consumers* [italics mine] make more informed choices; and measure and improve the quality of care" (43). Thus, the goals of POCR should be aimed at identifying those therapeutic modalities that positively influence the health of the individual citizen and can be maintained within the economic limits of the community-at-large. POCR necessarily is most appropriately accomplished within the community, using community-based hospitals, facilities, and physician-investigators. The AMCs are organized poorly to accomplish these goals and are better suited for the implementation of translational or basic biomedical research. It is an imperative that the collective and cooperative involvement of all concerned citizens, including physicians, nonexperts, patients, insurance companies, and managed-care organizations be encouraged as the specific aims of each new project are developed and methodologies of implementation determined. A template for construction of a geographic consortium to engage POCR trials suggested by the AHCPR focuses (*a*) on medical conditions that are common, costly, and associated with substantial variation in practice, and (*b*) on treatment modalities identified by groups for which evidence of effectiveness is incomplete or controversial (43). These clinical trials include quality and outcome-based assessments, epidemiologic and health services investigations, and evaluations of behavior modulation as related to prevention, as well as determining the efficacy of new treatments. Additional potential research initiatives now engaging POCR include an assessment of clinical performance and their relevance to improved quality of care (44, 45). These studies particularly are important as both purchasers and consumers demand accountability.

Any decision to initiate a clinical trial or to assess clinical practice is biased a priori, thereby indicating that the strategy in designing and implementing a POCR protocol is both complex and dubious (46–49). The bias results from the enthusiasm (or skepticism) of the physician-investigator and/or consumer-patient who is potentially impacted by the results of the project, from the pharmaceutical and technology company whose product is being evaluated and from the managed care organization and/or agency who must pay. Thus, the results of POCR studies should be publicized openly in popular as well as scientific venues, discussed and collectively judged before a treatment modality or strategy for altering access and performance becomes accepted as "valuable" by society-at-large. According to Parmar et al., most new treatments that have been tested for most diseases have been found to be ineffective or, at best, marginally effective, yet are championed by the medical establishment (50). Moreover, many POCR-related studies using the same procedure and/or in the same condition offer findings that are contradictory. Thus, the trick is to engage in POCR with therapeutic trials that are ethical, socially sensitive, and well designed "without reifying the method so as to suggest that such trials will provide degrees of certitude that they simply cannot do" (51).

Translational Biomedical Research

Advances in clinical medicine and biotechnology are dependent on the continued translation of information derived from basic biomedical research to therapeutic possibilities. Value in this discursive field is predicated principally on furthering the public good rather than on acquisition of proprietary or nonusable scientific information. It is the goal of translational research to rapidly recognize the applicability of new scientific discoveries to disease and to maximize the potential for implementation to improve society's health. Yet, translational research is an area of most concern as the discourse of reform redefines biomedical investigation. According to the AAMC (1995), only 5 to 7% of new faculty members [are] classified principally as translational research investigators who spent more than 50% of their time with clinical research (17). The effects of a decreasing number of investigators committed to translational research will be compounded as biomedical research in areas such as genetics and immunology accelerate and provide new avenues of potential therapeutic intervention. Additional factors of societal (consumer) demands and reduced funding sources join to threaten the future of translational research. These forces must confronted and reconstructed to ensure this research.

The formulation of General Clinical Research Centers (GCRCs) offers one model that incorporates the constrains of reform while fulfilling the goals of translational research and societal need (17). Formation of a network of regional GCRCs should provide a platform for conducting coordinated clinical research and accelerate the application of basic scientific discoveries to health and disease. This model offers a coordinated mechanism by which new and novel observations of basic biomedical research can be implemented and evaluated rapidly through phase I and phase II clinical trials. Furthermore, the rapidity and expertise required to develop and initiate these types of clinical studies demand ''centralization'' of translational research efforts within a system of designated and adequately funded institutions as opposed to the current status of decentralized research with its diminishing numbers of investigators, associated rising costs, and evolving cost constraints. Although these Clinical Centers may be ''freestanding'' or ''privatized'' in reference to governance and funding, it is paramount that all GCRCs be aligned closely with those elite AMCs that are consistent leaders and contributors to basic scientific and clinical research. These Clinical Centers, which serve as a ''national core of clinical research'' will be viable to the degree that they are funded adequately by biotechnology and pharmaceutical companies as well as by the federal government. The key to their success will be the merger of the market interests of biotechnology and pharmaceuticals with recent discoveries of basic science and the subsequent implementation of societally intriguing clinical protocols designed to met the demands of all.

Basic Biomedical Research

Basic biomedical research provides the infrastructure for all clinical research and potential improvements in the health of a society. Continuation of a vibrant and successful scientific effort is critical, not only from the perspective of improving health in general, but also for maintaining an international economic presence (17). Because its leadership role in biotechnology and biomedical science is so pivotal to the United States, basic biologic research must remain a top priority for federal support. Moreover, the ''neutrality,'' perceived or real, of federal funding of the basic life sciences avoids market-driven research in which the motivation of the individual is not necessarily social change but personal gain. In this manner, the social question of cost and expenditure once again reverts to attempts to identify a social solution to health and health care.

It is of value to examine more closely the basic biomedical research enterprise of AMCs as they now exist and to speculate on how they may look like in the not too distant future. The foundation of this enterprise is the basic research conducted primarily in the preclinical departments. For this discussion, basic scientists are defined as individuals who have doctorates, reside in preclinical departments (microbiology, pharmacology, biochemistry, etc.), and have no clinical obligations. Because there is a difference in how these departments and faculty are funded, particularly between private and public AMCs, we will investigate the University of Kentucky Medical Center as a representational model of a public institution engaged in medical education and research. The basic science departments have about 110 faculty whose salaries are fully funded by state funds (12-month appointments) and operate on a traditional ''7-year up or out'' tenure system which judges faculty on excellence in teaching, research, and service. There are an additional 3 to 5 administrative support positions per department whose salaries and benefits are derived from the state. Other than these monies, the remainder of the departmental funds for ''academic enrichment'' are derived solely from extramural grant support. The bulk of these funds come from indirect costs and salary reimbursement primarily associated with NIH grants. Thus, 10% of the total indirect costs received by the institution from NIH (approximately 48% of the award) and the salary reimbursements applied to these grants revert back to the departments. This sum approaches $300,000 to $500,000 per year. These monies are used to support the graduate program (about 20 students per department at $12,000 to $14,000 per year for each student), provide interim research support for faculty who are between grants, and provide for additional administrative functions, e.g., photocopying, shipping, postage, etc. Additional funds for ''start-up money'' for new faculty, matching funds for equipment and for interim research support may be obtained from the Dean or Vice-Chancellor for Research. The salaries of the basic scientists together with administrative support staff total about $10 million, which represents about 5% of the overall budget of the College of Medicine.

As managed care is implemented, it is inevitable that cost shifting will occur. For example, basic science faculty receiving federal funding may be asked to replace that portion of their state-based salary by NIH salary reimbursement. This could be implemented in several ways; the easiest of which is for the college to provide a reduced negotiated base salary with the remainder of the total salary derived from grant support. This is similar to that of clinicians who have a base salary supplemented by their clinical practice plan. Alternatively, all basic scientists at AMCs may be placed on 10-month appointments, similar to those faculty on the main campus, with the other 2 months of salary support coming from grant support when applicable. If such scenarios come to pass, it would have a dramatic effect on the monies available for academic enrichment in preclinical departments responsible for basic research. The loss of stipends for graduate students and interim research support for faculty between funding periods would limit continued postgraduate education and training as well as curtail the ability to pursuit a career in basic scientific research. The counternarrative holds that these cost constraints would abrogate the increasing numbers of students pursuing a Ph.D. in biological sciences in an uncertain job market that has resulted in many individuals being underemployed. This is not necessarily a problem unique to graduate education because the same events are occurring in many of the medical subspecialties where the market has become saturated.

The continued use of tenure to insure ''academic freedom'' is problematic and should be reinterpreted in the light of limited opportunities and projected curtailments of research funding, demands and obligations to society-at-large, and the necessity for the continued generation of young scientists. Is it cost efficient, or scientifically efficient, to maintain this system, given the constraints evoked by the market? Indeed, it may prove counterproductive to maintain tenured faculty who are unable to remain actively and competitively engaged in biomedical research in a research-oriented department. However, the research experience of these individuals should not be discarded; rather, it should be exploited to provide educational opportunities for students and information for nonmedical laity about the challenges and goals of biomedical science. These ''spokespersons'' should prove invaluable as the dialogue among those involved with health and health-care issues progresses in society.

Similar to the evolution of the principles establishing the GCRC, cost constraints imposed by reform of funding health care and related issues also urge a ''centralization'' of basic biomedical research. Current methodologies of funding basic research permit the diversion of diminishing federal funds to AMCs with no or poor records of productivity, insufficient numbers of investigators to provide an atmosphere conducive to scientific pursuits, and inadequate ancillary support required to successfully accomplish the goals of basic biomedical research. Granting awards to these institutions is an inappropriate use of health-care monies, particularly as budgetary constraints are imposed. Nevertheless, a restriction of funding must not restrain those individuals committed to basic biomedical investigation. The opportunity to become engaged in basic scientific research must be kept open to all qualified investigators, yet the locale for their efforts intrinsically must possess sufficient ''specific activity'' to assure a reasonable degree of certainty of fulfillment. It is interesting to note that 20 AMCs receive more than half of all the NIH funds awarded to the 124 AMCs in fiscal year 1996 (52). Comparing this list with that of fiscal year 1990 indicates that the same AMCs consistently appear among the top 20 research institutes. This is not a fortuitous occurrence, but, rather, it represents a rich tradition in research with a sustaining commitment for its support and maintenance. Interestingly, some of these AMCs have been moving toward the managed care delivery system with rather extensive health maintenance organizations (HMOs) or physician provider organizations (PPOs), yet have maintained their research competitiveness. Alternatively, the bottom 20 AMCs routinely garner less than 0.1% of NIH-awarded funding. This finding, in context with the fact that we may be training too many physicians and Ph.D.s, elicits the question: Do we need these 20 AMCs? Although we probably could do without them (and, thus, they should be closed), given regional politics, it is unlikely that this will occur.

Restricting funding for basic research to a limited number of AMCs will necessitate a reconstruction of the defining characteristics of AMCs. Do all AMCs need be involved in basic scientific research to accomplish their mission of educating health-care professionals? Do not the demands for advancements in biomedical research require exposure of students interested in pursuing a career in basic or translational research to "the best" researchers who typically are found in the "elite" AMCs? Some AMCs train better physicians than do other AMCs, which may be more successful in contributing to biomedical research. Both types of AMCs are necessary.

Educational Requirements for Reformed Biomedical Research

Medical education is not conceptually or practically designed to educate or train students to become research scientists. Although medical students are introduced to the scientific method during the first 2 years of medical school, by and large, they remain "scientistic," i.e., they believe they understand and appreciate scientific method; yet actually do not. They also have developed the "Dragnet Syndrome" ("Just give me the facts"). Unless students dedicate a year or two to postdoctoral fellowship training in biomedical-related research, they will join the AMC faculty or enter practice without any formal training in the scientific method and approach. This greatly hampers the ability to write grants that are hypothesis-driven and to perform research in a scientifically acceptable manner. Consequently in the current educational climate of AMCs, there are fewer clinicians who are capable, competitive, or have the desire to do basic or clinical research. As managed care makes greater inroads into the AMCs, clinical research is likely to diminish. Clinical investigators will have less time to perform research, and support for it by administrators may diminish as decreases in reimbursement call for increased productivity (volume) to maintain high clinical incomes. Additionally, translational research may become particularly vulnerable because it will be more cost effective to do outcome studies. Accordingly, the AMCs may become merely "medical centers," and a great era will have come to a close.

The goal of those AMCs successfully engaged in research should be to require additional postgraduate training for those wishing to pursue a career in biomedical research, while those AMCs less involved in basic or translational biomedical investigations may continue to train health-care providers to enter community practice. Those institutions aligned with managed care organizations and/or particularly interested in assessment of societal needs and outcomes of treatment must offer graduate programs specifically designed to address the economic, epidemiologic, and social issues of health and health care. Reformulation of the requirements and roles of postgraduate education for physicians and medical scientists holds the key to designing strategies for remaining competitive and successful in clinical and basic biomedical research.

Sources of Funding

Reformation of biomedical research necessarily requires a reconstruction and realignment of the sources of funding as discussed above. The NIH should continue to serve as the primary source for funding basic biomedical research. The link between biotechnology and pharmaceutical interests (private interests) and translational research is obvious. Managed care organizations should be looked to as a source for funding community-related research. Regardless of the funding agency, the key to procuring funding is education. The increasing demand by society in general and the nonmedical laity in particular to become instrumental in determining and clarifying health-related issues requires the opening of a dialogue among physicians, biomedical scientists, and the citizenry. Biomedical scientists must educate society about the relevancy of their particular research and strive to make obscure scientific observations understandable and exciting. The public, biotechnological or pharmaceutical companies, or a managed care organizations are much more likely to respond favorably to requests for biomedical research funding if their members are knowledgeable, interested, and engaged. Medical scientists, therefore, must view themselves as sponsored artisans rather than as authoritative aristocrats to whom society must pay its due.

SUMMARY

Our project has been to disentangle biomedical research from the current unfolding of reform in health care. To accomplish this goal, a new language is necessary, reconstructing relationships among physicians, scientists, and nonmedical laity; federal and private funding sources; and traditional venues of biomedical investigation. Remaining within the present parameters of discourse on health-related research based on authority and autonomy precludes the ability to understand the reformulation of biomedical research projects contingent on the instrumental and communicative characteristics of market and social paradigms. Biomedical authority is reinterpreted as stewardship; scientific autonomy is restructured in the context of democratization of science and individual uniqueness; and biotechnology and biomedical research emerges as socially responsive.

REFERENCES

1. Iglehart JK. Prepaid group medical practice emerges as likely federal approach to health care. Natl J 1971;3:1444.
2. Matherlee KR. The outlook for clinical research: Impacts of federal funding restraint and private sector reconfiguration. Acad Med 1995;70:1065-1072.
3. Genest J. Clinical research: Any future? Clin Invest Med 1993;16:237–246.
4. Starr P. The social transformation of American medicine. New York: Basic Books 1982, 19.
5. Best S, Kellner S. The postmodern turn. New York: Guilford Press. 1997. (in press)
6. Ezrahi Y. The descent of Icarus: Science and the transformation of contemporary society. Cambridge, MA: Harvard Univ Press 1990, 283.
7. Ezrahi Y. The descent of Icarus: Science and the transformation of contemporary society. Cambridge, MA: Harvard Univ Press 1990, 284.
8. Marx L. The idea of ''technology'' and postmodern pessimism. In: Technology, pessimism and postmodernism. Ezrahi Y et al., eds. Amherst: Univ Mass Press, 1984:11–28.
9. Saltman RB. Patient choice and patient empowerment in northern European health systems: A conceptual framework. Int J Health Serv 1994;24:201–229.
10. Singer MA. Community participation in health care decision making: Is it feasible? Can Med Assoc J 1995; 153:421–424.
11. Ezrahi Y. The descent of Icarus: Science and the transformation of contemporary society. Cambridge, MA: Harvard Univ Press 1990, 262–282.
12. Jasanoff S. Beyond epistemology: Relativism and engagement in the politics of science. Soc Studies Sci 1996;26:393–418.
13. Flexner A. Medical education in the United Sates and Canada, Bulletin no. 4. New York: Carnegie Foundation of the Advancement of Teaching, 1910.
14. Bush V. Science—The endless frontier: A report to the President on a program for postwar scientific research. Washington, DC: GPO, 1945.
15. Moore DB. What the 105th Congress portends for academic medicine. Acad Physician Scientist 1997;3:8.
16. The financing of medical schools. A report of the AAMC Task Force on Medical School Financing. November 1996, 15.
17. Interim report of the NIH Director's Panel on Clinical Research (CRP). Appendix B. December, 1996, 2.
18. Latour B. Science in action. Cambridge, MA: Harvard Univ Press, 1987.
19. Shapin S. Here and everywhere: Sociology of scientific knowledge. Ann Rev Sociol 1995;21:289–321.
20. Epstein S. Impure science: AIDS, activism and the politics of knowledge. Los Angeles: Univ Calif Press, 1996:15.
21. Pippin RB. On the notion of technology as Ideology: Prospects. In: Technology, pessimism and postmodernism. Ezrahi Y et al., eds. Amherst, MA: U Mass Press, 1994:94.
22. Ezrahi Y. The descent of Icarus: Science and the transformation of contemporary society. Cambridge, MA: Harvard Univ Press, 1990:70.
23. Epstein S. Impure science: AIDS, activism and the politics of knowledge. Los Angeles: Univ Calif Press, 1996:1–54.
24. Ahrens EH. The crisis in clinical research. New York: Oxford Univ Press, 1992:39.
25. Shapiro MJ. Reading the postmodern polity. Political theory as textural practice. Minneapolis, MN: Univ Minn Press, 1992:129–137.
26. Clarke A, Montin T. The many faces of RU 486: Tales of situated knowledges and technological contestations. Sci Technol Human Values 1993;18:42–78.
27. Epstein S. Impure science: AIDS, activism and the politics of knowledge. Los Angeles: Univ Calif Press, 1996:295.
28. Sclove RE. Democracy and technology. New York: Guilford, 1995:26–27.
29. Pardes H. The future of medical schools and teaching hospitals in the era of managed care. Acad Med 1997; 72:97–102.
30. Cozzens SE, EJ Woodhouse. Science, government and the politics of knowledge. In: Handbook of science and technology studies. Sheila Jasanoff et al., eds. Thousand Oaks, CA: SAGE, 1995:547.
31. Pippen RB. On the notion of technology as Ideology: Prospects. In: Technology, pessimism and postmodernism. Ezrahi Y et al., eds. Amherst, MA: U Mass Press, 1994:93–113.
32. Eisenhower DD. Farewell radio and television address to the American people, January 17, 1961. In: Public papers of the President of the United States, Dwight D. Eisenhower, 1960–1961. Washington DC: GPO, 1961:1035–1040.
33. Ezrahi Y. The descent of Icarus: Science and the transformation of contemporary society. Cambridge, MA: Harvard Univ Press, 1990:248.
34. Ezrahi Y. The descent of Icarus: Science and the transformation of contemporary society. Cambridge, MA: Harvard Univ Press, 1990:249–250.
35. Ezrahi Y. The descent of Icarus: Science and the transformation of contemporary society. Cambridge, MA: Harvard Univ Press, 1990:253.
36. Ezrahi Y. The descent of Icarus: Science and the transformation of contemporary society. Cambridge, MA: Harvard Univ Press, 1990:250.

37. Ezrahi Y. The descent of Icarus: Science and the transformation of contemporary society. Cambridge, MA: Harvard Univ Press, 1990:251.

38. Ezrahi Y. The descent of Icarus: Science and the transformation of contemporary society. Cambridge, MA: Harvard Univ Press, 1990:257.

39. Ezrahi Y. The descent of Icarus: Science and the transformation of contemporary society. Cambridge, MA: Harvard Univ Press, 1990:258.

40. Ezrahi Y. The authority of science in politics. In: Science and values: Patterns of tradition and change. Thackray A, Mendelson E., eds. New York: Humanities Press, 1974:215–251.

41. Freidson E. The impurity of professional authority in institutions and the person. Becker H et al. Chicago: Aldine Press, 1968:25–34.

42. Matherlee KR. The outlook for clinical research: Impacts of federal funding restraint and private sector reconfiguration. Acad Med 1995;70:1065–1072.

43. Gaus CR. Appropriations testimony by the administrator of AHCPR before a Hearing of House Labor, HHS and Education Appropriations Subcommittee, February 11, 1997.

44. Request for proposal: Evidence-based practice centers. AHCPR March 24,1997.

45. AHCPR funds projects which support medicine and public health initiative. Press Release. AHCPR March 3, 1997.

46. Eddy DM. Clinical decision making from theory to practice. JAMA 1993;270:520–526.

47. Richards E. The politics of therapeutic evaluation: The vitamin C and cancer controversy. Soc Studies Sci 1988;18:653–701.

48. Berry DA. Statistics: A Bayesian perspective. Belmont CA: Duxbury Press, 1996.

49. McDermott MM et al. Changes in study design, Gender issues and other characteristics of clinical research published in three major medical journals from 1971–1991. J Gen Intern Med 1995;10:13–18.

50. Parmar DS et al. Assessing whether to perform a confirmatory randomized clinical trial. J Natl Cancer Inst 1996;88:1645–1651.

51. Epstein S. Impure science: AIDS, activism and the politics of knowledge. Los Angeles: Univ Calif Press, 1996:345.

52. National Institutes of Health.1996 Extramural awards to medical schools. NIH/DRG/ISMS, 1996.

CHAPTER 12

Board Certification: Purposes, Issues, Dilemma, and the Future in Neurosurgery

SIDNEY TOLCHIN, M.D., JAMES R. BEAN, M.D.

THE NEW ISSUES AND THE DILEMMA

Before managed care, competition for specialty contracts and credentialing for managed care networks became commonplace, delay in board certification had little practical disadvantage. No limitation to practice was faced. The term ''board eligible'' was commonly substituted for certification. However, current neurosurgeons, completing training and entering practice in urban areas with numerous established neurosurgeons and high managed care penetration often find board certification a prerequisite for contract participation, even when joining a group practice. The requirement creates a dilemma, a Joseph Heller ''*Catch 22*.'' A new graduate can't practice until board certified, but can't be certified until after 2 to 3 years of practice. With the number of patients not included in some form of contracted managed care plan vanishing rapidly, the problem creates increasing economic impact.

WHAT DOES CERTIFICATION IMPLY AND WHY IS IT IMPORTANT?

The thirst for recognition of accomplishment has its roots in the earliest stages of social development. As children in kindergarten, we noted early that pasted gold stars or stamped smiley faces sufficed to distinguish efforts. That stamp of approval served as tangible acknowledgment of effort and could be declared to those who supervised activities to achieve reward.

Later, report cards served a similar purpose. Records of those reports were subsequently used to derive information for graduation. When approved, these records and other data allowed for conferring of a diploma that certified completion of a defined protocol of study. Accumulation of varied diplomas, when associated with satisfactory performance in college and graduate aptitude testing, was necessary in order to open doors for further study.

This procedure was repeated throughout the educational process. Concomitantly, activities such as scouting were rewarded by merit badges and certificates attesting to completion of or distinction in the performance of these efforts. Accumulation of medals or trophies has become a mark of the competitive nature of some, as has accumulation of diplomas and certificates to others. Napoleon affirmed to his political opponents, ''Give me enough ribbon and I will build you an army!''

Society has recognized the benefits of these tangible rewards. Industry and academia have acknowledged the need for track records in order to place competent individuals in positions in which they might excel. These records, diplomas and certificates are the tracks that can be used to derive a reasonable expectation of competence (1).

In fact, the same terminology is used by the American Board of Neurological Surgery (ABNS). One ''tracks'' toward certification in the education, training, and experience process. A framework of requirements for completion within a specific allotment of time permits this achievement in a reasonable manner.

All states have licensing requirements and most confer a license as physician and surgeon. Anyone with such a license may call himself or herself a neurosurgeon, with or without special training, and, except for a very few states, may legally advertise as such. Certainly, no state has, at this time, any requirement that the practice of neurosurgery demands special certification.

With diplomas, licenses, certificates, and fellowships, there exists more than a modicum of confusion among legislators as well as the general public. The layman equates licensure with adequacy, if not competency, and an atmosphere of caveat emptor prevails. Recently, led by attentive hospital medical staffs, more cognizant leaders of the community have reviewed these processes and have demanded proof of adequacy of ability and judgment.

Managed care executives have recognized the cost savings and the safety of quality provision of services and have required proof of proficiency before inviting participation on health plan panels now that the majority of physicians contract with managed care plans. Legal involvement in determination of standards of care by the use of tort liability has discouraged specialty practice in the absence of acceptable credentials.

Thus far, included in this review have been: adequacy, competency, safety; license, diploma, certificate; provision of service, reward, reimbursement; and Board, legislative and public activities. The chaotic nature of this taxonomy and these terms defies reason and creates part of the dilemma of understanding for participants, legislators, and the general public.

The limits of practice are the poorly-trained or untrained charlatan at one spectral end and the board-recertified surgeon with a spotless record in quality review, malpractice litigation, and patient satisfaction at the other.

Definitions are thus in order. A certificate is a document that attests to the truth of something and that can be issued to someone completing a course of study not necessarily leading to a diploma. It can also indicate some official franchise of a right to practice a profession. A license is an official or legal permit to do a designated action (or permission to deviate from ordinary activity). A diploma is a documentation of successful completion of a particular course of study. In the normal course of events, once gained, a diploma cannot be taken away unless fraud or other felonious activity that led to its award can be proved. A certificate or license, however, might be withdrawn or be issued for a limited time, after which it will no longer be valid (2).

COMPETENCY

Competence implies ability and infers quality. In this context, adequacy alone is disparaging when compared to excellence, but a competent neurosurgeon could be defined as one adequate to perform expected skills. Safety, however, should be the foundation, if *primum non nocere* preponderates. A technically and judgmentally qualified individual who does not depart frequently from recognized standards of care, who is careful and caring, and whose outcomes are positively measured might be considered safe.

The unfortunate reality is that certification or licensure is equated with competence by the uninformed. A diploma might be considered a license to continue learning ones profession, but a certificate, especially a board certificate in specialty medicine, is frequently misconstrued as a guarantee of competency.

Means to develop and measure characteristics of competency are legion. Written and oral examinations test knowledge and retention of facts, but these are only proxies for competency in that they do not necessarily measure performance. Personal, on-the-job assessments are expensive, impractical, and are subject to bias. Certification, recertification, and licensure all fail to measure competency, performance, or patient satisfaction.

THE AMERICAN BOARD OF NEUROLOGICAL SURGERY

One way the American Board of Neurological Surgery (ABNS) influences outcome and attains its quality goals is by defining, through interface with the Residency Review Committee (RRC) of the American Council on Graduate Medical Education (ACGME), the quality of, currently, ninety-nine neurosurgical residency training programs. Insistence on compliance with general and special program requirements is paramount in this evaluation. The RRC can recommend withdrawal of approval or probationary status for any program not meeting these requirements. However, the influence of: (*a*) managed care, (*b*) the increased workforce, and (*c*) the service needs of some institutions of training, has strained the attainment of these goals.

The legal profession has declared openly that its influence has improved the quality of medicine. Significantly, this has not been the case of training program accreditation. Because of the generous financial endowments, available funding for legal intervention allows some of these facilities to continue training activity in spite of unfavorable RRC reviews. This intervention is based on interpretation of Federal Trade Commission regulations and cannot be countered because of the limited resources of the supervising agencies such as the ACGME. Fortunately, the majority of training institutions meet the requirements or acknowledge the RRC analysis and take immediate steps to comply. A study comparing the quality of a group of neurosurgeons trained at one institution with that of a second cohort trained at another has not been undertaken, perhaps since tools for that form of evaluation are not valid or available.

The ABNS is a member of the American Board of Medical Specialties (ABMS). This is the only certifying organization recognized by the American Council of Graduate Medical Education (ACGME). ABNS-directed changes in curricula requirements in training, changes in definition of scope of practice, or requests for certification of added qualifications or special qualifications must all be reviewed by the ABMS prior to approval by ACGME. This negotiation and filtering process moderates problems generated by ''turf'' issues among specialties and serves as a policing agency, contributing to overall quality in training.

There are other ''boards'' and a few states have set up processes recognizing equivalency in training. California, for example, has gone through this process and recognizes ABMS equivalency in Plastic Surgery and Pain Management. These political techniques address the pressures to identify focused areas of practice by those who desire special recognition for specialized training. Although the external appearance of certification is most often directed toward uniformity and quality of training by instituting special requirements and testing measures, the practical effect is toward exclusion of others without such designated certification

from that sphere of practice. The pejorative term applied to these self-appointed and self-regulated agencies is that of ''bogus'' boards. The public, unaware of the differences between these and ABMS boards, perceives no difference when looking at letterheads, signs, or yellow pages. This form of certification is tacitly accepted by knowledgeable legislators recognizing that increased competition will help to drive reimbursement reductions.

The lack of recognition of these alternative boards by the ABMS and the responsible hesitancy in establishing focused subspecialties has created division within firmly established specialties. Maintenance of the philosophy of global training within the bounds of these already established specialties is important to assure quality without fragmentation of a specialty. All neurosurgeons eventually focus their practices to areas of special interest and, most often, take additional courses or fellowships to enhance these interests. The notion of further certification for recognition, and, therefore, exclusion of others so globally trained, carries not so much the assurance of quality as it does the mantle of self-interest. Fragmentation of any specialty, especially one so limited in scope and membership as neurosurgery, dilutes effectiveness, political and professional strength, and undermines the capacity to establish quality and uniformity in the practice of the specialty.

The ABNS certification process is rigorous and professional. Deviation from any segment in the training schedule, such as training in other than the primary institution, must have prior approval from the secretary of the board. Acceptance of the periods of training in neurosurgery, neurology, electives, and enfolded focused specialty preparation occurs only after intense individual review by committees of the board.

For almost its entire existence of over half a century, the ABNS has required professional practice data to be submitted in the evaluation of the candidate. Prone to bias, this facet of evaluation includes a primitive measure of outcome. Outcome assessment, if scientifically valid and reliable, appears to offer reasonable promise as a measure of competency. The instruments for use in validation in this process are still in the developmental phase and are themselves being tested. These instruments gauge function, well-being, patient and family satisfaction, and cost. They compare the scientifically based results of the activities of the potential certificant to accepted standards and determine actuarial factors such as morbidity and mortality, return to the operating room, etc. No current certification process incorporates this assessment method. Until scientifically validated outcome measures are available, it is doubtful that any should.

Peer review evaluation, during and for a short period following residency training, is an essential element of the certification process. Letters of recommendation are read for between-the-lines information as well as overt declaration. Some unsuspecting candidates have been nonselective in requesting these letters, naively dismissing the damaging effect of adverse recommendations from local competition.

Although not considered for the certification process until the written examination is passed prior to completion of residency, an applicant tracking toward board certification must incorporate careful documentation of operations performed and patients evaluated during the entire training period. In spite of the concentrated nature of this review, a preponderance of weight in evaluation is placed upon the recommendation of the training director, or in the event that multiple institutions were attended, all mentors participating in the training of the applicant. The enormous responsibility that this places on that director, especially in the case of a marginal candidate, is difficult to appreciate. Years of commitment by the trainee to service requirements of the program, rather than demonstrated ability, is occasionally rewarded by perfunctory approval for completion of training. Obvious misfits are most often discharged during the training program, and stars encounter no difficulty in completion.

The oral examination process very frequently identifies the poorly trained. The frustration and pain of the candidate in not being able to obtain certification after such protracted training and education is matched only by that of the Board itself: in self-reproach for not having been more instrumental and effective in being able to monitor the training program and to affect processes leading to that failure.

Board certification allows the recipient the title of diplomate. In itself, this designation implies a conferring of a diploma rather than a warranty or label of competency. Only extremely rarely, and even then only with absolute definition of felonious activity, is such certification withdrawn.

RECERTIFICATION

If, then, such an award carries no assurance of competency or ability, but rather a peer opinion of safety and an endorsement of completion of training, testing, and practice prerequisites, the misperception of society has not been addressed. However, should such certification be time-limited, and recertification ultimately attached to retrospective measures of individual outcome rather than testing measures for knowledge alone, a case for interpretation of competency and safety might be made.

Neurosurgery is blessed with a workforce of highly competitive individuals. As such, component practitioners have participated in voluntary continuing medical education to a degree not enjoyed by many other specialties in medicine. This participation is confirmed by the percentage of membership attending annual meetings, section meetings, specialty regional teaching conferences and local educational programs. Book sales, self-assessment programs, journal subscription, and electronic interaction are uniquely embraced by neurosurgeons. Professional development courses ranging from hands-on skull base technical interaction to practice management are usually filled to capacity. Neurosurgeons, generally, have demonstrated exceptional responsibility in recognition of the need for continuing education.

With full awareness of this continuing education effort and harboring reservations about the value of written recertification examinations in determining physician competency, the ABNS is the only major specialty of the 24 member boards of the ABMS that has no current active recertification process, mandatory or voluntary. All other specialties, except Anesthesiology, Otolaryngology, Pathology, and Preventive Medicine have time-limited certificates, most lasting 10 years (3).

ABNS policy exists that has been activated with the trigger of economic and legislative compulsion. This policy incorporates documentation of continuing medical education, evaluation of the health of the prior certificant, maintenance of licensure, and attestation as to existing credentials to practice neurosurgery locally without limitation, such as proctoring or continued quality review. State medical board regulatory action and malpractice history would also be considered in this process. A clean record at the end of the limited certification period incorporating these factors could certainly suggest, if not affirm, competency.

The need for knowledge testing, such as oral or written examination, remains controversial, but will undoubtedly play some role. Alternative methods, such as on-site practice assessment, notwithstanding the shortcomings previously noted, could be used in questionable cases.

The written examination has been shown to have only limited benefit in the recertification process. After 3 years in practice, scores drop measurably, and, after 7 years, scores drop precipitously. This does not imply a loss of knowledge base so much as it reveals a tendency to focus practice toward certain areas of interest, with an accompanying loss in retention of information not used persistently. A value exists, however, in requiring an applicant to review existing literature and textbooks.

One measure, used experimentally by the American Board of Internal Medicine (4), that seemed to have validity was local peer evaluation. This included not only physician peer confidential reporting but also nurse and administrative reporting. That the measure has not been put into use routinely is only a reflection of difficulty in obtaining consistent response rates. Recourse to the use of written and oral examination illustrates the expediency of using testing measures to satisfy popular demand for competency measurement rather than performance quality evaluation.

Recertification is time-consuming and expensive. The 7-year cycle of pediatrics has been most difficult to maintain. A few boards considered 3-year, time-limited certification but soon understood the impractical logistics of carrying out such a plan. Quality recertification cannot be accomplished on a short-term interval basis in neurosurgery. The problems with delay in initial certification have amply demonstrated the problems to be expected in any recertification process.

Little has been done in promotion of recertification to confront the enigma of lack of initial certification. Failure to complete the certification process in the restricted time allotted disrupts tracking. If certification has not been awarded in this window of opportunity, repeat written examination passage is required. The designation ''Board Eligible,'' in place for years, was discontinued when abuse in use of the title was noted. The ACGME has once again reinstituted this designation, with strict definition, as a response to managed care pressures. Practically, one is either board certified, tracking towards board certification, or one is not board certified. Unless limited in some way, a practitioner might, and frequently will, use the ''Board Eligible'' designation to achieve recognition for an entire professional career, once having completed any training program.

Osteopathic physicians not trained in residency programs accredited by the American Council of Graduate Medical Education are not eligible for board certification by the ABNS. Similarly, Canadian neurosurgeons starting Canadian residency programs after 1996 will not be eligible to sit for ABNS oral board examinations. There is no comparable Residency Review Committee activity currently in accrediting training programs in Canada.

Residents not passing the written primary examination prior to completion of ACGME-approved United States programs will not be eligible to sit for oral examination, and, indeed, will not be considered as having completed the residency program by the board. Some neurosurgeons, having completed their approved residency programs, have decided to not seek board certification at all, for reasons not associated with poor technical ability or questionable competency. A small percentage of neurosurgeons have never been able to pass the oral board examination process in spite of repeated attempts.

Some questions are immediately apparent. How does one recertify an individual who has never been certified in the first place? What happens to the person who has been certified initially, but fails in the recertification process? Are these persons to be considered abandoned as flotsam and jetsam, or are we bound to present alternatives if we wrest the opportunity to practice from individuals who stand to lose their livelihoods by the failure of certifcation or recertification?

A NEW ROLE FOR THE ABNS?

Detractors state unabashedly that it is not in the purview of the ABNS to concern itself with those who fail to meet the certification or recertification requirements, but only to ensure the quality (competency?) of those who are eligible. Pragmatic reasoning does not justify this position. If neurosurgery is to maintain its position of national and world leadership in medicine, the ABNS does bear partial responsibility for the quality of provided services, no matter the declarations of the provider. There has been no significant attempt to retrain those who cannot attain the gold star. There has been no alternative presented to the person who has dedicated many years of productive life in training, only to fail certification or to be denied entrance into the certification process. If certification is to be equated with adequacy, competency, or safety, then the lack of certification should be sufficient cause to limit the interaction of that unfortunate individual with the innocent population. Acceptable alternatives to such a wasted effort should be made available. If certification is not to be equated in this manner, then the entire process is sycophantic and shameful.

After series of successes in a remarkably competitive environment, characterized by repeated selection procedures, it is no wonder that most neurosurgeons completing the rigorous training and prerequisites of the board do satisfy those requirements and are certified as having done so. Equally, it is not astounding that almost all of these neurosurgeons remain safe and competent individuals during their entire professional lives, providing unparalleled quality neurosurgical services for our citizens.

Unfortunately, it is necessary to document what may be known to be true. If documentation of the competence of American neurosurgeons is to take the form of certification and recertification in the future, then it is the duty of the neurosurgical community to undertake that service just as it has provided those quality technical and cognitive services up to this time. It is the duty of our government to protect these activities in relief from trade restrictions and malicious use of due process against certifying agencies, such as the ACGME and the ABNS. It is the duty of the public to insist on this legislative relief if the perception of certification commensurate with competency is to be maintained.

THE CHALLENGES

The certification method and its process face several challenges in the immediate future. These challenges arise from change in practice requirements evolving with managed care contracting, and they are also affected by changing state licensure laws.

The major challenges and dilemmas of board certification fall into three categories:

- Recertification;
- Subspecialty certification;
- Delay in certification.

RECERTIFICATION

As described previously, the issue of recertification is clouded by several problems. Questions of the validity of the examination, the inadequacy of a written examination to confirm competency, a reduction in general scientific knowledge after years in practice, lack of actual performance measures, and expense of true practice assessment have all been reasons proposed for avoiding time-limited certificates and mandatory recertification. A majority of neurosurgeons have historically opposed recertification, even voluntary testing, because of these issues and also because of the inconvenience, time commitment, fear of failure, and the potential loss of practice.

However, three concerns drive neurosurgery to reconsider its resistance to recertification: state licensure requirements, competing specialties, and hospital/health plan credentialing. Of the three concerns, the first is the most compelling. Although New York State recently reversed its decision to hinge state licensure upon recertification, South Carolina requires an established physician who wishes to transfer licensure from another state to either take the standard state licensing exam or show evidence of recent certification or recertification in a specialty. If no recertification is offered—the strategy that neurosurgery formerly found successful—the state examination is required. In states where specialty recertification is or soon will be accepted as an alternative to state general medical licensure testing, either for interstate license transfer, or even for annual license renewal, the demand for available recertification process will rise.

Those neurosurgeons possessing a prior valid non-time-limited certification and not subject to mandatory recertification will have been "grandfathered (or grandmothered)" but will still face these licensure requirements, and, confronted with need, they will most likely undergo the recertification process voluntarily.

The second concern, competing specialties, is a theoretical problem. In an age of competition, advertising and exclusive contracting for service, specialties that can claim continued competence as proved by reexamination and updated certification may acquire a marketing advantage. Orthopedics, head and neck surgery, and general/vascular surgery all overlap neurosurgery in their boundaries and compete for similar surgical patients. In competition for spine referrals, recertification claims may give orthopedists a competitive marketing advantage.

The third concern, credentialing by hospitals and health plans, is a growing one as more and more institutions, insurers, and networks adopt timely board certification (or recertification) as part of credentialing, or recredentialing, criteria. So far, unavailability of an updated test or certificate from the specialty board has been an acceptable excuse. But the pressure to conform to what is rapidly becoming a professional standard (recertification) is mounting.

SUBSPECIALTY CERTIFICATION

Subspecialty certification was referred to earlier, in discussing political pressures to recognize specialty training, sclf-appointed boards, and a motive of competitive exclusion of fellow specialists. The traditional approach in neurosurgery has been to train every resident "globally," asserting competence in all areas of neurosurgical practice. The strategy has been to avoid fragmentation of the specialty by ignoring subspecialty training or qualifications.

When anesthesiology, general surgery, pediatrics, and internal medicine began offering subspecialty certificates in critical care (certificates of added qualifications, appended to the basic specialty certificate), neurosurgery felt threatened with exclusion from intensive care, and obtained approval for critical care subcertification in 1987. The feared exclusion never happened, the demand from neurosurgeons never materialized, the exam was never offered, and the approval was withdrawn by the ABMS in 1994.

However, the quest for subcertification did not die. In 1996, a group of neurosurgeons whose primary focus was in pediatrics incorporated an independent board for certifying pediatric neurosurgeons, using testing, training, and pediatric practice volume criteria. The board has no affiliation with the ABMS. The founders acted after long denial by the ABNS of the request for pediatric subcertification. The action

has sparked strong controversy within organized neurosurgery. Neurosurgeons specializing in pain management have supported another unaffiliated specialty board, the American Board of Pain Management. Unlike the neurosurgical pediatric board, this board draws members from multiple primary specialties and seeks recognition by the ABMS. It offers testing, but lacks rigid training criteria.

ABNS policy has been firm in opposing any subcertification requests, and the policy is widely supported among neurosurgeons. A resolution reaffirming opposition to subspecialty certification was approved by a wide margin by the Joint Council of State Neurosurgical Societies assembly in April, 1997, and the resolution was accepted by the Board of Directors of the AANS and the Executive Committee of the Congress of Neurological Surgeons.

Approval for subspecialty certification remains a small, but persistent demand, and it may increase as the number of subspecialty ACGME-approved or nonapproved fellowship-trained neurosurgeons grows. Recognition of subspecialty training and testing to confirm special technical ability, is a common appeal from subspecialty groups once a threshold number of trainees has been reached. This phenomenon accounts for the sixty primarily nonsurgical subspecialty certificates (Certificates of Added Qualifications: CAQ, and Certificates of Special Qualifications: CSQ) currently approved by the ABMS (5).

DELAY IN CERTIFICATION

Board certification in neurosurgery is commonly delayed 3 years or more following completion of residency. The delay fulfills a fundamental purpose of the certification process: to base at least a portion of the assessment on what is done in practice, i.e., actual performance. Although application for oral examination may be made in a timely fashion, 1 year of practice data, with a minimum of 3 months of follow-up is required. A 12- to 18-month delay frequently occurs between application and testing to allow for processing of the application, review of training, receipt of letters of recommendation, letters from local practicing neurosurgeons, and review of practice data.

The Board's practice requirement and delayed testing creates a financial hardship and added practice disadvantage for those just completing their training.

The solution lies somewhere in the Board's prerequisites. One solution suggested is the addition of a "provisional" certification for up to 5 years for graduates who have passed a written test and have verification of their completion of an accredited neurosurgical residency program. Another is oral testing at the completion of residency, thus eliminating practice data requirements. Neither solution satisfies all needs. Whatever the solution, the problem cannot be long ignored without handicapping finishing trainees.

THE FUTURE

Wherever there is a perception of nonaction or a vacuum of response to a set of circumstances, it is almost certain to be accompanied by the birth of new or contrived agencies to fill that need. This is certainly occurring in the process of economic credentialing or quality evaluation of performance, activity-based certification and recertification. A self-proclaimed assembly, made up almost exclusively by representatives of industry, and without portfolio from established government or medical agencies or associations, has been formed and has taken upon itself the role of evaluation. The National Committee for Quality Assurance, NCQA, has, in its embryonic phase, been able to accomplish what voluntary agencies, restricted by governmental and litigation actions, have not. Their mission is to serve payers through identification and credentialing of providers of medical care, primarily based on actuarial measures of efficiency and on their own definition of medical necessity, not necessarily on time-honored measures of medical quality. Exclusion from participation of those not meeting their criteria is their goal.

The American Medical Foundation, utilizing a panel of leaders in medicine, has established a review process for evaluation and credentialing. This incorporates on-site review of practice activities, supervision and monitoring of technical education, and on-site proctoring of new procedures. Hospital medical staff and administration or individual surgeons may request these services.

The American Medical Association, in a reactive mode, has introduced the American Medical Accreditation Program (AMAP) in a delayed attempt to moderate the effectiveness of the groups discussed above. The primary intent of this program is to credential the individual practitioner one time so that the myriad of approvals currently required by the varied managed care payers can be satisfied in a single review. Acceptance of the AMAP program by specialty societies has been marginal, primarily because of a perception that this program offers an unacceptable alternative to certification and credentialing when compared to that of the ABMS structure and process and that this form of individual accreditation, based on AMAP parameters of self assessment and review, will ultimately sanction equivalency to established certification methods.

The future of neurosurgery in the United States may hinge, not on our revered and respected institutions (fettered as they may be by inertia) whose activities are measured, proved in their protection of the public, and thoughtful in promoting growth and quality medicine, but on the iconoclastic activities of groups such as these. The destination of this aspect of neurosurgery in transition is yet to be decided.

REFERENCES

1. Newble D, Jolly B, Wakeford R. The certification and recertification of doctors; Issues in the assessment of clinical competence. New York: Cambridge University Press, 1994.
2. W W Webster Dictionary; Merriam–Webster Online. 1997. http.//www.m–w.com/dictionary. htm (8 Oct. 1997).
3. Annual Report and Reference Handbook 1995. Evanston IL: American Board of Medical Specialties, 139, 1995.
4. Lewis RP. Recertification—Its time has come. J Am Coll Cardiol 1996;28(1):260–262.
5. Annual Report and Reference Handbook 1995. Evanston IL: American Board of Medical Specialties, 1995: 135–137.

PART III

Other Issues

CHAPTER 13

"Throw Away the Scabbard": What Organized Neurosurgery Should Do Now

ROBERT E. DRABA, PH.D., MBA

INTRODUCTION

Barely noticed by the public, Colonel John R. Boyd died on March 9, 1997 at the age of 70 in a West Palm Beach hospital. A retired U.S. Air Force officer, Boyd developed theories of air combat that greatly influenced aerial tactics, jet fighter design, general military strategy, and even business planning. No mere theorist, Boyd was a highly skilled fighter pilot and instructor who helped establish the Fighter Weapons School at Nellis Air Force Base in Nevada. During the late 1950s, he was known as "40-second Boyd," because he could "shake" any pilot off his tail and have that pilot in his gun-sights within 40 seconds. Boyd offered to pay $40.00 if he failed to accomplish this amazing reversal of fortune within the prescribed time. Many top pilots challenged him over the skies of Nevada, but legend has it that Boyd never lost, and hence, never paid (121).

Boyd had limited combat missions during the Korean conflict, but they were sufficient to motivate him to ask, and eventually to answer with mathematical precision, why the slower American-made F-86 dominated the faster Soviet-made MIG-15. He correctly concluded that such dominance was due primarily to two important characteristics of the F-86: better visibility and a faster roll rate. He noticed that flying higher and faster was *not* necessarily better. How quickly a plane could begin to climb and how quickly it could turn were critical variables. Boyd also observed that air combat encounters involved four repeated cycles: observation, orientation, decision and action, collectively known as "OODA." He spoke of the "time/cycle loop" and "fast-cycle combat theory" to build an accumulated advantage in aerial combat. For him, the key to victory in the skies was to get inside the OODA "loop" of the adversary; doing so involved exemplary visibility and maneuverability (121).

Boyd's ideas about air combat endure today and have been reinforced in the Persian Gulf War by the performance of the F-16, a plane he helped to design. Also, his more general theory of "maneuver warfare" supposedly influenced the decision to use a flanking movement on the ground in the Persian Gulf war. So simple and powerful are his ideas about strategy and tactics in war, that some have adapted and applied them to the generic process of strategic planning (28).

Because organized neurosurgery has strategic challenges and opportunities posed by a rapidly changing health-care environment, Boyd's OODA cycle has been adapted as an organizing element for this chapter on professional medical organizations. In this chapter, there are four sections, which reach four conclusions. Namely, organized neurosurgery should:

- Make and implement good decisions, quicker;
- Recognize that deregulation of health-care delivery is the principal socioeconomic trend affecting neurosurgery now and in the future;
- Help neurosurgery act like a "niche player" in response to the deregulation of health care; and
- Consolidate and focus its resources.

OBSERVATIONS ABOUT ORGANIZED NEUROSURGERY

The phrase "organized neurosurgery" is frequently used to describe an array of professional organizations within the community of neuro-surgeons. The American Association of Neuro-logical Surgeons (AANS) and the Congress of Neurological Surgeons (CNS) are the largest of these professional organizations and perhaps most visible and influential. But, there is more, much more, to organized neurosurgery than the AANS and CNS. There are at least 10 other asso-ciations of neurosurgeons, including the Ameri-can Academy of Neurological Surgeons, The Neurosurgical Society of America, The Society of Neurological Surgeons, The Society of Uni-versity Neurosurgeons, and regional neuro-surgical societies like the Southern, New England, Western and Rocky Mountain. In addi-tion, there is the Council of State Neurosurgical Societies (CSNS), which represents so-called "grassroots neurosurgery." The CSNS has a policy council and governance relationships with the AANS and CNS. Growing in impor-tance are AANS/CNS Sections involving the specialties of spine, cerebrovascular, trauma, pain, pediatrics, tumor, stereotactic, and history. These sections elect officers, collect dues, and have meetings.

The phrase "organized neurosurgery" would not be completely defined without including such vitally important organizations as *The Journal of Neurosurgery* and *Neurosurgery*, both of which are admired for the independence of their editorial boards. Not to be missed are the Neurosurgery Residency Review Committee of the Accreditation Council of Graduate Medi-cal Education *and* the American Board of Neu-rological Surgery of the American Board of Medical Specialties. They are involved, respec-tively, with the training and certification of neu-rosurgeons. Finally, there are the Research Foundation and the Think First Foundation; the former funds research relevant to neuroscience, and the latter funds school programs on injury prevention. Other organizations could be named (e.g., North American Skull Base Society), but the foregoing makes the point that "organized neurosurgery" in 1997 is more than the AANS and CNS. It is a constellation of organizations, each of which meets specific membership needs, or they would not exist.

Often, within this constellation of organiza-tions, there are overlapping memberships, as is the case between the AANS and CNS, whose memberships overlap by over 75%. From time-to-time, leaders of one organization are leaders

or soon-to-be leaders of another organization. The currently serving (1997–1998) President, President-Elect, and Past-President of the AANS, for example, have strong and enduring ties with the CNS. And, it is very common to have leaders of one organization as committee members of other organizations. Hence, neuro-surgical organizations are often linked one-to-another by far fewer than "six degrees of separa-tion."

For all their linkage through membership and leadership, neurosurgical organizations have a great deal of independence. One Past-President of the AANS made this observation as well, and then added, "We like it that way." Deeply-held values involving research, education, and patient care seem to be forces which keep the "constel-lation of organizations" from pulling apart. There is, however, an unambiguous independ-ence about each organization that is unmistaka-ble—as unmistakable as the independence of stars in the sky. It is reasonable to speculate that one reason for this independence involves the origins of organized neurosurgery.

In 1919, the American College of Surgery de-clared neurological surgery to be a surgical sub-specialty. Five short months later, The Society of Neurological Surgeons was formed by Harvey Cushing with 11 members. Its purpose was to further establish the scientific and educational basis of the specialty. Consistent with this focus, it limited membership to just 45 "prominent ac-ademicians." Walter Dandy, who certainly qualified as a "prominent academician," was asked to join the Society, but he declined, due reportedly to "strained" relations with Cushing and Charles Frazier (42).

Because membership in The Society of Neu-rological Surgeons was limited and because there was a growing number of young neurosur-geons, The Harvey Cushing Society was formed in 1931. Much thought and care was given to establishing this second society, the mission and goals of which were remarkably similar to those of the existing society. Wisely, the founders sought Cushing's advice and counsel, and on May 6, 1932, Cushing welcomed to Boston 23 charter members of the new society bearing his name (42). The AANS is the successor to The Harvey Cushing Society, but more about that later.

Like the Society of Neurological Surgeons be-fore it, The Harvey Cushing Society limited its membership, first to 35 and then 50. This made inevitable the formation of yet a third organization, as Cushing had predicted. The American Academy of Neurological Surgeons was formed in 1938. It too limited membership and focused its mission on academic matters, but it also evaluated the ''interpersonal qualities of candidates.'' The Academy addressed, but did not solve, the problem of membership for a growing number of young neurosurgeons (42). Failure to do so made a fourth organization possible.

In 1948, The Neurosurgical Society of America was formed. It had several unique characteristics. It limited active membership to neurosurgeons under 45 years of age and made no distinctions between academic and private practice neurosurgeons. It also encouraged family involvement at annual meetings. However, it too limited membership, and when early members of this fourth society reached 45 years of age (and it was time for them to move out), the by-laws were changed to allow active membership after 45 years of age, thereby blocking membership for younger neurosurgeons (42).

It is important to pause here to emphasize that from 1919 to 1948, four separate neurosurgical societies had been established, or about one every 10 years. All had limited membership, and three were composed primarily of academicians. Hence, for the first 30 years, organized neurosurgery was composed of four independent, restrictive, and academically-oriented organizations. That, however, was about to change.

In 1951, the Congress of Neurological Surgeons (CNS) was established. It encouraged unlimited and broad-based membership. Seasoned or youthful, certified or not, academic or private practice, all neurosurgeons were welcome and all had a place in the CNS, which, like all other societies, focused primarily on academic matters. Virtually overnight, the CNS had a membership larger than all other societies except The Cushing Society, which was the predecessor of the AANS. It also imposed a restriction on the age of its leadership—45. It has been suggested that this was done to protect its open-door membership policies. For whatever reason, this policy has worked well for the CNS specifically and for organized neurosurgery generally (42).

In their comprehensive article, ''The evolution of organized neurological surgery in the United States,'' Hauber and Philips (45) describe the period after the CNS was established

as ''The era of parallelism.'' By this they meant that the CNS and AANS (still named ''The Harvey Cushing Society'') operated successfully side-by-side, not in competition. Both had journals and annual meetings that met at different times of the year. The CNS paid special attention to the needs of residents and young neurosurgeons, and even though certification was a requirement for active membership in the AANS, but not the CNS, the CNS made important contributions to preparing neurosurgeons for the certification examination. When neurosurgeons attained certification and joined the AANS, they frequently retained their membership in the CNS, which explains why the percentage of overlapping members of the AANS and CNS is so high. All in all, though, it was a very beneficial arrangement for organized neurosurgery.

By about 1960, there was a ''place'' for everyone in organized neurosurgery. Of course, some of these places were by invitation only, and the AANS maintained its requirement of certification for active membership, but the days of limited-access organizations as the only alternatives for neurosurgeons were finally over. All neurosurgeons had access to the benefits of membership in some professional organization, in some specific tent. However, there was more than one tent on the landscape of organized neurosurgery, and, from time-to-time, neurosurgeons, bound together by a common geographic region or common academic discipline, erected yet another tent. Towering above all were the tents of the CNS and AANS. Hence, back in 1960 there were a lot of tents (and the number is still growing), but there was really no central zoning commission to coordinate which tents got erected where and by whom.

In the early stages of a business, nation, or profession, there is often fragmentation and decentralized authority. Eventually there is consolidation and centralization, as with the development of the oil refining industry and the modern history of Germany. Professions go through this as well. Think of the early days of medicine, when there were multiple schools of medicine, such as magnetic healers and multiple training institutions, all of which made possible The Museum of Questionable Medical Devices in Minneapolis (77). Allopathic medicine (MD) and organized allopathic medicine (American Medical Association) consolidated the profession and defined for all what medicine was and was not, *and* who could practice medicine and who could not, *and* what constituted medical training and what did not. So there seems to be a tendency to replace fragmentation with consolidation in many areas of organizational development.

Unlike a business, nation, or profession, academic disciplines like neurosurgery seem to fragment over time as knowledge grows. Consider first the development of specialties within medicine and then think of the development of subspecialties within neurosurgery. Both follow a progression typical of so many fields such as biology, law, statistics, and even marketing. From the beginning (and now), neurosurgical organizations were so focused on education and research that it seems natural for there to have been a proliferation of discipline-oriented, decentralized organizations. In keeping with traditional academic values, it also seems perfectly natural for these neurosurgical organizations to maximize their organizational prerogatives and authority. From 1919 through 1960, this model of organizational development worked well for organized neurosurgery, but times were changing.

Once called "the conscience of neurosurgery" (120), Frank H. Mayfield graduated from medical school in 1931, the very year The Harvey Cushing Society was formed. By 1938, he had been invited to attend the meeting of The Cushing Society in Memphis. He had been "led to believe" that he and six others would be elected to membership that year. In Memphis, he and the others were informed that The Cushing Society had "changed course," and none would be elected. Like ducks to water and in the finest traditions of organized neurosurgery, Mayfield and the six other rejected candidates returned to a room at the Peabody Hotel and promptly formed The American Academy of Neurological Surgeons (68).

Mayfield was elected to membership in The Cushing Society in 1941, but of that election he wrote that "the experience was far less meaningful than it would have been to me in 1938 (68)." His first official assignment for The Cushing Society was membership on a committee studying how to meet the membership desires of a growing number of neurosurgeons, perhaps with provisional membership for noncertified neurosurgeons. In the prior year, 1940, the first board certification examination was given and then

used by The Cushing Society as a criterion for membership (68). Consequently, The Cushing Society rejected provisional membership for noncertified physicians in 1941. This decision, it seems, made the CNS inevitable.

Even though Mayfield was by then "active" in the affairs of The Cushing Society, he continued in a leadership role with The American Academy of Neurological Surgeons. At its tenth annual meeting held in 1947, Mayfield advanced a plan to combine the three existing societies into a single national organization that presumably could speak for organized neurosurgery. His suggestion, though, was referred to a committee for study (42). In 1965, some 18 years later, Mayfield was President of The Cushing Society and heading for its Annual Meeting in New York City to make "A Proclamation."

Throughout his long service to organized neurosurgery, Mayfield seemed to be guided by three principles: broad-based participation of neurosurgeons, unity among neurosurgical organizations, and official representation of neurosurgery through a spokes-organization. He touched upon all of these in his 1965 presidential address, but he is remembered most for saying, "I, Frank H. Mayfield, President, do hereby proclaim The Harvey Cushing Society, Inc., to be in fact the official organization representing the neurological surgeons of the United States (67)."

He also suggested that a subtitle be added to The Harvey Cushing Society, such as "American Association of Neurological Surgeons." Most likely, Mayfield suggested this change in name because John Stirling Meyer, M.D., who is quoted by Mayfield in his proclamation, thought "The Harvey Cushing Society ... sounds ... as though it were a private club honoring the outstanding American neurosurgeon. If it is in point of fact the national society representing American neurosurgery, it ... should be called something such as the American Neurosurgical Association (67)." In 1967, 2 years after the Mayfield Proclamation, The Cushing Society changed its name to "The American Association of Neurological Surgeons, founded as The Harvey Cushing Society in 1931 (42)."

It is interesting to note that Mayfield was not the first to suggest that The Cushing Society be a spokes-organization for organized neurosurgery. Hendrick Svein, Secretary of The Cushing Society, did so in 1962 (42). Why then did the "proclamation" take place in 1965 and not 1962? Like so many things, the answer involves timing.

In 1965, a federal program had just been approved to address issues related to heart, cancer, and stroke. Mayfield wrote to Doctor Michael DeBakey, President Lyndon Johnson's medical representative to the program, and mistakenly asked why no neurosurgeons had been involved with the deliberations, particularly with reference to stroke. In his letter, Mayfield also stated that he had never heard of the neurosurgical organization referenced in the final report. DeBakey called Mayfield immediately and referred him to John Stirling Meyer, quoted above, who was the Chairman of the Subcommittee on Stroke (68).

Meyer wrote Mayfield, saying, "there is a great deal of confusion in my mind and in the minds of everyone . . . as to just which of your societies represents what." Meyer also stated that he regretted the error in the final report which identified the Society of Neurological Surgeons as the American Society of Neurosurgeons, but he added "If in point of fact the Society of Neurological Surgeons does not represent American neurosurgery, just what does it represent (67)?" From his own account, Mayfield concluded that the Meyer letter "left no doubt that the federal government and major medical organizations such as the AMA, could not identify any neurosurgical organization that was capable of serving as the spokesman for neurosurgeons." This view, according to Mayfield, motivated the Board of The Cushing Society to authorize the proclamation made by him in 1965 (68).

Self-perception frequently influences the behavior of people. As it is with people, so it is with organizations. Not all members of the Board shared Mayfield's enthusiasm for the proclamation he made in 1965. Again, from his own account, Mayfield recalled that "Some were reluctant, for nostalgic reasons, to see the character of the organization change (68)." Mayfield knew, as did others, that the "character" of The Cushing Society would have to change, if it hoped to be an authentic, widely recognized spokes-organization for neurosurgeons.

Since 1965, The Cushing Society changed its name and governance structure and expanded its membership categories. In an iterative-like

process, the AANS has in the past 32 years taken small careful steps to broaden its base of representation on its Board and committees as ways to reinforce its claim and creditability as the spokes-organization for neurosurgeons. Such small careful steps illustrate the classic "big tent" strategy in action. By using that strategy, The Cushing Society grew from a group of 23 charter members in 1931 to The American Association of Neurological Surgeons with over 5000 members in 1997.

However, Mayfield did not make his proclamation to expand and change the AANS for its own sake. He had higher, more serious purposes in mind. By proclaiming The Cushing Society to be the spokes-organization for neurosurgery, he was pointing neurosurgery toward the external environment, which was changing rapidly in 1965, what with Medicare moving toward passage in The United States Congress, and Medicaid looming on the horizon. Emerging were magnificent academic health-care centers, fueled by federal dollars and loan guarantees to support research, education, and patient care. Medicine, and particularly medicine in academic health-care centers, numbering about 120 today and often called the "crown jewels" of American medicine, was becoming big business. This attracted entrepreneurs from the private sector to develop technologies and goods and services to be sold to health-care providers. Moreover, the pace of discovery in biomedical sciences was quickening, making big science big business, too.

Amid this swirl of activity, Mayfield, in his proclamation, saw a clear role for organized neurosurgery to play in education and research and even prevention. He also asserted that neurosurgery should "stake a claim in cancer, trauma, and stroke," and thereby further define the scope of practice for neurosurgery. He urged that more be done to foster participation of neurosurgeons on federal panels and other governmental and quasi-governmental agencies. He made all these points and more in his proclamation in 1965; however, they are not well remembered, nor well remembered is his impression that neurosurgeons "have permitted ourselves the luxury of being too parochial; that we have enjoyed talking to ourselves so much that we have as an organization isolated ourselves from the mainstream of medicine, especially from the body politic of medicine (67)." Read in its entirety,

The Mayfield Proclamation was much more than a simple statement about a spokes-organization. It was a plea for neurosurgery to stop being so preoccupied with itself and to stop standing on the shore watching others swim by—a plea for neurosurgery to get wet by jumping in the mainstream and swimming with the tide sweeping events along and transforming medicine. Like Shakespeare, Mayfield knew that there truly is a "tide in the affairs of men." And so, he closed his proclamation by urging neurosurgeons to "apply our resources to all issues with vigor. If we do, we will never miss another roll call."

Following the Mayfield proclamation, the bylaws of The Cushing Society were changed in 1966 to provide representation on the Board for the four sister organizations of The Cushing Society. In 1948, Mayfield tried to do something like this and failed. It is reasonable to speculate that this change in the bylaws was intended to provide broad-based representation and give meaning to the word, "spokes-organization." Perhaps, the proponents of this change also believed that it would provide cohesion and coherence among the organizations that defined at that point in history the phrase "organized neurosurgery." Such cohesion and coherence would allow the AANS to speak with authority and in a timely manner for neurosurgery. If these were the goals in 1966, then they have not been completely achieved in 1997.

Today, the four organizations no longer have "seats" on the AANS Board, and the CNS is considered to be a "partner" of the AANS in governing many aspects of organized neurosurgery, but not all. Other organizations like the Council of State Neurosurgical Societies and specialty sections have emerged to "stake their claim" on aspects of the agenda for organized neurosurgery. Rather than consolidating resources and centralizing authority for decision-making in the AANS as spokes-organization, authority seems to have been diffused over the past 30 years as more and more organizations emerge and assert their rights to set policy and represent organized neurosurgery. It seems everyone "wants to get into the act." Surveying the scene, one wag suggested that the phrase, "organized neurosurgery" is actually an oxymoron; better it be called "disorganized neurosurgery." The implication of these comments is that authority is now spread throughout organized neurosurgery, which makes most important decisions a result of multilateral negotiations.

Relations between the AANS and CNS are cordial, but complex. One long-time observer of organized neurosurgery described the relationship as "two behemoths circling each other while engaged in a fragile embrace of the Joint Officers, with each half still subservient to the final decision of the respective governing boards (90)." Well, they may not be "behemoths," but they do spend a great deal of time going back and forth between the leadership lines, as if there were some "no man's land" between them. And so much depends on the personal relations between the CNS and AANS leaders, because there exist significant differences between the organizations involving philosophy, operations, and mission. Such is the nature of partnership, but Mayfield did not contemplate a partnership to govern and manage the affairs of neurosurgery and to speak for it. He most likely envisioned a vertically integrated structure with clear lines of communications, command, and control. In this way, he would insure that neurosurgery would not "miss another roll call."

Because authority is dispersed widely in organized neurosurgery, it is difficult to reach decisions on a timely and consistent basis on what is to be done to whom, by whom, and when. So many pockets of authority slow the process down, and, some would say, bog it down. This is a consequence of the evolution of organized neurosurgery and is not uncommon in voluntary associations of physicians. Governance structures within organized neurosurgery specifically and organized medicine generally are intended to prevent hasty decisions. Working decisions through a board and its committees and sister organizations insures that ideas are thoroughly vetted before they are approved.

This is very much the university model, where careful consideration is a norm intended to protect values of academic freedom and collegiality. This process may be slow, but it is sure, in that few, if any, big mistakes are ever made or radical actions ever taken. It provides great stability for organizations which can *afford* to have long horizons and to preserve strong traditions, and can *afford* not to worry too much about the external environment. Because organized neurosurgery is so steeped in the academic tradition and emerged independent organization by independent organization, it too has a deliberate and, perhaps, cumbersome decision-making process. But can organized neurosurgery afford such a process?

John Boyd, the fighter pilot and military strategist, asserted that quickness and maneuverability were important variables in aerial combat specifically and warfare generally. Companies like Motorola, Compaq, and Intel have achieved great success because they have explicitly or implicitly applied Boyd's ideas about ''cycle time'' to their manufacturing operations. These companies have demonstrated the competitive advantage of being both quick and nimble in the marketplace. Others have emulated these companies, including health-care providers, where it has been observed that there are only two types of players, the quick and the dead. In the so-called global economy, ''being first with the most'' frequently separates winners from losers. All of this is perfectly consistent with Boyd's ideas about how an advantage is attained by moving more quickly than the opponent through the loop of observation, orientation, decision and action (OODA). From this very simple idea, a strategic planning literature has evolved, illustrating the importance of acceleration and of being quick, fast, and nimble. All of that literature can be summarized in but two words, ''speed kills.''

Reality is that the evolution of organized neurosurgery makes its decision making process deliberate, whereas the forces transforming medicine today are moving fast, very fast. Riding those forces are risk-taking entrepreneurs, whose cycle times are much quicker than organized neurosurgery's. These entrepreneurs, which include Catholic nuns, engineers, and investment bankers, frequently have sleek governance structures, permitting them to be ''up-tempo'' in their making of decisions and deployment of resources. And even though organized neurosurgery reaches very good decisions with its deliberate process, those decisions may not be timely. Success requires the right idea at the right time, which is then flawlessly implemented at the right time. The landscape is littered with businesses and organizations that could not act quickly enough on their good ideas. Remember Heath Kit? Now, think of Bose (14)!To advance its agenda in the fast-paced socioeconomic environment, organized neurosurgery should accelerate its cycle time for observation, orientation, decision, and action, so it can make and implement good decisions quicker. If not, it will ''lose,'' just as all those ''top-gun'' pilots lost to John Boyd over the Nevada desert.

ORIENTATION OF ORGANIZED NEUROSURGERY TO THE DEREGULATION OF HEALTH CARE

In December 1996, two neurosurgeons—department chiefs of different academic health-care centers in New York City—were invited to a ''beauty contest.'' It was not your typical beauty contest held in Atlantic City before a panel of lesser-known celebrities. Rather, it was a ''contest'' held in New York City before a panel exploring how these departments might be fused and, perhaps, which department would survive a proposed merger of their respective institutions. One neurosurgeon reportedly said, ''It is basically a question of who is No. 1a and who is 1b—we would consider ourselves to be 1a.'' The other neurosurgeon reportedly stated, ''I have never been the kind of person who gets up and tells people how great I am.'' In the end, though, the merger failed. Differences in culture between the medical schools could not be bridged and the debt of one medical school could not be assigned to a proposed hospital corporation. In February 1997, one potential merger partner bailed out. Hearing the news, a thrilled faculty member asked his dean whether the deal was ''truly dead—with a stake through its heart.'' The dean answered, ''Yes, it is (29, 59, 61).''

From a business perspective, the merger made sense. Together, these high-profile institutions in New York City would have had 2300 beds and $2 billion in revenues. Combined, they could achieve efficiencies, pushing costs lower and perhaps quality higher, and deal more effectively with managed care organizations, which have rapidly increased their market share to about 50% nationally and to 75% of those employed (45). In spite of the wave of hospital closings and mergers, there are still too many hospital beds, with 40% unoccupied on any given day (45). Had the merger gone through, surely there would have been downsizing of staff including senior nurses and physicians (95).

No strangers to mergers, acquisitions, and consolidations, members of the respective boards, though, did not anticipate the reaction of faculty to merging their medical schools. Perhaps, had these boards not put their schools in play, a merger of clinical operations would have succeeded. In California, for example, two high-profile institutions plan to merge their hospitals, not their medical schools (59). But the boards in New York City did not do this; now their institutions are traveling separate paths, where they will likely consider the merger question once again. They will do so because others have already done their deals and because the State of New York has just made a tough operating environment even tougher.

On January 1, 1997, the State of New York eliminated one of the last hospital rate setting programs in the country, thereby deregulating hospital prices and fostering competition among hospitals. Private employers in New York had lobbied hard to eliminate price controls and to allow greater flexibility in setting prices for hospital services among payers and providers. Major insurance companies and large employers expected to experience decreases in their costs for hospital-based services (127).

For many years, "pricing" of services for hospitals (and other health-care providers) in New York and elsewhere was based on a "cost-plus" reimbursement system. Providers were reimbursed for their "reasonable cost" of providing a service "plus" some margin of, well, profit. Such cost-plus systems, though, are not unique to health care. They are typical of pricing in regulated industries, like utilities. Because such pricing tends to be inefficient, there have been efforts to deregulate all kinds of industries, including health care. What happened in the State of New York with its hospital rate program, therefore, is but one sentence in a much larger story of deregulation.

Crandall and Ellig (24) studied the effects of deregulation in natural gas, long distance phone service, airlines, railroads, and trucking. They found that deregulation in these industries had price savings between $40 and $60 billion dollars a year. About deregulation, they conclude:

- Deregulation and customer choice lower price.
- Deregulation and customer choice align service quality and customer desires.
- Customers have experienced genuine benefits, not just reallocation of costs among customer classes.
- The lower the barriers to customer choice, the greater the benefits customers receive.
- Competitive markets continue to evolve in response to customer needs.

They also claim that "In virtually every case, the economic benefits from deregulation or regulatory reform have exceeded economists' pre-

dictions. The record shows that deregulation has led to lower prices, expanded output, and improved choices of service quality (24)." Because deregulation makes markets for goods and services more open and pricing more influenced by competitive forces, deregulation is *one* pathway health care is taking.

It is taking this pathway because health-care costs are simply too high and going higher, from 9% of gross domestic product (GDP) in 1980 to 11% in 1992, to a projected 15% by 2000 (27). In 1995, about $1 trillion was spent on health care or 14% of GDP (105); so the projected percentage for 2000 may actually be too low. For all the money spent on health care in America, about 40 million people are either uninsured or underinsured (91). These facts motivated President Clinton in 1993 to advance universal health-care coverage through "managed competition." While President Clinton failed, he may have stimulated and reinforced private sector actions to transform health care (126). There have been over 300 major health-care deals done from 1993 through 1996. One mergers and acquisitions specialist observed about this 3-year period that it is the "strongest period of consolidation I've ever seen (105)."

It is also taking this path of deregulation because America competes in a global economy, where the winners are companies with low costs and high quality. General Motors (GM), one example of a global competitor, is treating health-care providers like any other supplier and is actually sending GM efficiency experts to health-care facilities to find ways to reduce costs and increase quality. For GM there is a sense of urgency; its health-care bill for active and retired employees is $1200 for every car produced in America, which is $700 more than GM pays for steel to build the car. The health-care bill at Chrysler is $700 and at Ford, $510. Foreign manufacturers operating in American pay about $100 in health-care cost per car, because their workforce is younger and healthier. GM's global future depends in part on its ability to manage health-care costs; that is why GM is using its "clout" to make its health-care suppliers, better, faster, cheaper (11).

Finally, America is taking the pathway of deregulation because it is on the verge of an explosion in senior citizens. In 1997, 200,000 people will turn 65; 15 years from that date the annual increase will be 1.6 million (12). In 1970, Medicare costs were $6 billion; in 1997 they reached $200 billion and by 2030[125], Medicare may consume 7.5% of gross domestic product, up from 2.6% today. (125) While the 1997 proposed balanced budget deal between President Clinton and congressional leadership keeps the Medicare hospital fund solvent until the year 2008, nothing was done to address 2011, when baby boomers begin to retire in huge numbers (81). Most of the $115 billion in Medicare "cuts" negotiated in this budget deal come from hospitals, managed care organizations, and physicians, or the "usual suspects," as Department of Health and Human Services (HHS) Secretary Donna Shalala calls health-care providers (91).

It has been suggested that Medicare's long-term deficit may be as much as $9 trillion over the next 75 years (25). Faced with such unimaginable numbers, it has been proposed that managed care organizations bid on Medicare business, thereby establishing an average market price. Beneficiaries selecting a plan with a lower than average price could pocket the difference. Those selecting a plan with a higher than average price would pay the difference out-of-pocket (110). Whether this idea is politically viable is uncertain. Powerful organizations, like the 33-million member American Association of Retired Persons, have forcefully expressed concerns about higher deductible payments or contributions (81).

Looking at these same numbers, Senator Ron Wyden of Oregon really does not like what he sees. To combat adverse financial trends in Medicare, this Senator, thought to be a "liberal" by some, proposes a bill that would interject more market competition into the system by encouraging senior citizens to join lower cost managed care organizations (102). The future of Senator Wyden's bill is uncertain, but not uncertain is that in the years ahead there will be some very big fights about the future of Medicare (83, 89), including how best and how fast to deregulate the provision of health-care services under Medicare.

Due to costs, global trade, and demographics, there is an effort to deregulate health care. That process of deregulation, though, probably began as far back as 1983, with the implementation of a prospective payment system of diagnostically related groups for hospitals, followed in 1989 with the development of a fee schedule for physicians based on a resource-based relative value scale (5). Both of these were fixed-fee, not cost-plus systems. Since then, and because the private sector frequently follows the lead of HHS in pricing health-care services, deregulation has picked up speed in the non-Medicare sector as fixed-fee replaced fee-for-service plans, and more persons entered lower-cost managed care systems. Prospective payment systems replaced retrospective cost-based reimbursement systems, so common in regulated industries. This change interjected competition and market pricing in health care, which stimulated actions to rationalize the delivery of health care with systems, consolidation, integration, and risk sharing, developments also common in deregulated or deregulating industries. And so, the process of deregulation in health care is well under way, and developments in the hospital and managed care industries surely verify this.

A frequent effect of deregulation is merging and consolidating businesses to achieve size, power, and economies of scale. Formerly regulated businesses like airlines typically get bigger as one way to achieve efficiencies, reduce unit costs, and thereby compete effectively in the marketplace. Hospitals have been merging and consolidating and rationalizing services as ways to get more efficient in a deregulating health-care environment. As one expert said about a 1997 merger in the long-term care industry, "It's an indication that bigger is better. People are pursuing scale, partly to cope with managed care. When you have a greater number of facilities or a broader patient base, you have more negotiating power with managed care companies and suppliers (7)."

Columbia/HCA typifies this strategy. Called the King Kong of hospital chains, it has grown dramatically in the past 10 years through mergers and acquisitions. Today, Columbia/HCA is a $23 billion dollar empire, operating in 37 states. It has 343 hospitals, 136 outpatient surgery centers, and 550 home health-care operations, and is prowling for more (32). For $1.12 billion in cash, it bought Value Health to expand its reach into pharmacy benefits, mental health, and worker's compensation. Financial analysts believe that Columbia/HCA's $3 billion annual cash flow gives it $1 billion annually to "grab" even more health-care providers (32).

Recently, however, the Columbia/HCA juggernaut has been slowed by set backs in Ohio, where a proposed joint venture with Blue Cross and Blue Shield of Ohio was blocked; in California, where a joint venture with a not-for-profit hospital chain collapsed; and in Rhode Island, where another joint venture with a not-for-profit hospital has been delayed (73). At a field hearing in Providence about this Rhode Island hospital, Representative Pete Stark of California said of Columbia/HCA: "They are not good neighbors, they are not good practitioners, and they are not good people (73)."

Harsh words, but Representative Stark thinks that Columbia/HCA has grown rapidly by using certain business arrangements with some physicians that may violate the very physician self-referral laws he wrote. The federal government may think so too. This explains the 1997 investigation of Columbia/HCA operations in El Paso, Texas, where agents of the Federal Bureau of Investigation, the Internal Revenue Service, and the Department of Health and Human Services are reviewing records of physicians affiliated with hospitals and home health agencies operated by Columbia/HCA, to determine whether any of those relationships violate applicable rules regarding payments for physician referrals (39). The outcome of the investigation is at least months and perhaps years away, but this investigation gives new meaning to the Columbia/HCA tagline: "Health care has never worked like this before."

Representative Stark also describes Columbia/HCA as a "Pac man" and "giant octopus that is gobbling up American health care." About this Representative Stark may be right; the scale of its operations is unprecedented. Columbia/HCA treats about 125,000 patients a day, had 40 million patients in 1996, which is significantly better than its closest competitor, and operates 67,000 hospital beds. It has close ties to managed care organizations, which account for 32% of its admissions (66). So, Columbia/HCA is a huge player in the marketplace, but it is not alone.

Formerly known as National Medical Enterprises (NME), Tenet Healthcare is the second largest hospital company in the country. NME had its share of troubles, as recently as 1994, when it was fined $362 million for Medicaid fraud and paid another $230 million to settle other law suits. The NME board forced out the founder and CEO and installed a mortgage banker. From 1994 through 1997, he has completed deals worth $12.5 billion to resurrect

NME as Tenet Healthcare. One $3 billion deal to acquire OrNda HealthCorp in January 1997 was the second largest high-yield (read "junk") underwriting ever, with the largest being the leveraged buy out of RJR Nabisco in 1989 (104). All this "wheeling and dealing" made Tenet Healthcare big enough to achieve significant economies of scale in the marketplace. Like Columbia/HCA, Tenet Healthcare assumed a mountain of debt to achieve its size and scope, but like Columbia/HCA, it is poised to compete for business across geographic boarders.

On the 1996 Fortune magazine list of fast growing companies, (105) HealthSouth is the third example of consolidation and growth. HealthSouth operates rehabilitation clinics and outpatient surgery centers. It is a low-cost alternative to hospital-based services and is growing rapidly. In about 12 years, its 44-year-old CEO amassed over 1000 such facilities, creating $6 billion in shareholder equity. His personal 1996 equity position is $360 million, not bad for a onetime gas-station attendant, turned respiratory therapist, turned entrepreneur (107).

In 1996 he made $7 million in salary and bonus, and, between 1994 and 1996, he completed nine deals worth $2.6 billion. One analyst said of HealthSouth, "This company embodies nearly all the positive trends in this industry: consolidation, cost-efficiency, and good use of information." By 1996, revenues of HealthSouth reached $3 billion, with net income of $360 million. Its existing contracts cover over 130 million people for various health-care services. However, one of the most interesting ideas to emerge from HealthSouth is its desire to develop a brand identity, like McDonald's or Holiday Inn. Its CEO plans to do this with old-fashioned marketing and even co-branding products, like a HealthSouth athletic shoe (107). If he can establish HealthSouth as a household name, make it "top of mind," and then deliver high quality, cost-effective services, he will then have a powerful market position, which will only get stronger over time.

Such rapid consolidation is not limited to the for-profit sector. For generations, Catholic nuns have owned and operated hospitals throughout the country as a part of their religious mission. They are very good at what they do and generally enjoy a very favorable reputation for quality care. However, in this era of deregulating health care, where bigger is better, various Catholic orders are protecting their "turf" and becoming "players" in the game of mergers, acquisitions, and consolidations. Catholic Healthcare West (CHW) is a good example of this; its governing body is composed of 10 nuns from various orders. In 1989, CHW hired a new CEO, who, in 1996, was paid $500,000 plus a modest bonus. Over the past several years, he and the "good sisters" (as nuns are affectionately known by all who have ever worked closely with them) have implemented a plan of acquisitions and consolidation, and have even acquired non-Catholic hospitals by outbidding such rivals as Columbia/ HCA and Tenet Healthcare. CHW has a growth strategy that involves significant market share in 10 geographic areas of California and Arizona. It had 1996 revenues of nearly $3 billion and net income after charity care of $160 million. CHW is not an isolated example; in 1996 three religious orders came together to form the Denver-based Catholic Health Initiatives, which has 60 hospitals in 10 states (96). These non-for-profit Catholic chains, like their for-profit rivals, understand what it takes to compete in a deregulating health-care environment and act accordingly.

By getting bigger, hospitals, outpatient clinics, and extended care facilities hope to push costs down and quality up, and, thereby, compete more effectively for managed care contracts. Providers that can provide a range of services over a wide geographic area should be able to command more and better contracts from managed care organizations, insurers, and employers. Aetna, for example, wants to establish long-term relationships with as few as 25 integrated regional providers (40). Should Aetna achieve its goal, then very few small, unaffiliated community hospitals will be doing business with Aetna.

To advance its vision, Aetna made a huge bet on health care. Aetna paid $8.9 billion to purchase US Healthcare, described as "the nation's most successful health-maintenance organization (109)." It plans to fuse the companies and make Aetna a player in the managed care business. Like hospitals, managed care organizations understand that they must get larger, cover more lives, and compete over wider geographic areas, if they plan to compete in a deregulating health-care environment. They must also get more efficient, and, in Aetna's case, US Healthcare is very efficient in using technology, driving oper-

ating costs down, and bargaining hard with providers like hospitals. (109) US Healthcare typically pays hospitals significantly less than Aetna does, so it is not surprising that day-to-day operations of the combined entity will be the responsibility of former US Healthcare executives.

Overnight, Aetna's acquisition of US Healthcare made it one of the nation's biggest health care insurers. About a year later, Cigna took out Healthsource for $1.45 billion in cash and the assumption of $250 million in Healthsource debt, making the combined entity slightly larger than Aetna (31). At this point, and among publicly traded companies, only United Healthcare is larger than Cigna and Aetna, but that could change. In 1995 United Healthcare got larger when it bought for $1.6 billion MetraHealth, a joint venture of Metropolitan Life and Travelers (31). Proposed is PacifiCare Health's $2.1 billion purchase of FHP International (43). Still looking for a partner is Prudential, which is ranked among the 15 top insurers, but its managed care business is losing money. Soon it will have to acquire, or be acquired (31).

Like their counterparts in the health-care facilities industry, publicly-traded managed care companies want to be bigger to achieve efficiencies in operations and "clout" in the marketplace. As a result, there were $77 billion worth of consolidation involving health-care entities in 1996 (43). Because hospitals, managed care entities, and even pharmaceutical companies, are unable to increase prices, due to competition in the marketplace, they are looking for unit growth and cost cutting, which they hope to gain through mergers. As of January 1, 1996, two-thirds of all health maintenance organization (HMO) members belonged to just 15 national companies, some of which have subsequently merged, like US Healthcare and Aetna (119). In California, often considered the "tip of the lance" with respect to health-care trends, seven companies control 85% of the HMO enrollment (119), and some of those companies are making plans to expand into markets in the Midwest and East. If they do, they will encounter Oxford Health Plans, an innovative HMO whose CEO believes that "the customer will tell us what to do if we will only listen (44)."

Stephen Wiggins, CEO, Oxford Health Plans, has been listening to "customers" since 1984 when he started his company with $90,000. In 1991, he took Oxford public and eventually created a company whose 1997 market capitalization was $4.5 billion. At that capitalization, his 3% share was worth $150 million. As of 1996, its revenues were growing over 125% annually (105). This made Oxford Health Plans the fifth fastest growing company in America, and in less than 4 short years, its stock price zoomed from $4 to $47 per share. Earnings per share have grown 83% per year for 5 years. For one 3-year period, Oxford's growth actually outpaced such companies as Microsoft, Cisco Systems, and America Online. With 1.5 million members and 40,000 doctors, Oxford's 1997 revenues reached $3 billion. Because it listens to its "customers," Oxford plans to provide access to nontraditional medicine (51) and easier access to specialty care medicine (131), and even plans to use highly trained nurses for primary care medicine, a role traditionally reserved for primary care doctors (130). All of this illustrates that Oxford Health Plans has "figured out to take advantage of the changing nature of the business," as one writer observed (105).

Considering the changing nature of the health-care "business," the late-Cardinal Joseph Bernardin of Chicago did not like what he saw and said so before The Harvard Business Club of Chicago on January 12, 1995. In his speech, "Making the case for not-for-profit health care," Cardinal Bernardin presented a cogent, balanced, and clear case for not-for-profit health care (9). That case can be summarized best in his words as "the primary end or essential purpose of medical care delivery should be a cured patient . . . and a healthier community, not to earn a profit or a return on capital for shareholders." As he wove his argument, Cardinal Bernardin made an interesting observation: "Should the investor-owned entity ever become the predominant form of health-care delivery, I believe our country will inevitably experience a sizable and substantial growth in government intervention and control." Cardinal Bernardin may be right. Even though not-for-profit entities still dominate health-care delivery, there appears to be a movement to control and regulate managed care delivery systems and their partners in the health-care facilities industry.

In 1997, President Clinton appointed a 33 person panel called, the "Advisory Commission on Consumer Protection and Quality in the Health Care Industry" to study whether a patient bill of rights was needed to protect them during this period of continuity and change in health-care delivery (85). Composed of a cross section of interest groups, this panel held its first meeting on May 13, 1997 (88). Not unexpectedly, the panel will be sifting through much conflicting testimony on this topic before it can reach conclusions. However, the appointment of such a panel supports Cardinal Bernardin's observation about the potential growth in regulation. Clearly, a national bill of rights for patients would be government intervention writ large and perhaps would be a full-employment act for the nation's trial lawyers.

There is, however, speculation that Congress and state legislatures will not wait for the panel to provide a report. Both Democrats and Republicans have introduced bills in the 105th Congress which illustrate that there is bipartisan concern about such issues as patient access to emergency room services and specialists, the right of doctors to discuss treatment options with patients, and the right of patients to appeal the decisions of their health-care plan (72, 86). Most controversial in these bills is a provision that allows patients to bring medical malpractice suits against a managed care plan covered under the Employee Retirement & Income Security Act of 1974 (48). Enactment of this provision would remove the legal shield managed care plans now enjoy. Currently, providers and their insurance carriers assume all the risk of medical malpractice litigation. Perhaps, Congress will not pass comprehensive legislation, but it has already demonstrated a willingness to pass piecemeal legislation, as the 104th Congress did by requiring 48-hour maternity stays and a version of mental health parity. As one measure of congressional sentiment, an aide opined that "We could enact anti-managed care provisions every day and not meet the demand from members [of Congress] (13)."

While Congress has been talking, state legislatures have been acting. In 1996, 1400 pieces of legislation were introduced in the states to regulate managed care. Of those introduced, 56 were enacted into law in some 35 states (75). Perhaps this legislative activity has something to do with the "dim" view the public has of managed care companies and health insurers. In a recent poll, 80% of the respondents believe quality of care is compromised by insurers to save money (19). For whatever reasons, such actions at both the national and state levels may increase the costs of providing care, notwithstanding the fact that costs are already going up after being well behaved for several years (33 , 128). Some see dangers in the piecemeal approach being taken by the states and suggest that patients, doctors, managed care organizations, and hospitals get together to establish some parameters of cost-effective health-care all can understand and apply. If not this, then there may be a maze of conflicting laws, rules, and regulations, which will do little to advance quality patient care and a lot to increase costs (75). Regulation does cost something, because it frequently introduces inefficiencies in the allocation of resources.

While the federal ''drive through'' delivery law or state anti-gag-rule statutes may be tangible expressions of concern about the business of health care, one health-care futurist likens them to ''speed bumps'' and not impediments to the growth of managed care organizations (119). The real threat to their long-term growth is competition with other managed care organizations, and employer coalitions like Choice Plus in Minneapolis (20). Founded by 25 leading employers, Choice Plus cuts out the HMO middlemen, all of whom operate as not-for-profit entities in Minnesota. For a flat fee, an HMO handles paperwork for Choice Plus. Started in 1993 as an experiment, Choice Plus has reduced employers' health-care expenses by about 11% (114). Employer groups in Des Moines and St. Louis are replicating the Minneapolis model and trying to bypass insurers too. Their success in doing this has ominous implications for traditional HMOs. Physician-sponsored organizations could be another threat to traditional HMOs. One writer asserts that ''If doctors figure out how to find their own customers, insurers may find themselves simply processing claims—a low-margin affair (40).'' Another threat could emerge from physician practice management firms like MedPartners, PhyCor, and FPA Medical. These firms act as a liaison between groups of doctors and payers like HMOs, insurers, and employers. In just 3 years, MedPartners grew from nine physician members to 2600 and entered the pharmacy and disease management business (100).

Some predict that competitive forces, as those described above, will reduce the number of HMOs by 50% by the end of 1998 (119). Only the biggest, most efficient operators will survive the ongoing competition and the process of con-solidation. However, this is what happens during deregulation. A competitive market emerges, and entrepreneurs see opportunities and take them. And there are plenty of opportunities around, particularly in long-term care, chronic care, mental health, wellness, home health, disabled children, Medicaid, and Medicare. With these and other opportunities, the challenges are to reduce costs and increase quality. America has bet that more competitive health-care markets through deregulation can do both.

As a process, deregulation can occur quickly or over a protracted period of time. Airlines deregulated rapidly, whereas telecommunications is proceeding at a much slower pace. Efforts to deregulate telecommunications began as early as 1949, but, as late as 1997, the Federal Communications Commission issued new rules to strip away billions of dollars of subsidies and enhance free-market competition in telephone service (116). The variable pace of deregulation is important to keep in mind, because deregulation of health care will most likely be protracted. Perhaps as many as 150 million Americans have enrolled in some managed care organization, but this just may be the end of an initial phase involving the conversion of higher cost indemnity to lower cost managed care plans. Phases involving consolidation, price competition, and quality are just starting. However, once the process of deregulation begins, it is nearly impossible to stop or reverse. There may be new regulations or reregulation in an industry, as evidenced by the actions of the Congress and state legislatures with respect to health care, but the momentum of deregulation seems always toward freer, less regulated markets, simply because such markets provide, in the long run, better choice, access, quality, and prices. Any doubts about this should be dashed by the critical condition of the British National Health Service, a highly regulated health-care system on the verge of collapse (65).

There is, however, probably no such thing as absolute deregulation or a pure market economy. The economy generally combines both competition and regulation, and so does health care. There has been and will be an ongoing dialogue about what, when, and where to regulate, and about the extent to which competitive forces should operate freely. Efforts to close some small, rural hospitals involve elements of this dialogue, because such hospitals are casualties of a deregulating health-care environment (60).

Built in an era of cost-plus reimbursement and often with federal loan guarantees, these hospitals now have high costs and low patient volumes and, quite frankly, cannot compete for managed care contracts. They are like the "stranded assets" the economists write about when they describe investor-owned plants made expendable by deregulation in gas or electric utilities. Certainly, these small hospitals benefit the local community, but at what cost? And who pays that cost? And are there better and cheaper alternatives? These are the kinds of questions that have been asked and will be asked as society sets sail on uncharted waters, tacking between deregulation in health care and regulation of health care. Hence, professional organizations in neurosurgery must be able to advance their missions in two different, but related, environments.

One economist asserts that "greater reliance on market forces in imperfectly competitive industries turns out to require more of a regulatory presence, not less (58)." Health care is an imperfectly competitive industry, so it is reasonable to expect that efforts to deregulate health care will parallel efforts to regulate it. Recent actions of the Federal Communications Commission to deregulate long-distance telephone service had significant subsidies for schools, poor people, and those living in rural areas. The wisdom of granting those subsidies is not an issue here, but they illustrate that a regulatory agency in the same ruling can simultaneously achieve more competition and more regulation. Such actions have been called "regulated competition," a phrase that seems to apply to health care as it evolves.

Regulation in health care can involve matters quite specific or more global. Part of the 1997 budget deal cited above involves the provision of preventive services under Medicare. As a part of the deal, President Clinton agreed that Medicare beneficiaries would pay higher Medicare premiums over time, but insisted on additional preventive services as a benefit to be covered under Medicare, including screening for colon cancer. As the second leading cause of death from cancer, colon cancer kills 55,000 people a year. There are two ways to provide screening for colon cancer, a colonoscopy performed by gastroenterologists and a barium X-ray performed by radiologists. Which is best and which should be covered under Medicare as a screening

benefit are unanswered questions. But, because there are thousands of lives at stake and, quite frankly, billions of dollars of revenue for physicians and suppliers on the table, gastroenterologists have hired a high-powered lobbyist to make their case in Congress for colonoscopy and radiologists have hired one to make their case for barium X-ray. The professional societies are very much involved with this debate and have been so for years. The outcome is still uncertain, but this case illustrates how a very specific health-care matter can get tangled in the regulatory process and become "a shadowy, fierce battle to win the Government's imprimatur for some tests while denying coverage for others (82)."

On a global scale there is a battle under way involving care for 100 million Americans with chronic illness. The annual cost of providing such care is about $425 billion, which is a significant share of the $1 trillion dollars spent on health care in 1996. At issue is access to specialty care medicine. Involved in this issue is the American Medical Association. It wants a new designation called "principal care" physicians and wants managed care organizations to accept that specialists can be "principal care" physicians of first contact, who coordinate care for persons with chronic conditions. Primary care specialists, such as family medicine physicians, see the issue differently. They claim with some justification that their training and longitudinal care of patients make them uniquely qualified to detect subtle shifts in a patient's condition and then use specialists as appropriate (53). Access to specialists undoubtedly varies among managed care plans, which explains why proponents for greater access seek relief in the form of rules, regulations, law, and statues. Neurosurgery is also a minor player in this drama, as a member of a coalition to advance access to specialty care medicine. Working largely out of Washington, DC, this coalition of 130 specialties and affiliated groups has "worked" this issue for years and uses many modern techniques of communications to reach decision makers and opinion leaders. That both Republicans and Democrats sponsored bills to enhance access to specialty care is either one measure of success or an illustration that "An invasion of armies can be resisted, but not an idea whose time has come."

Whether the regulatory issue is specific or global, neurosurgeons, through their professional organizations, should be ready to represent the interests of their patients. Staying focused on the interests of patients in these regulatory battles and "tiffs" is consistent with neurosurgery's traditional mission: "to provide the highest quality of neurosurgical care to the public." Moreover, staying focused on patients is the moral high ground that allows organized neurosurgery to see all regulatory issues as involving but two fundamental issues: access to and quality of neurosurgical care. When HHS proposed to reduce significantly reimbursement for the practice expenses of neurosurgeons in the 1998 Medicare fee schedule, organized neurosurgery argued that such a drastic reduction would reduce quality and access to care, just as such reductions in reimbursement reduced access and quality in the Medicaid system. By standing for their patients, neurosurgeons stood for themselves, because if their patients have no rights to access and quality, then neurosurgeons have no prerogatives. Such rights and prerogatives are two sides of the very same coin. Hence, what is good for their patients just so happens to be good for neurosurgeons.

However, standing for their patients can be expensive for neurosurgery. Specialties adversely affected by proposed revisions in practice expense reimbursement contributed about $1.6 million in 1997 to advance their common cause in Congress and relevant agencies. It seems like a lot of money, but $1.6 million does not go very far in Washington, DC, where "can-do" lobbyists command multiple six-figure fees. Organized neurosurgery committed $100,000 to the coalition. That, too, seems like a lot of money, but that contribution, combined with ongoing efforts to represent the interests of patients in Washington and elsewhere, represents less than 5% of the combined operating revenues of the AANS and CNS. The $200-billion-a-year electrical power industry is about to undergo serious deregulation. Sides are forming in Washington, DC for the battles that lie ahead. It is estimated that on a combined basis, both sides will spend $50 million in the first year on lobbying and advertising (99). That figure makes the coalition's $1.6 million and organized neurosurgery's $100,000 seem minuscule by comparison.

Neurosurgeons, though, should not expect their professional organizations to have significant influence with regulatory matters. In politics, there are two sources of power: people and money. Organized neurosurgery has neither of those; so, in the bigger scheme of things, neurosurgery is really a very small player. It can never have the kind of close and cozy relationships with its regulators that the insurance companies purportedly have with theirs (122). Neurosurgeons who go to Washington to advance an agenda for neurosurgeons and their patients soon learn that their challenges are greater than they imagined and their ability to overcome those challenges less than they imagined. Compounding their difficulties is a constituency, neurosurgeons, who are often more interested in science than regulation and much more interested in patient care than health-care policy. At nearly any annual meeting of neurosurgeons, planners rarely, if ever, schedule socioeconomic and science/patient care presentations at the same time. They know in advance what the result will be—a mostly empty room for the socioeconomic presentation.

Attempting to achieve favorable regulations in Washington is not easy. Everything starts with access, but easy access, at least to Congress, takes big money. For $250,000, the Republican Party offered a "season pass" to elite donors, with the promise of special staff to help them throughout the year with their problems. At least 75 corporations and individuals anted up the $250,000 in 1996 (123). But organized neurosurgery does not have that kind of money to toss around. Even if it did, political money typically buys access, not results. As one health-care association executive stated, "I have never seen money tied to favors, but access is critical. I can't make my points if I don't have access. Would I have less access if we didn't make contributions? There is no question that a willingness to participate in the electoral process, including financial participation, does help insure access (84)."

Bankers are not shy about using their money and network of contacts to advance their point of view in the regulatory environment. Accordingly, they make perfectly lawful contributions to both political parties and to individual politicians. In May 1996, some of the nation's most important bankers attended a Democratic Party-sponsored coffee at the White House with President Clinton to discuss administration-supported regulations some bankers thought were onerous. Treasury Secretary Robert E. Rubin attended this coffee as did a top banking regulator. In January 1997, well after the presidential election, this coffee klatch was reported in the press. Responding to a question about it at a news conference, President Clinton indicated that he used such events to provide a hearing for supporters about issues important to them, but no promises or commitments are made and no results guaranteed (97). While powerful interests were involved and billions of dollars at stake, the current record suggests that no deals were made either before, during, or after that coffee with President Clinton. This illustrates that even big-time players often get a fair hearing and nothing more for their money.

Of course, there are exceptions to this generalization. One involves a case of a top environmental regulator from Utah, who over a 10-year period received $600,000 in cash, gifts, and real estate from a nuclear-waste disposal company near Salt Lake City. Payments stopped 2 years after the regulator lost his job in 1995. In 1997, the former regulator filed suit claiming that the company breached its verbal agreement with him and claiming further that the company owed him some $5 million for services rendered while he was a regulator (94). Trial is pending, but Utah has an unambiguous law prohibiting regulators from accepting more than $50.00 from people they regulate, a fact which makes this suit a "10" on the chutzpah scale. Back in the nation's capitol, a second case involves a Congressman who pressured an official to delay, and perhaps abort, an effort to "crackdown" on standards of eligibility for loans to students attending off-shore medical schools. Turns out the operator of one of those schools contributed $1000 to that Congressman and promised to find a seat at the school for his daughter (49). Effective as they may seem, these crass examples of "capturing" the regulatory process are far beneath the dignity of organized neurosurgery. None of its leaders—past, present, or future— would stoop so low to conquer.

Over 30 years ago, Doctor Mayfield urged neurosurgeons to get involved with the "body politic of medicine." He understood that regulatory affairs, particularly at the federal level, would affect the future scope and practice of neurosurgery. Unfortunately, Doctor Mayfield did not proclaim how organized neurosurgery might do this effectively, given its rather limited resources. In fairness, though, Doctor Mayfield

could not have anticipated the explosion in the size and scope of government. Nor could he have anticipated how costly and frustrating it would eventually be to do "business" with the Congress and its agencies.

In spite of these difficulties, organized neurosurgery has a small office with three professional staff in Washington to track legislation and regulation, and to respond as appropriate. Working closely with Washington staff is a group of highly knowledgeable and dedicated neurosurgeons, who give freely of their time and talents. However, the current complexity of regulatory affairs and demands on practicing neurosurgeons motivate organized neurosurgery to consider doing what other physician associations have already done, namely, to develop a center for socioeconomic affairs. This proposed center would have professional staff who could address matters like reimbursement, state regulations, and agency policy more completely than the existing staff who focus primarily on federal matters. Recall John Boyd; he observed that visibility and maneuverability were *the* critical variables in aerial combat. A center for socioeconomic affairs would help organized neurosurgery see better and move quicker in regulatory "combat."

Well known are the tragic tales of airline pilots so focused on an indicator light of one kind or another that they failed to realize that they were flying their plane into a mountain or the ground. Just like those unfortunate pilots, organized neurosurgery should not get overly focused on events in Washington. Beyond the Beltway, there is a merger mania under way, pushed on by deregulation and competition. In 1996 there were $1 trillion in mergers and acquisitions on a world-wide basis (64), and $77 billion of that $1 trillion involved health-care mergers and acquisitions in America. This wave of mergers seems mostly about efficiency and market power; hence, what is happening in health care is happening in other businesses and for precisely the same reasons.

When this urge to merge will end is uncertain. Shifts in the regulatory environment seem to favor efficiency. No longer is big necessarily bad. Competition makes it nearly impossible for firms to achieve pricing power in the market, so they must lower their costs by merger or acquisition. Traditional antitrust analysis no longer impedes such mergers and acquisitions for all kinds of industries, including health care (80). It seems, therefore, that this trend will proceed unabated for some time to come. While neurosurgery is a small, unique specialty, it can neither run nor hide from more deregulation, competition, and consolidation, and cannot easily achieve favorable regulations to preserve its prerogatives. Organized neurosurgery should orient neurosurgery and neurosurgeons to this environment and then decide how best to protect and advance its traditional missions in research, education, and patient care. Doing these will not be easy. About this environment, one health-care executive said, ''It's rough out there.''

DECISION OF ORGANIZED NEUROSURGERY TO BE AN EFFECTIVE NICHE PLAYER

Along with more competitive markets for major players, deregulation creates opportunities for small entrepreneurs to grab and defend a piece of the action. Since airline deregulation in 1978, there have been two waves of new, small carriers seeking to occupy market niches (24). Most of them failed, partly because they started to emulate larger carriers in costs and operations. One small carrier, though, was wildly successful—Southwest Airlines. It is the poster child for airline deregulation, with its low fares, low costs, customer service, and employee relations. It has become so successful that it now challenges more established players.

But Southwest Airlines is a very special story of how a niche player in a deregulated environment can get big and rich almost overnight, because it does what it does better than anyone else, meets a market need, and provides terrific value. For many years Alaska Airlines was considered to be that special niche player in the airline business, but for different reasons. Serving the Pacific Northwest, Alaska Airlines, unlike Southwest Airlines, had high fares, high operating costs, and a much-deserved reputation for exceptional passenger service. Because it had limited competition and a loyal market segment that could afford its fares, Alaska Airlines had a very good deal in the Pacific Northwest and parts of California. But then, enter Southwest Airlines and United Airlines' West Coast Shuttle. Alaska Airlines could not compete with them and started to hemorrhage cash. Its costs were simply too high; therefore, Alaska Airlines

moved aggressively to cut its costs through consolidation of operations, better labor agreements, and modification of its passenger services. After going through a near-death financial experience, Alaska Airlines emerged from its make-over much more competitive and dominant in its major markets. It beat back Southwest Airlines with strategies invented by Southwest Airlines and thereby survived this battle in deregulated skies (17).

A battle in deregulated skies for hegemony in the Pacific Northwest is not an isolated event. Similar battles have been going on in America for nearly 20 years, and by nearly every measure Americans have benefited from them in that they are flying more and paying less. Such battles, though, are just starting in Europe. Airline deregulation of 1993 in Europe made low-cost airlines like Virgin-Express popular. As one person observed, ''Europeans are just like Americans: They'll fly more if the price is good.'' And just like in America, many small European start-up carriers have already failed. Nonetheless, the airline deregulation genie is out of the bottle in Europe, and it is reasonable to expect stable competitive patterns to emerge after the final phase of deregulation in the European Union (EU) settles in. In April 1997, any EU carrier will be able to fly anywhere within the 15 nations of the EU (38). Sensing dangers ahead, European carriers are looking to hire airline executives from America having experience with deregulation. A 'brain drain' of sorts may be starting; both Swissair and Lufthansa have just hired top executive talent from America (117).

In both America and Europe, airline deregulation creates opportunities for entrepreneurs willing to bet *their* house to be a player, albeit small. This is what deregulation does: it creates opportunities. In telecommunications, resellers of long-distance phone service have captured nearly $1 billion of a $73 billion market. Using what has been described as guerrilla marketing techniques, resellers have stimulated companies like AT&T to lower their rates (37). However, they have not lowered their rates enough, because leading resellers are getting ready to make public offerings in their fast-growing, fast-moving companies. Deregulation made competition possible, which gave resellers an opportunity to occupy and defend a niche. Freer markets do this, creating vibrant competitors in such divergent areas as fast-food (36), peeled mangoes

(79), cellular phone chips (78), grocery stores (21), and health care. Yes, health care!

A recent *Wall Street Journal* article proclaimed: "Start-ups in health care are booming; Change in nation's medical care provides openings (52)." This article observes that recent mergers and consolidations in health care created opportunities to start businesses not possible even 5 years ago. Companies targeting patients with chronic disease and those developing special managed care products for senior citizens are but two examples. Many start-ups will fail; in spite of this, they attracted $1.2 billion in capital in 1996, twice the amount start-ups attracted in 1995. Some entrepreneurs are betting they can organize physicians into large networks and can help them use information systems to provide better and more efficient patient care. In Nashville alone, there are 10 such companies including UniPhy, Inc., and there are so many small health-care start-ups around Nashville that the supply of right-sized office space for these ventures is getting tight. On a national basis, the demand for executive talent is strong, so strong that one venture capitalist said that "There is too much money chasing too few proven executives." This is not surprising, though; health-care occupations will be among the fastest growing in the next decade (18).

Another sure sign that there is real opportunity in health care is that organized crime is getting into the business. Investigators discovered that 12 members of a New York City "family" established a company that arranged or brokered health-care services for one million persons. Using traditional "mob" methods of intimidation and "skimming," these mobsters hoped to transform medical insurance into an "underworld treasure trove." Authorities uncovered this activity and indicted "family" members on fraud. No surprise, they pleaded "not guilty (93)." Concerned, federal authorities are hiring more people, increasing budgets, and creating multiagency teams to combat fraud and abuse and other regulatory infractions (3).

On the sunnier side of opportunity, an insurance company has developed a "member-to-member" program for senior citizens in its HMO product, where members help one another with such simple tasks as shopping, minor home repairs, and telephone calls to home-bound seniors. Participants acquire credits for performing these services, which they can use for services they may need. It is a good, old-fashioned barter system made relevant to today's health-care market. It is difficult to value this innovative program, but it may keep people out of expensive nursing homes. America spends about $75 billion a year on nursing homes and is projected to spend $180 billion in 2005. Yet, from 10 to 20% of persons in nursing homes really need not be there. Using these figures, a significant savings in health-care costs could be imputed should member-to-member programs become pervasive (70).

Beyond venture capitalists, mobsters, and senior citizens, there are many more examples of how a deregulating health-care environment creates opportunities for niche players. One entrepreneur wants his company to be the drug distributor of choice among hospitals (35). Another established clinics for women that combine traditional medicine and spa treatments (22). A third plans to develop a network of hospitals that only provides care for long-term acute cases (41). A fourth provides contact lens through the mail (124), and a fifth wants dental braces for the masses (26). And one academic health center plans to export its expertise in transplant surgery (8). Whether any of these ventures will succeed is uncertain. Markets provide opportunities, not guarantees, and some think that the market will eventually provide terrific opportunities for specialized practices that focus on particular niches in health care (46).

There are probably no more than 3500 actively practicing neurosurgeons spread throughout the country, and they represent less than 1% of all physicians. Because the group is so small and unique, a business economist would surely observe that neurosurgery is a niche player. However, small size is rarely an inherent advantage in the market. Good, small niche players have specific characteristics, which organized neurosurgery should emulate, so it can advance "the specialty of neurological surgery in order to provide the highest quality of neurosurgical services to the public."

Successful niche players work very hard to define and defend their niche in the market. Organized neurosurgery defines its place in the market as a scope of practice, which, in turn, is defined by residency and continuing medical education programs. But, it is not enough to define a scope of practice; neurosurgeons should defend that scope through patterns of practice.

Through its programs, meetings and publications, organized neurosurgery provides knowledge and skills that neurosurgeons need to keep their practices dynamic and current. Education, then, is a key activity in an ongoing effort to define and defend neurosurgery's niche.

Because neurosurgeons are among the highest paid specialists, a business economist might also say they are high, value-added, niche players. Their services can really make a difference, and they operate in high risk areas with leading-edge technology. Society is willing to pay neurosurgeons well for what they do, for the risks they take, because what they do can add so much value to a person's life. But, the ability of neurosurgeons to add high value in patient care and receive above average compensation for their work is linked to advances in neurosurgery. This means research.

In business, companies invest heavily in research and development, and in new plant and equipment; these allow a business to do whatever it does better, faster, or cheaper. On a world-wide basis, as much as $1 billion a day is spent on research. Such investments are intended to provide a competitive advantage in the market. As a high technology, leading edge specialty, neurosurgery's interest in doing basic research, pioneering minimally invasive techniques (47, 129), and using computers for planning and guiding surgical procedures (54) help neurosurgeons defend their niche in the market place. That it does protect their niche explains why organized neurosurgery promotes *both* education *and* research, and spends most of its financial resources doing so.

Highly successful niche players receive favorable pricing for their products and services over a long period of time by minimizing substitutes. Minimizing substitutes is particularly germane to neurosurgeons, because it is difficult to find a substitute for what neurosurgeons do. No trauma center, for example, can operate without neurosurgeons. Of course, there have been encroachments on the traditional scope of practice by other specialties in such areas as spine surgery and stroke, but relative to other specialties, neurosurgery occupies a very favorable place in the health-care delivery system. This enviable position is made possible by rigorous training and a commitment to education and research. Hence, there exists a symbiotic relationship between the town and gown in neurosurgery, which should be strengthened in the years ahead.

Strengthening that relationship reinforces a key asset of neurosurgeons, namely, their brain power. Intellectual fire power is the source of good ideas and their application. Bill Gates, Chairman and CEO, Microsoft, understands this, and that is why Microsoft hires only the very best people. Although about 120,000 people send resumes to Microsoft each year, only a small fraction of that number is hired. They are the "super smart," people who are creative, grasp ideas quickly, and can extend the hegemony of Microsoft. Gates believes so completely in intellectual capital that he said in 1992, "Take our twenty best people away, and I will tell you that Microsoft will become an unimportant company (115)."

Bill Gates is not alone in his assessment of the importance of brain power (113). One controversial economist thinks that the long-term prosperity of nations depends on their good ideas, not necessarily their money and land (132). Good ideas in America are powering its exports with such high technology as gamma detectors and global positioning systems (108). Some suggest that hiring smart people is a very sound business strategy, because intelligence matters in every job, including "sweeping up after the programmers go home (103)." Organized neurosurgery already has the brain power others seek, but like any asset, it must be nurtured. For neurosurgeons, that means life-long learning and research. Both help neurosurgeons define their niche, defend their scope of practice, and create barriers to entry for others.

Good niche players also make every effort to control the channels of distribution for their goods and services. Business battles have been won and lost over control of key distribution channels. It is not enough to have a great product or service; it must get through the distribution system and to the customer. Computer retailers learned this lesson in 1996 when their sales of personal computers dropped on a year-to-year basis (74, 112); yet, overall sales of personal computers increased during this same period. It turns out that direct marketers like Dell have created a new channel of distribution and are capturing more of the market. Channels of distribution matter: they matter very much. And that is why Eli Lilly & Co. paid $4.1 billion, and Merck paid $6.6 billion, to buy pharmacy benefits managers as a way to get more of their products to consumers (15).

In the past ten years, integrated health care delivery systems have created new channels of distribution. Traditional channels of distribution, called referral patterns, have been altered forever. Because they have, the American Medical Association and its allies worked for many years to create a more favorable regulatory climate to foster physician-sponsored health-care plans. That has been achieved with new federal guidelines, which may not encourage, but clearly do not discourage physician involvement in the ownership, management, and control of joint ventures (63, 71).

Most likely the trend toward consolidation of channels of distribution in health care will continue, as will trends toward physician group practice and ever larger physician groups. This will set the stage for specialty carve outs, where large groups of neurosurgeons will assume risk contracts to provide services within an integrated health-care delivery system. As physician groups consolidate and get larger, they will have the financial and human resources to assume such contracts. If they do this, then they will have greater control of the distribution system. Several neurosurgical groups have gotten large enough to assume risk contracts. They are part of a larger trend that involves physicians assuming risks and operating managed care organizations.

The environment for neurosurgeons to do this may be just right. Some believe that Richard Scott, former Chairman and CEO, Columbia/HCA, has it all wrong. Health-care delivery systems will not be vertically integrated behemoths, providing cradle-to-grave services. Rather, they will be virtually integrated networks of providers, which are loosely coupled but nimble and quick enough to react to market opportunities. In a larger context, theorists suggest that businesses of the future will create networks of customers, partners, and suppliers, creating an ecosystem that will compete and cooperate with other ecosystems across vast territories (76). Such systems are perfectly congruent with the virtually integrated health-care systems starting to form in places like California (30). In such health-care networks, or ecosystems, good niche players will have a place at the table and partners to leverage. However, to join such a network, neurosurgeons need some structure to organize, finance, and market their scope of practice.

Physician-organized delivery system (PODS) is one way to do this. Usually, PODS are small, multispecialty individual physician associations (IPAs) which require limited capital and can be profitable fast, all of which means that barriers to entry are not high. One Nashville-based firm specializes in developing PODS and helps physicians manage capitation contracts. PODS require some collective risk-taking, which focuses attention on the financial implications of medical care. Heretofore, PODS have been organized mostly by primary care physicians with some specialty care physicians participating as either partners or contractors (118).

This structure might be one of several vehicles neurosurgeons could use to group up and to connect to larger networks of providers. Doing so will prepare neurosurgeons for something Richard Scott may be absolutely right about, namely, a trend toward disease management groups(106). If this trend accelerates, neurosurgical groups should be the prime managers of diseases associated with their scope of practice. If not, then they risk being cut out of the system, just as so many independent pharmacists were put out of business in Massachusetts by a smart drugstore chain with tight relationships with managed care entities (6).

Neurosurgeons, indeed all physicians, face stark choices. Defined in simple terms, they can be owners or employees of a health-care delivery system. With rapid consolidation, more physicians have decided to be employees. In 1983, 24% of nonfederal physicians were employees; by 1995, 45% of them were employees, and there is no meaningful difference between the percentage of primary care (48%) and nonprimary care (43%) physicians who are now employees of a hospital, HMO, or other physicians (2). As more physicians become employees, they are beginning to look to unions to represent their interests (2). There is already one active union in Tucson, and others may follow.

Several neurosurgeons who are "solid citizens" and active in the affairs of organized neurosurgery are exploring whether a union makes sense for them. An alternative for neurosurgeons might be publicly-traded physician-practice-management (PPM) companies, which are emerging to consolidate physicians into ever larger groups. One analyst thinks that PPM companies are not only here to stay but that they will also become "the new center of the health-care universe (10)." Strong words, but PPM companies do provide an option for neurosurgeons to develop bargaining power with managed care companies. As such, they are worth thinking about as alternatives to unions or doing nothing at all.

It is better, though, for neurosurgeons to get in the game. There are a variety of ''ownership'' models to consider, and because markets for health-care services are so different, what makes sense for one market may not make sense for another. There are issues to be addressed involving antitrust and fraud and abuse regulations (4), and those involving capital structure, governance, business development, and management (133). But, individually and collectively, neurosurgeons are smart people. With technical assistance from organized neurosurgery, they should have little difficulty navigating toward safe harbors and safety zones as they work to own and operate channels of distribution for their scope of practice. Can neurosurgeons do this? Of course they can. After all, surgeons helped build the first health-care delivery system, called ''hospitals.'' They can surely help build the next one, called ''provider networks.''

Through education and research, and with channels of distribution, neurosurgeons can occupy a niche in the health-care market as it is today. To occupy that place over time and to eliminate all substitutes for their services, neurosurgeons will have to demonstrate their services are superior to other providers and add significant value. Today, cost seems to be the key performance variable, but, in the future, value will be the key performance variable, where value = quality/price. When the period of consolidation ends, new performance variables for hospitals, managed care organizations, and physicians will emerge. These will involve dimensions of quality (34).

There are difficulties in measuring quality, which involve what is to be measured, how measures might be adjusted for the severity of illness, how much and what kind of data are needed, and how best to analyze and then use those data. Organizations involved with the accreditation of hospitals (the Joint Commission on the Accreditation of Health Organizations or JCAHO), managed care organizations (National Committee on Quality Assurance or NCQA) (50), and physicians (American Medical Accreditation Program or AMAP) are groping for answers. Nonetheless, some entities are disseminating what information they have to help con-sumers make informed choices about health-care plans. Usually their information is more descriptive than quantitative. Moreover, reports about health-care plans, and even report cards about physicians, are being developed and disseminated. About these reports, one writer opined, ''Given the limitations of these rating systems, it's a wonder employers use them at all (69).''

Starting in 1997, the Health Care Finance Administration (HCFA) will require performance data from managed care organizations doing business with Medicare. They do not plan to do anything with these data, yet. To begin with, HCFA wants so-called customer-satisfaction data, but such data may have little relationship to quality (92). A study of 17 HMOs in Massachusetts reached this conclusion. HMOs with the lowest quality had very high patient satisfaction ratings; whereas, HMOs recognized for their quality were among the lowest in customer satisfaction. While such ratings may have nothing to do with quality, annual guides are being published with these data (111).

Accreditation organizations provide some kind of credential to hospitals, managed care organizations, and physicians, but these are not necessarily certificates of clinical quality. Typically, they are not linked to valid and reliable measures of clinical outcomes. Among intelligent persons there is a debate about how to define and then measure outcomes in medicine generally and in neurosurgery specifically. To resolve theoretical and methodological issues, medicine generally and neurosurgery specifically need to do as Harvey Cushing did, namely, take small, careful steps and then evaluate thoroughly before taking more small, careful steps. Following this method, Doctor Cushing made a lot of progress in neurosurgery, and the same can be done with outcomes studies.

With greater frequency, neurosurgeons will be asked, ''How are you doing?'' Organized neurosurgery should help them answer that question, such that when value is the criterion of evaluation, neurosurgeons are truly the high quality, low-cost providers of services. Organized neurosurgery should get moving while there still remains so much confusion about outcome measures. Economists and others are starting to do their own outcomes analyses, which ask serious questions about the allocation of scarce health-care resources (23), about ''our inalienable right to health care (87);'' and about the value of money spent on health care over the past 50 years (57). Because there will be pressure to reduce health-care spending, neurosurgery should have outcomes data to demonstrate its value. Having such data is the best way to defend its scope of practice, its niche, now and in the future.

With such data, organized neurosurgery could develop a targeted communications plan to market its scope of practice at the local level, in managed care organizations, and with decision-makers and opinion-leaders of the regulatory arena. Good niche players have good marketing plans to complement an overall strategy. They advance their niche in the marketplace to acquire and retain a spot in channels of distribution. With respect to health-care channels of distribution, neurosurgery should be ''top of mind'' with reference to its scope of practice.

To start this process, organized neurosurgery sent a team to the annual meeting of the American Association of Family Physicians held in New Orleans in 1996. That team had a booth on the exhibit floor and talked with over 500 family medicine specialists. It was a good learning experience for family medicine specialists, but a better one for organized neurosurgery. First, family medicine physicians were happy to see neurosurgery represented at the meeting. Second, they asked for clear referral guidelines from neurosurgery. Third, they wanted neurosurgeons to be more visible and available to them in their local community. Stated more plainly, they wanted better service from neurosurgeons. What organized neurosurgery learned in New Orleans and from ''grassroots neurosurgery'' stimulated a marketing plan, which focuses on lumbar stenosis. Hopefully, it is the first of many targeted campaigns intended to increase awareness about what neurosurgeons do.

The trip to New Orleans and the targeted marketing plan that emerged after it are merely the beginning of a more comprehensive marketing plan needed to reinforce the scope of practice of neurosurgery at the local level, in managed care organizations, and with officials in the regulatory arena. Frequently, though, marketing to officials in the regulatory arena is overlooked. Unlike patient-oriented campaigns, campaigns designed for decision-makers and opinion-leaders in the regulatory arena are not expensive and can pay huge dividends. While organized neuro-

surgery cannot easily affect the regulatory process, there are, from time-to-time, issues important to neurosurgery and to hardly anyone else. By communicating with officials on a regular basis, a context is created in which specific issues can be placed. Creating this context is a special kind of marketing called public affairs. It and other forms of marketing are tools that organized neurosurgery should learn to use, so it can advance the specialty and provide the highest quality of care to its patients.

In summary, then, deregulation of health care has created opportunities for niche players of all kinds including neurosurgeons. To seize its opportunities, organized neurosurgery should:

• Define its scope of practice in unambiguous terms,
• Defend its scope of practice through education, research, practice patterns, and outcomes studies,
• Control the channel of distribution for its scope of practice, and
• Use communication plans to reinforce its scope of practice with well-defined market segments.

These four objectives are easy to state but hard to achieve. Achieving them requires commitment, cooperation, focus, hard work, and a burning desire to do what organized neurosurgery does better, faster and cheaper than anyone else. But time is slipping away, and because there really is ''a tide in the affairs of men which, taken at the flood, leads on to fortune,'' organized neurosurgery ''must take the current when it serves, or lose [its] venture.''

ACT TO CONSOLIDATE AND FOCUS THE RESOURCES OF ORGANIZED NEUROSURGERY

Neurological surgeons are facing a two-front war. One involves the impact of deregulation of health care, while the other involves the impact of reregulation of health care, as managed care entities and health-care facilities corporations get larger and more business-oriented. In response to these changes, neurosurgeons should be adroit niche players, who dominate the delivery of services for their scope of practice. To do this, neurosurgeons will have to group up and affiliate with entities seeking hegemony over vast territory and patient panels. Where possible, neurosurgeons should assume risk contracts within delivery systems and thereby become owners, not employees, of those systems. In addition, neurosurgeons should anticipate that emerging delivery systems will be subjected to regulatory pressures and anticipate further that others will attempt to use the regulatory process to achieve a competitive advantage over neurosurgeons. Hence, neurological surgeons should get ready to succeed in the market and at the table where regulators of all kinds gather to establish the rules by which the market will operate. In other words, neurological surgeons should be able to fight a two-front war.

As neurosurgeons grapple with this two-front war, organized neurosurgery can pursue its traditional missions in research, education, and patient care in the traditional manner. Or, it can modify its traditional missions and take measures to assist neurosurgeons to succeed on both fronts. Doing the latter keeps organized neurosurgery relevant, protects the traditional scope of practice for organized neurosurgery, and extends traditional missions. Doing the latter effectively will not be easy, though. Other physician organizations with many more members and a lot more money have similar strategies in mind for their members and their traditional scope of practice. So, it is not as if neurosurgeons have an open field (62). However, it is important to remember the lessons taught by John Boyd about aerial combat. Being faster and flying higher are not as important as visibility and maneuverability. Because the F-86 had better visibility and a faster roll-rate than the MIG-15, it dominated the MIG-15 in aerial combat. From this, it can be concluded that, although organized neurosurgery has limited resources, it can be successful in its two-front war. It can do this if it has better information and acts faster than other organizations seeking to occupy neurosurgery's niche in the marketplace or to displace it at the regulatory table.

There is an interesting analogy to the challenge facing organized neurosurgery with respect to this two-front war. It involves America's two-war strategy. America's military force structure is based on the assumption that America might have to fight two wars simultaneously, as it did in World War II. Following that conflict, military planners developed a two-war strategy to meet perceived threats from the former Soviet Union in the West and from the People's Republic of China in the East. Now that the Soviet Union has collapsed and Russia has a relationship with NATO, and now that China is a most-favored trading partner, the importance of a two-war strategy is somewhat diminished. Moreover, maintaining a two-war strategy is expensive, very expensive, during a period when a balanced budget seems to be a shared political value. Yet, some see enduring value in this strategy. It reassures our allies in the West and East and prevents opportunistic warfare in one region should America, operating with a one-war strategy, be engaged in another region. Stated another way, a two-war strategy provides stability throughout the world, as it has for the past 50 years.

Several military analysts wonder whether it is possible to maintain a two-war strategy and modernize the force structure without busting the budget (56). They think so, if six action steps are taken, which they admit "will be politically difficult to implement." These six action steps seem to apply to organized neurosurgery, if it plans to prevail in a two-front war involving both market and regulatory competition. These steps would also be "politically difficult to implement" for organized neurosurgery, but if they were implemented, then organized neurosurgery would consolidate and focus scarce resources and gather better information and use it faster.

First, organized neurosurgery should eliminate all unnecessary costs of doing its business. There are duplication of services and programs among organizations and, within these duplicative services and programs, there are opportunities to trim expenses. Where possible, organized neurosurgery should consolidate its services, so that economies of scale can be achieved and the unit costs reduced. The President of Harvard University, for example, has a long-term plan to end a tradition allowing Harvard's twelve schools to operate independently (16). Because this tradition is so much a part of the history and culture of Harvard, achieving this goal will not be easy. And it will not be easy for organized neurosurgery; but maintaining separate, uncoordinated services and programs within organized neurosurgery is expensive. Close coordination could achieve savings better spent on new programs and services targeted on the real-world issues with which neurosurgeons must deal. Close coordination can be accomplished by developing a meaningful partnership among neurosurgical organizations, based on shared values, good faith, and fair dealing. This partnership could be a "virtual network," like emerging health-care networks or "ecosystems" in business. Such a network is a viable alternative to merging and integrating existing organizations, which would be difficult if not impossible to achieve anyway, due to the independent nature of neurosurgical organizations.

Second, organized neurosurgery should eliminate services and programs that are nice to have, but produce no direct benefits for neurosurgeons. Programs, services, and committees have proliferated over time and use resources better spent elsewhere. Hard questions should be asked across organized neurosurgery about the cost at which neurosurgeons benefit from services and programs and from committee activities. Surely, sunset provisions should be routinely attached to new programs which would ensure that, absent explicit refunding, they would end on a date certain. Professional staff should be scrutinized, too. Often, staff are hired to support programs approved year-after-year without a needs analysis. Because resources are so limited within organized neurosurgery, criteria of evaluation should be applied to programs and services, and outcomes studies should be done.

Third, organized neurosurgery should enhance the capability of retained programs, services, committees, and staff. By eliminating unnecessary overhead and duplicative and/or ineffective programs, services, and committees, organized neurosurgery should have additional resources to make what remains more effective. Really effective organizations focus their resources on a handful of critical areas. They do not spread their resources around, trying to be everything to everyone. American business went through a phase where conglomerates were greatly admired. Soon American business realized that conglomerates were not the most efficient way to enhance share-holder value. Quite often, the parts were worth more than the whole; as a result, the great conglomerates of the 1960s were broken apart in one spin-off after another, allowing the new entities to focus on their core business. One modern "conglomerate" remains—General Electric (GE). It, however, is quite special, in that it operates companies in related (not unrelated) businesses. Moreover, it applies rigorous performance standards to its businesses; business units that fail to be profita-

ble market-leaders are sold. Hence, GE has achieved its status as one of America's most-admired companies, because it focuses its resources on related businesses it can operate very effectively. Organized neurosurgery should follow this example. Invest in what it does well for its members and jettison the rest.

Fourth, organized neurosurgery should be masters of information through technology. Whether it realizes it or not, organized neurosurgery is in the information-handling business. Much of what it does involves creating, gathering, and disseminating information. Think of the money spent by organized neurosurgery on meetings, journals, and research, all of which involve the transfer of information. To manage these and other information activities, organized neurosurgery should make ongoing investments in technology—technology which can be used to gather data as well as ascertain relationships among data sets, and can be used to transmit information to members electronically. This is why the AANS and CNS investment in a web site is so important.

Organized neurosurgery cannot exist without dues-paying members; therefore, it should have a comprehensive understanding of its members, which includes not only extensive demographic data but also information about attitudes, preferences, and consumer patterns. In a very real sense, neurosurgeons are the "customers" of organized neurosurgery. Organized neurosurgery should get close to its members (its customers) by meeting their needs and satisfying their expectations. Getting close to members begins with technology. Consumer-oriented companies understand this and are using their information infrastructure to mount "micro-marketing" campaigns tailored to the demographics and preferences of smaller and smaller market segments. Modern computers make this possible. Finally, expectations of members about how organized neurosurgery should handle information are formed by their experiences with for-profit entities like first-class hotel chains, big-time investment companies, and well-established mail-order firms. Their transactional records are usually correct and instantaneously available. When members call organized neurosurgery, they expect the same fast, accurate response. Without ongoing investments in technology and data bases, organized neurosurgery cannot meet member expectations.

All are familiar with stories about how advances in technology have made workers more efficient. Not-so-old neurosurgeons can testify to how advances in imaging and computer-guided surgery have revolutionized the practice of neurosurgery. Neurosurgery is a high technology specialty, and so neurosurgeons are early adopters of technology and new devices. And, in many cases, they help develop technology and devices. Think of the Mayfield clip. Hence, advances in technology and increases in productivity tend to proceed side-by-side. Some speculate that this side-by-side relationship made possible the "right-sizing" of American business, where powerful information systems eventually made layers of employees unnecessary. Because organized neurosurgery really cannot afford more professional staff, it should make its existing staff more productive and efficient. This can only be accomplished through more and better technology and aggressive training.

Most important of all, the battles organized neurosurgery will fight in the future will involve information. The central issue to be decided in the market and at the table of regulators will be whether neurosurgery provides the highest value for services associated with its scope of practice. Stated more bluntly, the fights will involve whether neurosurgeons are the high quality, low-cost providers of services. To win, neurosurgeons have to be the first with the most and best information about their services. Having a comprehensive network to gather information about these services across geographic areas will provide organized neurosurgery the information needed to advance their interests in the market and regulatory environments, as well as to establish benchmarks for cost and quality. To create such a network will not be cheap. It takes a can't-miss plan, a financing mechanism, and a well-trained staff.

In August 1996, the United States Air Force published a report which examines what would be required for the Air Force to remain dominant in the air and space in the year 2025 (55). It is a futuristic look at warfare, and an eye-opening report with lessons for organized neurosurgery. Based on current trends, the Air Force anticipates that in the year 2025 "influence increasingly will be exerted by information more than by bombs." The report discusses the importance of information operations and even the possibility of information warfare. It speculates that warfare in 2025 will involve the control of knowledge and, increasingly, advantage will be "achieved through investments in information systems, decision-making structures, and communication architectures."

This emphasis on information and on the idea that "knowledge is power" relates to having total battle space awareness. Commanders in 2025 will know precisely where the adversary is at all times and deploy effective and appropriate force. A preview of such warfare was the Persian Gulf War, where coalition forces first destroyed the capacity of Iraq to gather and process information related to the battle space, and then used their information about the battle space to formulate and implement the much-admired flanking maneuver of the ground war. Because "victory smiles upon those who anticipate changes in the character of war," organized neurosurgery should anticipate that the character of war in health-care demands total battle space awareness. To achieve this requires information systems.

Fifth, organized neurosurgery should distribute tasks to partner organizations. There is a tendency in organized neurosurgery to come together, stay together, and work together on a wide variety of projects. This is done to share resources and, perhaps, to keep organized neurosurgery from fragmenting. There are, however, only a handful of issues where joint operations are really necessary. Within the context of an explicit partnership (or "virtual organization"), partners in organized neurosurgery ought to be assigned tasks with criteria of evaluation and allowed to get the job done. This approach in business usually stimulates innovation and efficiency, and, more importantly, fixes responsibility.

In organized neurosurgery, though, where responsibilities are not explicitly shared, organizations often address similar issues and have similar programs. In the context of an explicit partnership, a better approach would be to assign specific tasks to specific organizations. The Society of Neurological Surgeons, with its many program directors, is the most likely organization to study workforce issues. The CSNS, given its origins, seems well suited to set and execute an agenda in socioeconomic affairs. The CNS with its youthful but seasoned leadership who have many more years of active practice seems right to tackle outcomes. And the AANS could give renewed meaning to the word, "spokes-organization," by acting aggressively and systematically to seat qualified neurosurgeons on governmental and quasi-governmental entities, where the interests of neurosurgery are at stake. Other examples could be given, but these are sufficient to illustrate that organized neurosurgery could distribute many tasks to partner organizations. This just might foster innovation, accountability, and efficiency, and might reduce the number of joint operations to a minimum. Quite frankly, joint operations diffuse responsibility rather than focus it.

Whether this distributive, partnership approach would work is not certain. Merging all the organizations, as Doctor Mayfield wanted to do 50 years ago, is a nonstarter. Even if it were possible to merge them, it may not be desirable. Having so many organizations provides multiple opportunities for service and leadership and provides multiple opportunities for cooperation and competition. This keeps organized neurosurgery dynamic and fluid. So, organized neurosurgery needs to play this ball where it lies. It can do so by developing a partnership which has unambiguous rights, responsibilities, and obligations for all.

Sixth, organized neurosurgery should be selective about what it does. Currently, the AANS is engaged in a strategic planning process. There are some 45 strategic areas in this plan 1. That's too many. Organized neurosurgery is facing some well-defined challenges in the health-care market and regulatory arena. It needs to focus

on them. In this regard, the AANS Board of Directors, CNS Executive Committee and Chairpersons of the AANS/CNS specialty sections completed a survey that ranked the importance of the 45 strategic areas cited above. There were several interesting outcomes. First, results were statistically equivalent among the three groups. Second, in spite of the small number of respondents, results were highly reliable. Third and perhaps most interesting, the 15 strategic areas ranked highest by leaders within organized neurosurgery seem relevant to advancing the scope of practice in the health-care market and regulatory arena. These 15 strategic areas are listed below (Table 13.1) and are grouped by "rough" categories.

These 15 areas represent a good starting point for an action agenda for organized neurosurgery. Another round of ranking priorities could provide a tight, focused action agenda of seven or eight areas. Coupled with a "distributive partnership," it is easy to see how seven or eight critical strategic areas could be assigned to organizations within organized neurosurgery. On behalf of the entire partnership, organizations would be responsible for making operational their assigned strategic areas and providing regular reports of progress to the partnership.

If organized neurosurgery implements these six steps, it would consolidate and focus its resources, an important task, given that it has limited human and financial resources. Organized neurosurgery would also align its partner organizations according to a shared agenda and provide

TABLE 13.1
AANS Strategic Categories

Research	Encourage funding for outcomes and quality-of-life research.
	Encourage member participation in and awareness of outcomes research.
Communications	Better communicate the scope of practice and quality of neurosurgical outcomes to other disciplines, agencies and gatekeepers.
	Develop collaborative relationships with other organizations to enhance their recognition of neurosurgery.
Representation	Advocate quality of care as the primary goal of health care.
	Become the leading informational resource for neurosurgeons to the government, private agencies, and businesses.
	Represent neurosurgeons in the managed care debate.
	Develop a "single-voice" representation.
	Improve communications with regulatory and certifying bodies.
	Champion medical tort reform.
Patient Care	Expand areas of clinical involvement within the scope of practice.
	Position AANS as leading resource in the evaluation of neurosurgical manpower issues.
	Ensure high quality graduate and post-graduate educational programs.
	Advocate that the intererst of patients be foremost in the minds of neurosurgeons.
Education	Increase the attractiveness and effectiveness of the annual meeting.

meaningful opportunities for partners to develop real expertise in critical strategic areas. This, in turn, should foster gathering more and better information and acting in a more timely manner for the commonweal. Finally, these six steps allow organizations to retain their traditions and unique missions. A distributive partnership with shared responsibilities is not a merger; it is a virtual network of organizations pooling their resources to advance neurosurgery and provide high quality care. Of course, good-faith accommodations must be made to make any partnership work, but if everyone gives a little, everyone gets a lot, including a greater capacity to wage a two-front war.

It is interesting to note that Imperial China was once far ahead of the West in the arts of war. When the Greeks were using the single tactic of mass collision, China had developed various formations and ways to deploy them. Yet, China declined in military affairs and in science. Why it declined is one of those questions often debated by scholars. Despite its innovations in war, Imperial China tended not to use military solutions to repel aggression. Its rulers and ministers believed that China's superior culture would mitigate the war-like tendencies of barbarians. If China's superior culture failed to impress, it resorted to bribes. If both culture and bribes failed, it hired other barbarians to fight barbarians. One historian observed that Imperial China had a "doctrine of cultural superiority that entailed the ideal of subjugating external enemies solely by Virtue (98)."

Over 30 years ago, Doctor Mayfield observed that neurosurgeons "have permitted ourselves the luxury of being too parochial; that we have enjoyed talking to ourselves so much that we have as an organization isolated ourselves from the mainstream of medicine." He urged neurosurgeons to confront challenges and seize opportunities of a rapidly changing health-care environment. But Doctor Mayfield knew that neurosurgeons needed more than their personal and intellectual "virtue" and "superior culture" of patient care to secure their place and advance their missions. Today, the health-care environment is changing rapidly again, and, unlike the rulers and ministers of Imperial China, neurosurgeons cannot use virtue, "superior culture," bribes, or barbarians to subjugate the "hordes" threatening their scope of practice.

Because the stakes are so high and time so short, and because there really are people "out there" whose job is to put physicians out of business, organized neurosurgery should seek counsel not from Confucius, but from Thomas J. Jackson, a Christian soldier, known to all as Stonewall Jackson. Fearless under fire and a devout Christian, Stonewall Jackson was a professor at Virginia Military Institute (VMI) when the Civil War started in 1861. Although he was not a very good teacher, he understood fighting and how serious the Civil War would be. About *their* War, Stonewall gave his VMI cadets some advice organized neurosurgery should follow in *its* war: "Draw the sword and throw away the scabbard (101)."

DEDICATION

Dedicated to the memory of James S. Todd, M.D. (1931–1997), Executive Vice President, American Medical Association (1990–1996).

REFERENCES

1. AANS. A comprehensive AANS long-range strategic plan. Park Ridge IL: The American Association of Neurological Surgeons, 1996.
2. Adelson A. Physician, unionize thyself. The New York Times. 1997, Apr 5:Y21–22.
3. Anders G, McGinley L. Feds attack fraud in health care. The Wall Street Journal. 1997, May 6:A8.
4. Anders, G. Hospital-doctor ties can be a legal quagmire. The Wall Street Journal. 1997, Apr 24:B1, B7.
5. Committee on Ways and Means, U.S. House of Representatives. 1994 Green Book: Medicare reimbursement to hospitals. Appendix D, E. 1994, Jul 15: 947–1043.
6. Auerbach, JG: CVS grows rapidly, using shrewd tactics and ties with HMOs. The Wall Street Journal. 1997, Feb 24:1, A12.
7. Bagli CV. Another health care merge set, for $1.8 Billion. The New York Times. 1997, May 9:C1.
8. Baker S. Transplanting the transplant biz. Business Week. 1996, Nov 25:128–130.
9. Bernardin, J: Making the case for not-for-profit healthcare. [Speech to The Harvard Business School Club of Chicago] 1995, Jan 12.
10. Bianco A. Doctors Inc. Business Week. 1997, Mar 24: 204–210.
11. Blumenstein R. Auto makers attack high health-care bills with a new approach. The Wall Street Journal. 1996, Sept 9:1.
12. Broder DS. Gramm's Medicare prescription. The Washington Post National Weekly Edition. 1997, Mar 31:4.
13. Budetti PP. Health reform for the 21st century? JAMA 1997, 277(3):193–198.
14. Bulkeley WM. How an MIT professor came to dominate stereo speaker sales. The Wall Street Journal. Dec 31, 1996, 1.

15. Burton TM. Eli Lilly's lack of success with PCS may soon lead to a major write-off. The Wall Street Journal. 1997, Jun 5:A3, A6.

16. Butterfield F. Dismay at Harvard as provost decides to move. The New York Times. 1997, Mar 7:A8.

17. Carey S. How Alaska Airlines beat back challenges from bigger rivals. The Wall Street Journal. 1997, May 19:A1, A5.

18. Chartrand S. Aging baby boomers will mean a big surge in health care jobs. The New York Times. 1996, Jul 7. http://search.nytimes.com/web/docs-root/library/jobmarket/9707sabra.html

19. Church GJ. Backlash against HMOs. Time. 1997, Apr 14:32–36.

20. Church GJ. Twin Cities' friendly plans. Time. 1997, Apr 14:36–39.

21. Coleman CY. How grocers are fighting giant rivals. The Wall Street Journal. 1997, Mar 27:B1, B18.

22. Conlin M. Massages while you wait. Forbes. 1996, Dec 30:132–133.

23. Coy P. Quality of life vs. longevity. Business Week. 1997, May 5:30.

24. Crandall R, Ellig J. Economic deregulation and customer choice: Lessons for the electricity industry. Washington DC: The Brookings Institute and Center for Market Process.

25. Dentzer S. Spend now, tax whenever. U.S. News & World Report. 1997, Feb 24:56.

26. Dolan KA, Feldman A. Braces for the masses. Forbes. 1996, May 20:260–262.

27. Edmondson B. Finding tomorrow's health-care consumers. Ithaca, NY: American Demographics, 1992: 1–20.

28. Fallows J. "A priceless original." U.S. News & World Report. 1997, Mar 24:9.

29. Fein EB. 2 New York hospitals abandon merger plans. The New York Times. 1997, Feb 15:A20.

30. Forum for Medical Affairs. The 1996 Forum Reclaiming Control of Medical Practice. Marriott Hotel, Atlanta, Georgia.1996, Dec 7.

31. Freudenheim M. Cigna to buy healthsource, vaulting ahead in H.M.O.'s. The New York Times. 1997, March 1:21, 23.

32. Freudenheim M. Columbia/HCA makes new, cash offer for Value Health. The New York Times. 1997, Apr 16:C3.

33. Freudenheim M. Health care costs edging up and a bigger surge is feared. The Wall Street Journal. 1997, Jan 21:A1, C20.

34. Fromberg R. Measuring up under managed care. Healthcare Executive. 1977, Jan/Feb:6–11.

35. Galuszka P. The $9 billion company nobody knows. Business Week. 1997, Mar 3:88–90.

36. Gegax TT. Fast-food fast tracker. Newsweek. 1997, May 26:57.

37. Goldblatt H. The guerrilla attack on AT&T. Fortune. 1996, Nov 25:126–127.

38. Goldsmith C. No-frills flying gains altitude inside Europe as barriers fall away. The Wall Street Journal. 1996, Dec 17:A1, A10.

39. Gotlieb M, Eichenwald K. Biggest hospital operator attracts federal inquiries. The New York Times. 1997, Mar 28:1, C15.

40. Hammonds KH. Health care. Business Week. 1997, Jan 13:114–115.

41. Hammonds KH. Medical lessons from the Big Mac. Business Week. 1997, Feb 10:94–98.

42. Hauber C, Philips C. Organized neurological surgery in the United States. Neurosurgery 1995;36(4): 814–826.

43. Hayes JR. Health: The merger frenzy continued, and HMOs got burned by some unexpected cost increases. Forbes. 1997, Jan 13:166–168.

44. Hayes JR. Ya gotta give 'em what they want. Forbes. 1997, Jan 27:62.

45. Anonymous. Health-care inflation. Business Week. 1997, Mar 17: 28.

46. Henkoff R. Why HMOs aren't the future of health care. Fortune. 1997, Jun 9:38–40.

47. Hilts PJ. Surgeons step inside device that gives them a clearer view. The New York Times. 1997, Mar 25:B13.

48. Holland K. HMOs may lose a legal shield. Business Week. 1997, May 5:48.

49. Hunt AR On campaign financing, everybody does do it. The Wall Street Journal. 1997, May 15:A23.

50. Iglehart JK. The National Committee for Quality Assurance. N Eng J Med 1996; 335:995–999.

51. Jackson S. Alternative medicine: Not so alternative anymore. Business Week. 1997, Jun 2:150–151.

52. Jaffe G. Start-ups in health care are booming. The Wall Street Journal. 1997, May 23:A9A.

53. Jeffrey NA. Doctors battle over who treats chronically ill. The Wall Street Journal. 1996, Dec 11:B1, B6.

54. Junnarkar S. Virtual reality guides surgeons' hands. The New York Times. 1996, Oct 25. http://search.-nytimes.com/web/docs...ibrary/cyber/week/1025 surgery . html

55. Kelley JW. Executive summary: 2025. Air University Press, 1996. http://www.au.at.mil/au/2025/mono-graphs/E-S/e-s.htm#CHAPTER7

56. Khalilzad Z, Ochmanek D. An affordable two-war strategy. The Wall Street Journal. 1997, Mar 13: 1.

57. Koretz G. The impact of better medicine. Business Week. 1997, Jan 13:30.

58. Kuttner R. Everything for sale [book excerpt]. Business Week. 1997, Mar 17:92–98.

59. Lagnado L. Elite medical schools seemed perfect mates, except to the doctors. The Wall Street Journal. 1997, Mar 21:1.

60. Lagnado L. Small town erupts over plan to close its ailing hospital. The Wall Street Journal. 1997, Jan 13:A1, A6.

61. Lagnado L. Hospital merger in New York falls through. The Wall Street Journal. 1997, Feb 18:B7.

62. Lauter B. Giving internists a competitive advantage is ASIM's new mission. ASIM News Release, 1996, Oct 10–13.

63. Letter: Seward PJ. American Medical Association, Sept 13, 1996.

64. Lipin S. Corporations' dreams converge in one idea: It's time to do a deal. The Wall Street Journal. 1997, Feb 26:A1, A12.

65. Lyall S. For British health system, bleak prognosis. The New York Times. 1997, Jan 30:A1, A6.

66. DJM. The King Kong of hospital chains stays on top by gobbling up everything in sight. Money Magazine, 1997, April.

67. Mayfield FA. A proclamation. J Neurosurg 1965; 23(2):129–134.

68. Mayfield FA. The years of growth and refinement: Reminiscences. History of The American Association of Neurological Surgeons Founded in 1931 as the Harvey Cushing Society. Chicago IL: AANS, 1981: 41–46.

69. McCafferty J. The rating game. CFO 1997 March: 73–77.

70. McCarry C. Old and frail and on their own. Expand barter systems for elderly health care. U.S. News & World Report. 1996, Dec 30:72, 74.

71. McGinley L, Gurley B. Antitrust rules eased for physician networks. The Wall Street Journal. 1996, Aug 29.

72. McGinley L. HMOs face tough reform from the GOP. The Wall Street Journal. 1997, April 23:B8.

73. McGinley L. Liberal Democrat pursues feud with Columbia/HCA. The Wall Street Journal. 1997, Apr 7: A16.

74. McWilliams G, Burrow P. Deck the halls with unsold PCs. Business Week 1996, Dec 23:36–37.

75. Meyer M. Bound and gagged. Newsweek. 1997, Mar 17:45.

76. Moore J. The death of competition. Fortune. 1996, Apr 15:142–144.

77. Anonymous. Not covered by any H.M.O. Time. 1997, Mar 17:15.

78. Palmeri C. Chips ahoy! Forbes. 1997, Apr 7:48.

79. Palmeri C. Mango tango. Forbes. 1996, Feb 12:84–86.

80. Passell P. A Sea change in policy by the trustbusters. The New York Times. 1997, Mar 20:C1, C2.

81. Pear R. Negotiators move to rein in Medicare, Medicaid and Social Security. The New York Times. 1997, May 2:A12.

82. Pear R. Backers of rival health tests fight to get Medicare dollars. The New York Times. 1997, Mar 26: A1, A12.

83. Pear R. Battle lines form in Medicare fight. The New York Times National. 1997, May 27:A1, A10.

84. Pear R. Big donors from nursing homes had access. The New York Times. 1997, Apr 23:A16.

85. Pear R. Clinton picks panel to draft bill of rights in health care. The New York Times. 1997, Mar 27: A14.

86. Pear R. Congress weighs more regulation on managed care. The New York Times. 1997, Mar 10:A1, A11.

87. Pear R. Harsh medicine. The New York Times Book Review. 1997, May 11:31.

88. Pear R. Health care panel considers need for patient bill of rights. The New York Times. 1997, May 14: A12.

89. Pear R. Medicare rift is now sequel of first budget agreement. The New York Times. 1997, May 7: A17

90. Pevehouse BC. Commentary of Hauber, C and Philips, C: Organized neurological surgery in the United States. Neurosurgery 1995;36(4): 826.

91. Pretzer M. What Washington has in store for you in 1997. Medical Economics. 1997, Jan 13:34–43.

92. Quinn JB. Is your HMO OK–Or not? Newsweek. 1997, Feb 10:52.

93. Raab S. Officials say mob is shifting crimes to new industries. The New York Times. 1997, Feb 10:A2, A10.

94. Richards B. A Nuclear-waste firm is sued—For paying a regulator too little. The Wall Street Journal. 1997, Jan 27:A1, A6.

95. Rosenthal E. Older doctors and nurses see jobs at stake. The New York Times. 1997, Jan 26:1, 16.

96. Rundle RL. Catholic hospitals, In big merger drive, battle industry giants. The Wall Street Journal. 1997, Mar 12:A1.

97. Sanger DE, Labaton S. Billions at stake as Clinton and bankers met. The New York Times. 1997, Jan 31: A1, A14.

98. Sawyer RD. The art of the warrior. Boston: Shambhala Pub Inc, 1996.

99. Schmitt E. Sides square off on decontrolling electricity sales. The New York Times. 1997, Apr 14:A1, A13.

100. Schonfeld E. Doctors unite. Fortune. 1997, Mar 3:200.

101. Sears SW. Onward, Christian Soldier. The New York Times Book Review. 1997, Mar 16. Http://search.nytimes.com/search/d...christian % 29 % 26AND%26 %28soldier%29

102. Seib GF. Wyden Wonders: Why dither now over Medicare? The Wall Street Journal. 1997, May 7: A20.

103. Seligman D. Keeping up. Fortune. 1997, Jan 13:38.

104. Serwer AE. Drexel's heir. Fortune. 1997, Apr 14:104. http://www.pathfiender.com/@@39uwFQ...KyZnA/fortune/1997/970414/dlj.html

105. Serwer AE. Health care stocks: The hidden growth stars. Fortune. 1996, Oct 14:74–82.

106. Sharpe A, Jaffe G. Columbia/HCA plans for more big changes in health-care world. The Wall Street Journal. 1997, May 28:A1, A8.

107. Sharpe A. Medical entrepreneur aims to turn clinics into a national brand. The Wall Street Journal. 1996, Dec 4:1, A11.

108. Siekman P. Brains are powering U.S. exports. Fortune. 1997, Feb 3:70[B]–70[L].

109. Smart T. Moving Mount Aetna. Business Week. 1997, Feb 10:100–101.

110. Spiers J. Medicare's bad prognosis. Fortune. 1996, May 27:57–58.

111. Spragins EE. The numbers racket. Newsweek. 1997, May 5:77.

112. Steinhauer J. Computer retailers reel from slow holiday season. The New York Times. 1997, Jan 8. http:www.nytimes.com/yr/mo/day/news/financial/computer-sales.html

113. Stewart TA. Brain power. Fortune. 1997, Mar 17: 105–110.

114. Stodghill R. Minnesota's HMO-ectomy. Business Week. 1997, Jan 13:115.

115. Stross RE. Microsoft's big advantage—Hiring only the supersmart [book excerpt]. Fortune. 1996, Nov 25: 159–162.

116. Anonymous. Sweeping changes in phone industry approved by F.C.C. The New York Times. 1997, May 8:A1, C6.

117. Tagliabue J. American aces of the foreign sky. The New York Times. 1997, Jun 6: C1–C2.

118. Terry K. Are PODS the way to go? Medical Economics. 1996, Oct 14:91–106.

119. Terry K. You can thrive under managed care. Medical Economics, 1997, Apr 7:12–25.

120. Tew JM. How Dr. Mayfield influenced aneurysm surgery. In: The History of Aneurysm and Microneurosurgery. AANS 1995 Annual Meeting Archives Exhibit Brochure. 1995:9. privately published

121. Thomas RM. Col. John Boyd is dead at 70: Advanced air combat tactics. The New York Times. 1997, Mar 13:C24.

122. Updegrave WL. Stacking the deck. Money. 1996, Aug: 50–63.

123. Van Natta D, Fritsch J. $250,000 buys donors 'best access to Congress.' The New York Times. 1997, Jan 27:A1, A10.

124. Weber J. Contact lenses: Focus on open markets. Business Week, January 13, 1997, 39.

125. Anonymous. Will Medicare sink the budget? The Economist, February 1, 1997, 27–28.

126. Wines M, Pear R. President finds et advantage from failure of health-care effort. *The New York Times*, July 30, 1996, http://search.nytimes.com/web/docs-root/library/politics/0730clinton.html

127. Winslow R. Health reform in New York triggers taxes. The Wall Street Journal, December 31, 1996, 9.

128. Winslow R. Health-care costs may be heading up again. The Wall Street Journal, January 21, 1997, B1, B6.

129. Winslow R. Hope and hype follow heart-surgery method that's easy on patients. The Wall Street Journal. 1997, Apr 22:A1, A10.

130. Winslow R. Nurses to take doctor duties, Oxford says. The Wall Street Journal. 1997, Feb 7:A3, A8.

131. Winslow R. Oxford to give more control to specialists. The Wall Street Journal. 1997, Mar 25:B1.

132. Wysocki B. For this economist, long-term prosperity hangs on good ideas. The Wall Street Journal. 1997, Jan 21:A1.

133. Yang C. Money and medicine: Physician, disentangle thyself. Business Week. 1997, Apr 21:40.

CHAPTER 14

Neurosurgery and Politics

RUSSELL L. TRAVIS, M.D., KATHERINE O. ORRICO, JD

"Me this uncharted freedom tires; I feel the weight of chance desires: my hopes no more much change their name, I long for a repose that ever is the same."

Ode to Duty, 1807
—William Wordsworth

INTRODUCTION

Change we have had and change we will have. Indeed, change is implicit in medicine, whether it be in education, science, or technology. The question is, "On balance, has change accelerated in recent time, and has it taken a positive or negative turn? Or, has what we conveniently term 'change' been, in fact, a series of essential subtle transitions?"

The American medical care system has evolved by responding to changing perceptions and, indeed, by changes in government oversight, the way many of our national institutions have evolved. The federal government has assumed a greatly expanded role in fashioning the health-care delivery system, and organized medicine has reacted to the extended reach of government. The forces of change have altered practically all previous assumptions about our health-care system. We have witnessed a kind of historical *pas de deux*, in which two dancers seem to continually bicker over who is going to lead.

By the standards of today, the pre-World War II physician had few weapons to help him in the fight against disease. There were a few vaccines, antitoxins, vitamins, liver extracts for pernicious anemia, and insulin for patients with diabetes. There was arsphenamine for syphilis, the botanical drugs digitalis and quinine, aspirin, and opium for pain. There were no medicines that attacked the real source of the disease and some treatments were as agonizing as the disease symptoms.

In the early 1940s, all began suddenly to change. Over a short period of several years, a succession of therapeutic discoveries transformed medicine, and lives—at least a million by one estimate—were saved and suffering markedly relieved (1). Surgery blossomed, as antibiotics reduced the risk of surgery, and newer techniques expanded the benefits achieved. "Surgery before the war was all big surgery," recalled H. Thomas Ballentine, a prewar surgical resident at the Massachusetts General Hospital and a neurosurgeon at the hospital after the war. Dr. Ballentine also served as an AMA trustee (2). From this period on, the American public slowly, but progressively, began believing in the powers of medicine; and one of the dramatic changes was a shift from resigned acceptance of suffering to an expectation of cure and relief of suffering.

Before War World II, the Federal government spent less than 1% of its annual budget on health and, by 1940, financed only 20% of the total national health bill. In 1995, however, the Congressional Budget Office (CBO) projected that by fiscal year 2000, Medicare and Medicaid alone would account for 22.5% of the $2.2 trillion amount of Federal spending (3). It has been estimated by several agencies that the government now finances, either directly or indirectly, from 55% to 60% of the total dollars spent in the United States on health care. In the early 1940s, both for Congress and the general public, health-care issues were politically a low priority. Congress was not spending much, and the general public did not expect much.

The system in those years, with the government financing only 20% of the total national health bill, was overwhelmingly private. Oden W. Anderson, Ph.D., the University of Chicago sociologist, pointed out that the United States system of medical care grew up in a climate of laissez-faire economics and in the presence of the largest, most affluent middle class the world has ever known. He pointed out that the large, middle-class income group, unique to the United States, was the only available mass purchasing power at the time (4).

However, characteristic of medicine, as times changed, medicine adapted. By 1945, the private character of the American medical care system was being pressured to adapt to a changing economic scene. The affluent middle class had temporarily lost its affluence during the Great Depression. Pulitzer prize-winning author, David Halberstam, in *The Powers that Be*, described the extent and suddenness of political change as President Roosevelt ushered in the New Deal to reduce postdepression unemployment rates as high as 25%. He said "The federal government's taxing power increased as its mandate increased; and as its taxing power increased, so did its real power (5).

President Roosevelt believed in wider federal participation in medical care. He held the belief that "necessitous men are not free men." That is, men who lack the necessities of life could be forced to trade their freedom to attain them.

The combination of Roosevelt's philosophy at the end of the Depression, the availability of antibiotics, new technological advances, and the return to prosperity, all increased the demand for access to medical care; and medicine had to adapt to a society that was developing a moral claim to medical care and a government with taxing powers to provide the access.

In the early 1940s, a group of Southern Democrats and Northern Republicans forged a powerful voting block in Congress, and a more conservative attitude slowed, for a time, the progression of federal participation in the provision of access to medical care.

However, during the 20th century, American health politics has been characterized by a succession of attempts at federal legislative health-care reform. Reformers have, on repeated occasions, made unsuccessful all-out drives for expanded or universal health insurance. Each time, after defeat of the drive for universal coverage, there has followed in its wake a significant change in the patterns of health-care financing and delivery. Political pundits in the late 1940s predicted that President Truman's campaign for "compulsory health insurance" could

not be derailed. Although his drive was defeated, many felt Truman's struggle for national health insurance propelled the eventual passage of Medicare and Medicaid in 1965. From the 1940s on, the share of Americans with private or public health insurance grew consistently, leveling off in the 1970s at approximately 85%. Since at least 1980, however, the number of people excluded from health insurance coverage has steadily increased, now exceeding 40 million.

As federal health-care spending exploded in the years after Medicare's passage, the alarmingly rapid growth of the federal budget deficit in the 1980s began to focus Congressional attention on the growing entitlement programs, especially Medicare and Medicaid. In 1981, Congress began the budget reconciliation process and, in 1982, began to pass legislation to clamp down on Medicare payments to medical providers. From 1981 to 1993, an cumulative total of $39.1 billion was taken from Medicare reimbursements to physicians by Budget Reconciliation Acts (6). These measures signaled a dramatic change, from open-ended spending on programmatic expansion to strict budgetary control, the single most important change in American health politics in the last quarter of a century.

As the decade of the 1980s wore on and tax revenue failed to keep pace with rising spending on mandatory entitlement programs, the budget deficit emerged as the dominant domestic policy issue in American politics. Medicare and Medicaid, as opposed to defense and Social Security benefits, became the focus of attack by politicians, as well as the media, on what they described as "spendthrift entitlements that threatened to bankrupt future generations (7).

The fundamental problem with Medicare has been its rapid growth. Total program disbursements increased 3377% between 1966 and 1994. A number of factors, such as inflation (medical care inflation was 702% over that period), can be cited in that growth (8). Demographic change, marked increased in the rate of use of services, marked addition of entitlements and benefits, and technological progress were all factors in this growth.

The End-Stage Renal Disease Program is a prime example of the evolution of medicine, with the explosion of benefits followed subsequently by restrictions and limitations. To paraphrase a biblical quote "What Congress giveth to voters, Congress taketh not away." The Seattle Artificial Kidney Center, founded in 1962, pioneered the development of dialysis treatment centers. Following 10 years of medical activity, Representative Wilbur D. Mills (D-Ark), a powerful legislator with presidential ambitions, in December 1971 put on a dramatic demonstration of an actual patient undergoing dialysis during a public hearing of the House Ways and Means Committee, which he chaired. Senator Vance Hartke (D-Ind) later successfully amended a broader measure that President Richard M. Nixon signed into law on October 30, 1992. This act officially created the Federal End-Stage Renal Disease Program (9).

The End-Stage Renal Disease Program typifies the problems faced by Congress, past, present, and future. This program, like many others, started with lofty ambitions to help a needy and vulnerable group of people. Also, typically, the impetuous action often is driven more by emotional empathy and political expediency than by rational, budgetary planning.

When the program was created, eligible beneficiaries numbered about 10,000. At that time, it was assumed that, by 1995, enrollment would level off at about 90,000. However, by 1993, there were 165,000 Medicare patients with end-stage renal disease; and it is projected that by the year 2000, enrollment will exceed 300,000, with over 85,000 incident (new) cases in that year (10).

For 20 years, the government has essentially frozen the level of payments to facilities and physicians providing dialysis treatment. As all of medicine, like dialysis centers and dialysis physicians, faces such fiscal constraints with expanding numbers of patients, attention will focus ever increasingly on whether the quality of care is maintained, with little regard for physician reimbursement.

Government has been described as shifting in the 1980s from a "provider of health services" to a "prudent purchaser of health services." This shift in role began a sharp decline in government's willingness to yield to professional authority, and it marked a new attitude that medical care should be considered simply another type of market good, subject to the same type of competition and quality control as any other commercially purchased good or service.

THE WASHINGTON COMMITTEE

In 1975, in the midst of this rapidly changing medical political environment, the AANS and CNS made a decision to become involved in the federal government's rapidly expanding role in formulating, legislating, implementing, and regulating health-care policy at every level of society. Dissatisfied with representation on a number of issues by the primary umbrella organizations, namely the American Medical Association and the American College of Surgeons, neurosurgical leadership felt that more direct involvement in Washington would give neurosurgery more influence on positions taken by the AMA and the ACS. It was felt that, at a minimum, the two organizations should monitor broad, emerging issues, such as national health insurance, the malpractice crisis, the National Institutes of Health (NIH) support for science, and medical manpower reform.

The pioneer committee consisted of Dr. Lewis Finney, Dr. Donald Stewart, Dr. Russell Patterson, and Dr. Charles Fager. After diligent research and after interviewing a number of individuals on the Washington scene and from medical societies with a Washington office, this group reached an agreement with Charles Plante, a former Senate Administrative Assistant, and opened a Washington office in 1976.

The original agreement with Charles Plante was to provide part-time services with a small six-member committee (11). One of the major philosophical decisions in the early 3-to-5 years was deciding what issues the Washington Committee for Neurosurgery should take on. The Committee early on developed a philosophy that would limit its activity to specialty-specific issues.

After the first 10 years of an ever expanding agenda, the small Washington Committee faced criticism for "elitism" and was reorganized. The relationship between the Board of the AANS, the Executive Committee of the CNS, and the Washington Committee was formalized; the President and President-elect of both parent organizations became official members of the Committee, with the Committee Chairman and the Washington representative formally responding in person to the governing bodies of the parent organizations at least semi-annually.

With the new structure, the Washington Committee became an innovative force in formulating ideas and programs for the benefit of neurosurgical membership. Many program ideas, such as "Think First," "Decade of the Brain," and the "Current Managed Care Symposium" were first generated by the Washington Committee and subsequently approved and implemented by the parent organizations. The agenda gradually changed to include nonneurosurgical issues with an indirect secondary impact on neurosurgery.

Continued pressures by the federal government and private health insurers on the practice of medicine, particularly in areas of reimbursement and managed care, have heightened the need for a proactive presence in Washington, D.C. Neurosurgical leadership recognized that without involvement by a combined effort of organized medicine, certain basic medical principles, such as the physician/patient relationship, physician autonomy, and access to specialty care, would be eroded. These bedrock principles are being controlled by the "managers" of the matrix, since they increasingly are the arbitrators of the access, quality, and cost of medical care. Nearly all health-care public policy proposals that are considered by the Washington Committee, directly or indirectly impact these fundamental issues. In 1996, the leadership of the AANS and CNS made the decision to move from a part-time to a full-time Washington, D.C. presence. Now, in 1997, organized neurosurgery has a permanent, full-time Washington, D.C. office, with a staff of three.

The Washington Committee has an ambitious agenda, including issues such as physician payment, managed care, national health insurance, professional liability, biomedical research, graduate medical education, Food and Drug Administration actions, and guidelines and outcomes research. In addition, the Committee continues to review its working relationships with the AMA, the American College of Surgeons, and the individual medical speciality society organizations.

Having a full-time Washington representative and full-time office to maintain a proactive Washington, D.C. presence is one of the key components of an effective public policy program. Other vital methods and activities by which the Washington Committee enhances its role in Washington are: (*a*) building coalitions, (*b*) grass-roots lobbying, and (*c*) political action committees.

COALITION ACTIVITY

To a certain degree, neurosurgery is a niche player in the world of health policy; and while it usually does well when it focuses on those areas that exclusively affect neurosurgeons (e.g., revision of the neurosurgical CPT codes and funding for the National Institute of Neurological Disease and Stroke), the high-paced change of the current health policy debate means that it now must be able to influence policies of more global issues. For example, the debate over managed care and direct patient access to specialty care is driven by big business and the health insurance industry. These groups are highly organized and well funded. In the 1996 Congressional debate over tort reform, medicine lost the fight to insurance and other corporate big business, and medical liability was dropped from the liability reform bill in the Senate. Corporate business did not wish to risk veto of the product liability bill with the controversial malpractice liability reform attached, and, while medical reform was deleted, product liability reform survived. In the past, the AANS and CNS had participated in few coalitions, preferring instead to focus on those areas in which neurosurgeons have a particular interest or expertise. Over time, however, it became apparent that the AANS and CNS alone had little influence in the larger debate unless they forged relationships and built broad coalitions with other interested groups to support principles consistent with organized neurosurgery's philosophy. Membership in a number of coalitions allows organized neurosurgery to leverage its influence not only in the United States Congress, but also on the policies of other medical organizations, such as AMA and ACS.

The AANS and CNS are leaders and founding members of the following coalitions: the Practice Expense Coalition, the Patient Access to Specialty Care Coalition, the Coalition for American Trauma Care, and the National Medical Liability Reform Coalition. Each of these groups has achieved modest legislative successes that would not have been possible had each individual medical society championed the issues alone. For example, the National Medical Liability Reform Coalition has contributed to the passage of Federal tort reform legislation in the House of Representatives, and the Patient Access to Specialty Care Coalition has succeeded in passing federal legislation in the Senate guaranteeing patients direct access to specialty care and managed care plans. Most recently, participation with the Practice Expense Coalition was helpful in preventing the immediate implementation of the health-care financing administration's (HCFA) arbitrary scheme to reimburse physicians for their practice expenses based on flawed data (which would have reduced neurosurgical Medicare incomes by 30 to 40%).

The AANS and CNS have also expanded the role of neurosurgical representatives and liaisons to other medical organizations to broaden organized neurosurgery's influence in the health policy debate. Organizations in which neurosurgery has a very active presence include: The AMA, the ACS, the American Tort Reform Association, the Association of American Medical Colleges, and several institutes at NIH.

GRASS ROOTS LOBBYING

The term "grass roots" originated in a speech by Senator Albert Beveridge of Indiana to a delegation of the 1912 Bull Moose Convention. Senator Beveridge stated that theirs was the party of grass roots . . . "grown from the soil of the people's hard necessities." Today, the term "grass roots" has evolved to mean organized efforts by special interest groups, particularly at the local level, to promote support for or against specific issues. Thomas P. "Tip" O'Neill's point that "all politics is local," emphasizes the need for interest groups to organize at the local or "grass root" level.

The AANS and CNS have long recognized the need to involve grass roots neurosurgery in the development of organized neurosurgery's national health policy agenda. In the early 1970s, the Joint Socioeconomic Committee (JSEC) was formed to help the parent organizations deal with the expanding role of socioeconomic matters in the practice of neurosurgery. In 1984–1985, JSEC was reorganized as the Joint Council of State Neurosurgical Societies (JCSNS); and in 1994–1995, the Chairman of the JCSNS became an official member of the Washington Committee.

More recently, the AANS and CNS have established programs to further involve grass roots neurosurgeons. In 1992, the "key person program" was initiated to establish a network of neurosurgeons with personal contacts with members of Congress. Over 300 neurosurgeons participated in this program and have helped to promote organized neurosurgery's legislative agenda with their Congressional contacts. In 1997, the Washington Committee, working with the JCSNS, hopes to further expand its grassroots lobbying and education capabilities by establishing "State Action Teams."

POLITICAL ACTION COMMITTEES

Organized neurosurgery operated its legislative affairs activities without a political action committee (PAC) for over 20 years with a high degree of success. Through the political contacts of neurosurgery's Washington representatives (in particular, Charles Plante) organized neurosurgery has generally enjoyed access to key members of Congress and their staff. The Key Person Program has also been used to enhance access to members of Congress. In spite of the philosophical distaste felt by many to the idea of a PAC, the neurosurgical leadership, after extensive debate, identified several practical reasons, relating to current Washington political activity, that necessitated establishment of a PAC.

The Republican-controlled Congress has changed the way Capitol Hill operates. Republican leaders, particularly in the House of Representatives, have made it apparent that those who financially support Republican candidates will have greater access to members and their issues will be given priority consideration. The old political parable applies: "The Golden Rule— Them what has the gold, makes the Rules." Many members keep detailed lists of contributors, and their policy decisions are often affected by these lists. Organizations not on the list, either because they contribute primarily to Democrats or do not have PACs, find it difficult to advance their legislative agendas in the current Congress. Congressional legislators, however, cannot be effective if not elected and then reelected. A campaign for the House of Representatives commonly costs $2–3 million, with a Senate race even more expensive.

In 1995, the House and Senate enacted gift ban rules that prohibit virtually all gifts to members and staff. In the past, the lobbyists and organizations were able to cultivate relationships with staff members by taking them out to lunch, giving them tickets to events, and sponsoring out-of-town trips. These gifts and favors are now prohibited, making it much more difficult to establish contacts on Capital Hill. At the time the gift ban passed Congress, most Washington lobbyists concurred that much more emphasis would fall on the fund raising and PAC process and would drive people toward campaign contributions and "ticketed events" as a way of gaining access to members of Congress.

With these issues in mind, the Washington Committee in 1996 responded to a resolution from the JCSNS to form a PAC and, after considerable debate, recommended to the parent organizations that neurosurgery seek to form a PAC.

In April 1997, an independent group of neurosurgeons formed the American Neurological Surgery Political Action Committee (AN PAC). AN PAC was formally incorporated in the District of Columbia, and a founding Board of Directors was appointed. AN PAC is now fully operational and has begun contributing to key Congressional candidates. AN PAC is dedicated to protecting the interest of neurological surgeons and their patients by backing candidates for federal office who support the goals of the neurosurgical community. The creation of the PAC, along with a full-time lobbying presence in Washington, has complemented the retooling of the public policy activities of the AANS/CNS.

Neurosurgeons stand to lose much (e.g., cuts in Medicare reimbursement and restricted patient access to specialty care) if they are not well represented. In addition, neurosurgery has a unique legislative agenda to promote (e.g., the "Quality in Graduate Medical Education Act," which gives antitrust relief to the Accreditation Council on Graduate Medical Education and Residency Review Committees when they discontinue residency programs based on quality). These changes in the *modus operandi* of the Washington Committee are invaluable in accomplishing neurosurgical political goals.

THE PRESENT AND FUTURE POLITICAL SCENE

Although President Clinton's proposed Health Security Act failed resoundingly in 1994, attempts at federal health-care reform did not end there. The defeat brought dramatic political reversals in the 1994 elections; and the new conservative Republican majorities in both halls of Congress have pursued an aggressive course to cut taxes and balance the Federal budget, primarily at the expense of Medicare and Medicaid. President Clinton outmaneuvered the new Republican majority by using his veto to kill the Republican "balanced budget" initiative and re-

claim the White House in the 1996 Presidential election. However, during the budget battle, both President Clinton and Congressional Democrats committed themselves to the Republican initiative to balance the Federal budget in the near future. Traditionally, such efforts to control spending carry serious consequences for the federal government's large health entitlement programs, Medicare and Medicaid. These two programs are invariably subject to the most intense budgetary scrutiny, because they are among the largest and fastest growing of the federal spending programs.

The Congressional Budget Office (CBO) projected that total Federal spending from 1995 to 2002 would grow at an average rate of 5.5% over fiscal year 1995 spending levels (12). Mandatory spending—entitlements—accounted for 51.8% of the total spending in fiscal year 1995. Mandatory spending is dominated by three major programs: Social Security, Medicare, and the Federal share of Medicaid.

The mandatory programs are the largest and fastest growing component of the budget, but growth rates differ among the programs. The three programs, Medicare, Medicaid, and Supplemental Security Income (SSI) for the aged, blind, and disabled have projected growth rates of about 10% per year during this 7-year period. These three programs are growing nearly twice as fast as the total Federal budget (5.5%), consuming an ever-growing percentage of available tax funds.

The federal deficit was projected to reach $3.6 trillion in fiscal year 1995 and $5.6 trillion by 2002, the earliest year policy makers set to balance the federal budget. The budget deficit not only focuses on Medicare spending, but has had a chilling effect on any new programs, particularly since the introduction of new budget procedures in 1990. Under current budget rules, the CBO must report to Congress on the budgetary consequences of any proposed tax revenue or spending legislation prior to passage. Special procedural restrictions apply to legislative initiatives that the CBO estimates will increase the deficit in any years subsequent to passage.

Characteristic of all past drives at health-care reform, American medicine continues to change following defeat of wholesale legislative reform. The transformation since Clinton's health reform defeat has had a number of catalysts. One important factor driving legislative change is the fiscal constraint created by the Federal budget deficit, with consequent dramatic reductions in the Medicare and Medicaid budgets. Even more dramatic, however, are the changes in the private health insurance market that are moving unprecedented numbers of Americans into managed care. The percentage of workers and private firms who are enrolled in some form of managed care grew from 29% in 1988 to 70% in 1995 (13).

The dynamics of health system change today are quite different from those of recent decades. During the period of open-ended, fee-for-service insurance payments, factors such as technology, demographics, physician and hospital supply, and physician decision making were usually identified as key drivers of change.

Private sector employees have now become the key drivers of health system change. They have achieved this influence by shifting their purchasing power from paying for open-ended, fee-for-service health insurance benefits to buying health-care coverage from managed care plans that pay out on a capitation basis. Employers have developed a firm belief that enormous savings are possible in health spending without reducing the quality of care, and the consumers depend on providers to maintain that quality regardless of cost-cutting. Employers now expect, even demand, that instead of the annual double-digit premium increases of the "golden 80s" and early 1990s, health insurance premiums should fall, or rise only modestly.

Although managed care has come to dominate health-care services and the popular press is filled with articles about health care, the public remains poorly informed and suspicious of the new system. Nearly two of three respondents —67% of them enrolled in Preferred Physician Organizations (PPOs)—said they have a poor understanding of the difference between traditional fee-for-service and managed care plans (14). One of three Americans has not heard the term HMO (health maintenance organization) or does not know what it means.

This lack of information and the movement of the private insurance market toward highly restrictive forms of managed care will inevitably revive public desires for more government activity in health-care financing and regulation. Managed care utilization restrictions have already spawned passage of Federal legislation requiring insurance to provide coverage of at least 2 days of hospital care to women at childbirth.

In the past, failures at comprehensive health-care reform were followed by incremental, but substantial, government measures to expand health care to vulnerable groups of citizens not already covered by other means. Reformers now doubt a repeat of the detour to Medicare and Medicaid after Truman's failed effort between 1948 and 1950. The years after the demise of Clinton's Health Security Act have been marked by a new agenda. The political upheaval of 1994 generated a new strategy for incremental reforms, such as modest insurance market reforms as contained in the Kassebaum-Kennedy Bill (Health Insurance Portability and Accountability Act) signed into law in 1996.

The public, however, seems to be reacting against a Republican public policy that many Americans see as divisive, mean-spirited, and favoring the well off. There are still millions of uninsured citizens, and Americans remain as concerned about the availability of affordable health insurance as they were before Clinton's Health Security Act (15).

It is likely that an opportunity for comprehensive health-care reform will come again in some form or another. There is no question that health-care policy will change dramatically as America enters the next century, and controversies will boil to the surface again in some major crisis.

The 1997 Congress continues to struggle with strategies to restructure the 31-year-old Medicare program. Debate about reengineering the Medicare program focuses on managed care. Enrollment in Medicare risk programs more than doubled between 1987 and 1995 and grew by 30% in 1995 (16).

The rapid shift of 37 million Americans toward managed care plans will occupy much of future government and public scrutiny. As enrollment grows at 25 to 30% annually, tens of billions of dollars will shift to the bargaining power of health plans (17), while reducing providers' fee-for-service revenues and payment support for charity care, graduate medical education, and rural hospitals. Providers that have borne these social costs face dire consequences; government action will likely be called for to provide other financing.

Managed care has thus far "cherry picked" the young and healthy. HMOs do not advertise for chronically or seriously ill patients. Consumers' concerns, particularly those of disabled and chronically ill patients, have been felt strongly in state legislatures. More than 1000 state legislative consumer protection bills were introduced in 1995. While few have passed to date, they will be a serious concern in the future.

Last, but not least, medicine, and neurosurgery, must continue to deal with changes within its own ranks. The face and characteristics, and thus the political desires, of the individual neurosurgeon continually changes. Current trends in the United States health-care system are rapidly changing the career opportunities of patient-care physicians, and hence, physicians' choice of practice arrangements. Between 1983 and 1994, the proportion of patient-care physicians participating as employees rose from 24.2% to 42.3% (18). The proportion of physicians self-employed in solo practices fell from 40.5% to 29.3%, while the proportion of self-employed in group practices fell from 35.3% to 28.4%. Although the proportion of employee physicians is lowest in the surgical subspecialties, the referral base of neurosurgery is changing dramatically.

Women in neurosurgery now number 295. As the characteristics of the individual neurosurgeon and the referral base change, the political philosophy of neurosurgical leadership must adapt to meet the needs of a diverse and changing membership. The agenda of the Washington Committee must continue to revise, expand, and diversify to meet the needs of all its constituents.

CONCLUSION

The dramatic change in neurosurgery's Washington, D.C. presence demonstrates that the AANS and CNS have moved in part from the ivory towers to the trenches. It also suggests that physicians need to recognize and accept that certain changes are inevitable in a pluralistic society, which sees medicine in a more pragmatic way today than it did 2 decades ago. Writing to a friend in the 4th Century, Basil The Great observed, ''I have abandoned my life in the town as an occasion of endless troubles, but I have not managed to get rid of myself.'' To paraphrase, medicine, particularly neurosurgery, must rid itself of its provincial and often cynical view of government, as well as its lofty view of itself.

Politics is not a spectator sport. Legislatures must answer to constituents, and unless physicians do ''hands-on politics'' they will not be ''constituents.'' Politicians, like all people, re-

member and respond to the people who are there when times are tough. This means involvement in campaigns, not only by contributing money, but by manning phones and pounding the pavement. ''Hands-on politics'' is essential to modern day public policy, but not really new to neurosurgery.

Harvey Cushing played a key political role in federal health-care policy. As a famous neurosurgeon, author, and teacher, he was one of the most respected men in American medicine in the 1920s and 1930s. Harvey Cushing became one of medicine's most effective voices against national health insurance.

In 1934, the federal government created the Federal Committee on Economic Security and drafted what would become the Social Security Act. Harvey Cushing was appointed to an advisory committee on medical matters to the Committee on Economic Security. Cushing urged his strong anticompulsory insurance feelings on Frances Perkins, the Secretary of Labor and the person appointed by President Roosevelt to oversee the development of the new legislation. Dr. Cushing wrote to the Secretary, ''Most of the agitation regarding the high cost in medical care has been voiced by public health officials and members of foundations, most of whom do not have a medical degree, much less any firsthand experience with what the practice of medicine and the relationship of doctor to patient means (19).''

Although Harvey Cushing was a man of great renown and influence as a neurosurgeon, he resorted to ''hands-on politics'' in this debate. Unknown to the general public, Dr. Cushing had a direct pipeline of communication to the White House. Betsy Roosevelt, wife of the President's oldest son, James, was Harvey Cushing's daughter. Being an astute politician, Dr. Cushing relied not on his medical reputation, but on this relationship, to bring his arguments directly before the President.

The challenge for the new neurosurgical Washington presence is, and will be, the ability to keep faith with the basic principles of essential quality care for patients and access to specialty care. Neurosurgeons must be party to forming a new enlightened health-care delivery system through issue-driven coalitions, grassroots lobbying, and focused, effective political action. Each of these components broadens the base of a small specialty, such as neurosurgery, by working in concert with other groups, encouraging and facilitating doctor-to-legislator discussions regarding key issues, and supporting candidates for public office who share professional views for an improved health-care system.

In the end analysis, change will continue, both on the political scene and in the make-up of medicine and neurosurgery. A presence at the table is imperative whenever important decisions are made shaping the future of the health-care system. The effectiveness of neurosurgery's presence will depend in part on how the leadership of neurosurgery responds to the ever constant change within its own ranks. Neurosurgery must ''circle its wagons,'' but not shoot inside! The single most important determinant, however, to neurosurgery's future success in the political arena will be the extent to which individual neurosurgeons personally get involved in the political environs of their own Congressional legislators.

Neurosurgery, not politics, must remain each neurosurgeon's *raison d'etre*. However, each must face the cold reality that neurosurgeons can no longer maintain the quality of their profession without active involvement in the political process.

Acknowledgment

With appreciation to Charles L. Plante: mentor, friend, and a guiding light to neurosurgery for over 20 years.

REFERENCES

1. Prescription drug industry fact book. Washington DC: Pharmaceutical Manufacturing Association, 1976:1.
2. Campion FD. AMA and US health policy since 1940. Chicago: Press Chicago Review, 1984:21.
3. Source book for medicare reform. Center for Health Policy Research and American Medical Association, June 1995.
4. Anderson OW. Blue Cross since 1929. Cambridge MA: Ballinger, 1975:16–17.
5. Halberstam D. The powers that be. New York: Alfred A. Knopf, 1979:12.
6. Source book for medicare reform. Center for Health Policy Research and American Medical Association, June 1995:C35.
7. Hacker J et al. The new politics of U.S. health policy. J Health Polit Pol Law 1997;22(2):323.
8. Source book for medicare reform. Center for Health Policy Research and American Medical Association, June 1995.
9. Iglehart JK. Health policy report: The American health care system, The end-stage renal disease program. N Eng JMed 1993;367.
10. Eggers PW. Projections of the end-stage renal disease population to the year 2000. In: Proceedings of the 1989 Public Health Conference Records and Statistics. Washington DC: 1990,121–126. (DHHS Publications No. CPHS)90-1214).
11. Watts C, Plante C. The neurosurgeon and health care policy. In: Philosophy of neurological surgery. 189–195.
12. Health Policy Alternatives, Inc. Primer on the federal budget. Washington DC: Henry J. Kiser Family Foundation, 1995.
13. Etheridge L, Jones SB, Lewin L. What is driving health system change: The new fundamental forces for change as seen by health care leaders and market watchers. Health Aff 1996;15(4):94.
14. Isaacs SL. Consumers information needs: Results of a national survey. Health Aff 1996;15(4):40.
15. Wines M, Pear R. President finds he has gained even if he lost on health care: Proposal was midwife to swift transformation. New York Times, 1996, Jul 30: A1, B8.
16. U.S. General Accounting Office. Managed HMOs: Rapid enrollment growth concentrated in selected states. (GAO/HEHS-96,63) Washington DC: GAO, 1996.
17. Zarabozo C et al. Medicare managed care: Numbers and trends. Health Care Financ Rev, 1996; Spring: 243–261.
18. Cooper RA. Prospective on the physician workforce to the year 2000. JAMA 1995;274(19):1534–1560.
19. Campion FD. AMA U.S. health policy since 1940. Chicago: Press Chicago Review, 1984:7–8.

CHAPTER 15

Ethical Issues in Neurosurgical Practice

JOHN J. ORO', MD

"Moral dilemmas are often generated by conflicts among moral principles."

—*JF Childress*

INTRODUCTION

Ethics is the field of inquiry concerned with the principles which guide us in determining what is right and wrong. Bioethics or biomedical ethics is the application of general ethical theories, principles, and rules to problems of medical practice, health-care delivery, and medical research. Prior to considering the ethical issues facing neurosurgeons today, we must have some understanding of the major ethical theories, the principles derived from those theories, and the guidelines derived from those principles.

THEORIES AND PRINCIPLES OF MEDICAL ETHICS

As described by Ronald Munson (1) in Intervention and Reflection: Basic Issues in Medical Ethics, there are five major ethical theories: natural law ethics, Kant's ethics, utilitarianism, Ross's ethics, and Rawls theory of justice.

Natural Law Ethics

Among the oldest ethical theories, natural law ethics was expounded by Roman philosopher Cicero and 13th century philosopher and theologian St. Thomas Aquinas. Natural law ethics holds that moral principles are objective truths present in nature and open to our discovery "by reason and reflection." Through reflection, for example, we can discover that living things by nature act to preserve their own lives. Thus, we should work to preserve our life and the life of others. From this, it follows that we should maintain our health, as well as the health of others. Natural law ethics would encourage us to rely on ordinary, not extraordinary, means and would rule out euthanasia.

Kant's Ethics

Immanuel Kant, the 18th century German philosopher, proposed an ethical theory based on the "categorical imperative," which, in essence, means that all human beings should be treated as an end to themselves, and never as a means. Every rational creature should be recognized as having inherent worth. This theory is the foundation of the principle of autonomy (discussed below), which has become a primary ethical principle during this century.

Utilitarianism

The 19th century British philosophers, Jeremy Bentham and John Stuart Mill, proposed the ethical theory of utilitarianism (1). Utilitarianism is based on the principle of utility, which is also called greatest happiness principle: "those actions are right that tend to produce the greatest happiness for the greatest number of people." Happiness itself is the intrinsic good. By itself, utilitarianism lacks justice: it could be used to support harm to a few for the good of the many, such as in human experimentation without consent.

Ross's Ethics

W.D. Ross, the 19th century English philosopher, believed that we posses the capability to know right and wrong. Our moral intuitions can reveal moral rules. However, these rules are not absolute, but depend on the situation and on reason. Ross's duties, according to Munson (1), include duties of fidelity (telling the truth), reparation (righting the wrongs we have done to others), gratitude (recognizing services others have done for us), justice (preventing a distribution of pleasure or happiness that is not in keeping with the merit of the people involved), beneficence (helping to better the condition of other beings with respect to virtue, intelligence, or pleasure), self-improvement (bettering ourselves with respect to virtue or intelligence), and nonmaleficence (avoiding or preventing an injury to others).

The difficulty with Ross's theory is the claim that we should know our duties through reflection. Ross believed that if we do not know, we should continue to reflect until we do. Another difficulty is that it may be difficult to determine which action to take if we are faced with conflicting duties. When duties conflict, Ross suggests that we do the more "stringent" of the duties—the duty that has "greatest balance" of rightness over wrongness (1).

Rawls' Theory of Justice

The Theory of Justice, proposed by Harvard philosopher John Rawls in 1971, is considered to be one of the most important works of moral and social philosophy of this century (1). Rawls asks us to make decisions for a group of individuals as though we were under a "veil of ignorance." Before making a decision we should consider ourselves as part of the group but ignorant of who we are within that group. Rawls believes that this would lead to a decision that would provide fair opportunity. Applied to society, the theory of justice indicates that in order to have a just society there must be an equal right to liberty and fair opportunity.

However, since we are usually not in a "veil of ignorance," deciding as if we are may be difficult. In addition, the theory excludes from the decision process morally relevant knowledge about the situation itself. This type of decision making may by itself result in doing everything for everyone and thus would require enormous social resources.

PRIMARY PRINCIPLES

From these theories come four primary principles that apply to medical ethical decision making: beneficence, nonmaleficence, autonomy, and justice.

Beneficence

Beneficence is defined as "the doing of good." It is the central duty of the physician—to cure when we can, to alleviate pain and suffering when we cannot. As quoted in Munson (1), the Hippocratic writings state "As to disease, make a habit of two things—to help or at least to do no harm." Physicians are expected to make reasonable sacrifices to help.

Nonmaleficence

Nonmaleficence is the avoidance of doing harm. As stated in the Latin injunction "*Primum non nocere*" (Above all, do no harm), nonmaleficence has been one of the primary principles of medical practice since ancient times. In practice, we exchange a small harm, for example, the making of an incision, for the larger good, the removing of the tumor.

Autonomy

The principle of autonomy has achieved a central role in medicine during this century (2). From the Greek words "*autos*" meaning *self* and "*nomos*" meaning *rule*, autonomy was first used by the Greeks to describe their self-governing city-states. Autonomy can best be thought of as personal freedom. As rational individuals, we have the right to decide for ourselves what is the best for us.

Autonomy is based on Kant's ethics that people have an inherent unconditional worth and on natural law ethics. Our duty is to respect others' autonomy. When we violate or limit autonomy, we treat the individual as less than a person.

As important as autonomy has become to modern medical ethical thinking, it is not absolute or unconditional and can be restricted. However, limitations of autonomy should be based on principle. The harm principle allows us to restrict an individual's autonomy, if it is necessary to prevent harm to others. Restricting an addicted physician from practicing medicine would be justified under the harm principle. The welfare principle allows us to limit someone's autonomy in a small way, if by doing so we bring a much greater good to the group. In practice, we may require vaccination against certain diseases, in view of the much greater good to the society, even though the individual may not want this.

ISSUES

Informed Consent

Throughout most of history, medicine has been paternalistic (3). The physician decided what was best for the patient and would often not involve the patient in decision making. Early in this century in malpractice cases decided in civil courts, the concept of informed consent began to be applied to medical decision making. In these cases, "touching competent patients without consent" was found to be unacceptable, irrespective of value of the care provided (2). In 1914, Justice Cardozo stated that (as quoted in Beauchamp (2): "Every human being of adult years and sound mind has the right to determine what shall be done with his own body; and a surgeon who performs an operation without his patient's consent commits assault, for which he is liable in damages. . . . . This is true except in cases of emergency."

To better understand informed consent, we must consider its two components. In order for the patient to be "informed," relevant choices must be disclosed. We cannot make a choice if we are not given the options available to us. Withholding information or being deceptive is destructive of autonomy. Likewise, a health plan that does not provide viable options constrains autonomy.

When giving "consent," the patient must not be coerced and must be competent. In order to judge someone's competence, we must take context into account. While many of us are competent to drive a car, most of us are not competent to fly a plane. Thus, judgments about competence should be made with reference to the area in which the decision is being made. A patient who is generally incompetent may still be competent to make some important decisions, such as those regarding medical treatment.

One is competent if, as quoted in Beauchamp (2) one can "comprehend and process information and reason about the consequences of one's actions." In practice, a patient must be able to have some understanding of the options presented, and the risks and benefits of those options, and be able to make a decision based on this understanding.

The American Medical Association Code of Medical Ethics reflects current thinking on informed consent in stating that "the patient's right to self-decision can be effectively exercised only if the patient possesses enough information to enable an intelligent choice. The patient should make his or her own determination on treatment. The physician's obligation is to present the medical facts accurately to the patient or to the individual responsible for the patient's care and to make recommendations for management in accordance with good medical practice."

The Future of Informed Consent

Informed consent is likely to continue to evolve. Various trends can be identified that will likely impact informed consent including governmental regulations, multicenter trials, outcomes measures, and case law.

Governmental Regulations

The Food and Drug Administration (FDA) is becoming increasingly active in the regulation of devices it deems investigational. To what extent should a physician disclose to the patient the status of a product within the FDA?

Judge Louis C. Bechtel, as reported by Muehlbauer (4), who was overseeing the pedicle screw litigation, ruled on March 8, 1996, that a physician cannot "be held liable under the doctrine of informed consent for failing to advise a patient that a particular device has been given an administrative or regulatory label by the FDA. The law of informed consent obligates a physician to advise a patient of the medical risks, benefits, and alternatives directly related to the patient's operative procedure. The term 'Class III,' 'investigational,' and 'significant risk' device are terms adopted by the FDA for administrative or regulatory purposes and cannot be said to be risks of a particular surgical procedure."

Whether this view will be upheld in future remains to be seen. While this decision would seem to limit the scope of informed consent, other trends point toward a widening of the scope.

Multicenter Trials

The increasing number of well-designed multicenter trials will likely impact informed consent by more specifically defining the natural history of diseases and the results of treatment. For example, the North American Asymptomatic Carotid Endarterectomy Trial (NASCET) defined the risk of stroke in patients with greater than 70% internal carotid artery stenosis treated with aspirin alone or aspirin and surgery (NAS-

CET). Since the risks of stroke with and without endarterectomy are now more precisely known, patients will expect more accurate information as to the risks and benefits of a specific treatment.

Outcomes Measures

Another developing trend, outcomes measures, will allow individual surgeons to know their own morbidity and mortality figures for the treatment of many neurosurgical disorders. Computer software programs are increasingly available that allow such tracking. In the future, a neurosurgeon seeking to become a provider for a managed care company may be at a disadvantage in negotiations if another neurosurgeon, or neurosurgeons, can document better outcomes. This concern will increase as the use of outcomes becomes more prevalent and likely becomes a routine part of neurosurgical practice.

How will outcomes measures impact informed consent? As neurosurgeons know their own specific risks and benefits for a procedure, this knowledge will become material to the patient in making an informed decision, thus expanding the expected disclosure during informed consent.

Case Law

Another trend that is also likely to widen the scope of informed consent was identified by Dr. Donald A. Shumrick in 1994. Dr. Shumrick (5) analyzed two cases: *Hidding v. Williams* and *Beherenger v. The Medical Center at Princeton, New Jersey*. In *Hidding v. Williams*, the court ruled in favor of the plaintiff, when information that the surgeon suffered from alcohol abuse was not disclosed. The patient had not been fully informed about material risks. In *Beherenger v. The Medical Center at Princeton, New Jersey*, the plaintiff, a surgeon with AIDS, won a judgment against the medical center based on discrimination against him. However, the hospital won the right to require the doctor to inform his patients that he had AIDS, so the patients could make an informed decision on choosing to proceed with the surgeon. A third, more recent, case, *Faya v. Almaraz*, also found negligence in the physician's failure to inform patients of the physician's HIV-positive status (6). Together, these cases expand the definition of disclosure to include physician-related factors that may materially affect the patient's risk.

In 1996, a landmark case was decided by the Minnesota Supreme Court that expanded the required disclosure within Minnesota (7). A patient undergoing clipping of a vertebral artery aneurysm developed permanent quadriparesis postoperatively. While there were many issues contested in the case, such as the risk of morbidity and mortality as it was presented to the patient, the thrust of the Supreme Court decision was that the surgeon should have informed the patient that a specialized center to clip the aneurysm (the Mayo Clinic) was available 90 miles away. The court ruled that the specialized center had higher capability and could offer lower morbidity and mortality, and thus the patient should have been informed of this option. The court tightly limited this extension of disclosure to very specialized cases such as aneurysms of the posterior fossa (the Court did not believe that this standard should be applied to aneurysms of the anterior circulation).

As we have seen, informed consent is based on autonomy, which, with its respect for individual self-rule, is a powerful force in modern society and will likely continue to expand. However, concerns about a possible over-reliance on autonomy at the expense of the physician/patient relationship have been raised (8):

- "Does the health care provider tell the patient everything he or she can determine relative to the treatment or surgery? Or does the physician look at the patient as an individual, decide what the patient actually needs to know, and then obtain consent in a way that is comprehensible and consistent with the person's language, custom, and culture?"
- Is there a risk of causing "emotional damage" from "the recitation of so many details about what may happen in surgery?"
- Does the presentation of an "exhaustive list of information . . . confuse patients and adversely affect the physician/patient relationship, and create barriers to communication and truth?"

The physician should strive to apply the reasonable person standard. Is the disclosure of specific information material to the decisions of the patient? The patient, or the patient's surrogate, is the decision maker and needs "all information relevant to a meaningful decisional process (*Canterbury v. Spence*)." In the few cases in which patients do not want the information, it is best for the physician to provide treatment based on the principles of beneficence and non-maleficence.

Finally, the environment within which informed consent is obtained may be as important as the process. For years we have focused on the information delivered during the informed consent process: the risks, benefits, and alternatives. In the future, we will see an increased emphasis on the "environment" within which informed consent is obtained. Have we presented information in a fashion that allows an open interaction with the patient and family, that encourages questions and the expression of concerns or fears by the patient or family? Providing an appropriate setting to allow open interchange will be increasingly important.

When the neurosurgeon is uncertain about informed consent, it may be helpful to keep the following hypothetical letter in mind:

Dear Neurosurgeon,

We are all autonomous individuals inherently worthy of respect. At times we must balance our needs with the needs of others; in the medical realm, our needs should be paramount.

If I am ill, inform me, give me my options, be truthful, guide me in understanding, so I can make my best decision.

Keep yourself clear thinking and fit for the complex practice you perform. Always continue to learn. Your skills will give me or my family a better chance to heal and live. Help others in your profession to do the same.

If I am brain injured beyond repair, respect my wishes as I have made them known to my family or friends or through my directive. If my wishes are unclear, ask yourself what a reasonable person would want if so afflicted.

If my brain has died, respect the rules of my state and let my body pass on.

Always remember that as far as our searches indicate, we remain the only conscious life in the universe. You, as my neurosurgeon, are the guardian of that consciousness. Take good care of me.

Your Patient

Critical Care and End of Life Issues

Critical care issues present the most common ethical dilemmas that face neurosurgeons. These include issues of pain management, advanced directives and substituted judgment, futile care, palliative care, the persistent vegetative state, and brain death.

Pain Management

The fact that the public is disappointed with the treatment of pain is not well understood by many neurosurgeons. This failure to control pain, as perceived by the public, may be a factor in the majority opinion favoring euthanasia. This undertreatment of pain may be the result of physician's fears about shortening patients' lives, litigation, or medical board sanctions.

The greatest assistance to a physician treating terminal pain comes from moral theology and the *principle of double effect* (US Catholic Conference). The basis of this principle is that actions can produce both good and bad effects. If a patient dying of terminal cancer is suffering from pain, giving that patient analgesics may relieve suffering, but hasten death. Whether the action is ethical depends on the intent of the physician. According to the principle of double effect, if the intent is to hasten death, it is wrong. If the intent is to relieve suffering, it is right, and death is the unintended consequence. Other ethical principles are also relevant to the management of terminal pain. Unalleviated suffering in the face of terminal illness goes against beneficence and autonomy.

Advanced Directives and Substituted Judgment

As we have seen, in order to protect patients' autonomy, we must inform them of their options and the associated risks and benefits, and allow them to make their own decision. Many neurosurgical patients, however, are unable to make those decisions, due to depressed level of consciousness or coma. How do we assure that we are acting in a way that respects the individual's autonomy?

We must attempt to determine what the patient would have wanted in such a circumstance. The advanced directive may range from a written form designed specifically for the purpose to a simple hand-written note by the patient conveying his or her wishes regarding health care.

In many cases, advanced directives are not specific to the medical situation at hand. The physician should then seek the family's impressions as to what the patient may have wanted. Did their family member make a statement or statements to them that would be helpful in making the decision? When no such information is available, the physician can also turn to the primary care practitioner, who may know the patient well, or to clergy or nurses caring for the patient, who may have discussed such issues with the patient.

Other patients will have court-appointed

guardians that have been given durable power of attorney to make health-care decisions when they are unable to do so themselves. The court appointed individual becomes the surrogate decision maker for the patient.

Futile Care

Neurosurgery finds itself at the center of social change regarding the deliberate withdrawal of support systems from patients who are terminally ill. Two types of cases have dominated the debate of futility: (a) patients in their final stages of a terminal illness in intensive care units, and (b) patients in the persistent vegetative state (PVS). We will focus on futile care in the ICU and discuss PVS later in the chapter.

Traditionally, physicians treating patients in intensive care units have been resistant to withholding or withdrawing care. The principle of beneficence has led to application of complex and often high technology care, even when such care has appeared futile. However, dramatic progress has been made in this conflict. Studies on the high cost of critical care provided at the end of life and the futility of some treatments previously offered uniformly, such as CPR, have now led physicians to a greater awareness of the proper role of critical care. In neurosurgical practice, more precise diagnosis offered by computed tomography (CT) and magnetic resonance image (MRI) scanning has allowed a better assessment of prognosis.

The progress made by the medical profession in understanding futility is documented by a study of 1719 patients admitted to two intensive care units at the University of San Francisco. Approximately half of the patient deaths in those two units from July 1987 to June 1988 resulted from the withholding or withdrawing of life support from critically ill patients. Care was withheld or withdrawn in 115 patients (7 %) (9). Eight of these patients were brain dead, 99 were incompetent, and only 5 patients made the decision to limit care themselves. Of the 110 patients who were brain dead or incompetent, 102 had families that participated in the decision to withhold or withdraw care. A large majority (93%) agreed with the physicians to limit care. Of the 10 families initially disagreeing with recommendations to withhold or withdraw care, 8 families agreed with the recommendations within 2 to 3 days. Thus, this study demonstrates that joint decisions by the physician and family only infre-

quently result in disagreement, and, in those, the issue is resolved most frequently with time.

Ironically, while physicians have been gaining a better understanding of futility and have been less reluctant to withdraw care, an opposing conflict occurs: patients for whom the physician believes further care is futile have family members who disagree and who wish to continue with care. Although the numbers are few, as noted in the San Francisco ICU study above, these disagreements create conflict between the physician and the family. At the center of this conflict are several issues: the definition of futility itself, who should decide, and whether utilization issues have been allowed to enter the decision process (3, 10, 11).

Although definitions of futility have ranged from a narrow physiologic definition—"treatment is futile when it is known with a high medical certainty that it cannot produce the physiological effect that is being sought" (3) to more expansive—a treatment is futile if it "merely preserves permanent unconsciousness or . . . fails to end total dependence on intensive medical care" (11), in this latter definition, while treatment may provide some physiological benefit (maintaining life), the benefit is seen as too little in view of the care required. This definition raises the concern that futility can be used by the "acolytes of cost containment," in their quest to reduce health-care expenditures, according to Capron (10).

In these conflicts, the physician should focus on the patient and the family. If the physician perceives that care is futile, open frank discussions with the family will often allow them to appreciate the futility. The patient's CT or MRI scans, or brain models or diagrams, may be useful in exploring the basic concepts. The physician should allow adequate time for this discussion and provide an environment that allows the family to ask open questions of the physician's perspective on the case and to express their own concerns and fears. The bedside, the hall, or the waiting room will not do. In the case in which disagreement persists, the physician should continue treatment and seek assistance from others, such as the institutional ethics committee or legal counsel, although this last should be an unusual step.

New approaches are being developed to resolve issues of futility (Gatter). By developing a "triage planning framework," communities would become involved in establishing criteria for prioritizing access to chronically scarce medical resources. While "communities" are not defined by the authors, it could be argued that managed care (discussed below) is potentially creating new communities. The large numbers of individuals within a health plan are a community in the sense that they share a type of coverage of health care among themselves. These "communities" could become more actively involved in what type of health care they want from their health plan and in decisions on the limits of care.

Palliative Care

With the increased utilization of futile care, how does a physician then care for someone that will have care withheld or withdrawn? In the dying patient, beneficence, doing good, guides us to shift from attempting to treat an illness or injury to providing comfort and alleviation from pain and suffering. To this end, palliative care programs have been developed.

The Palliative Care Program at the University of Missouri has provided a new avenue for care providers and families to care for the dying patient. The goal of palliative care is to help the patient and family be as comfortable as possible. The focus shifts from treatment to comfort. The palliative care team, which includes nurses, social workers, and clergy, are on call to assist the families and the care givers in this transition. Patients and families are provided a more comfortable environment away from the intensive care unit, where they can have 24 hour visitation. All medical therapy is discontinued except for pain control and comfort measures.

Persistent Vegetative State

The ethical concerns regarding persistent vegetative state (PVS) frequently focus on the continuation of nutrition and hydration. In many states, these issues are decided between the physician and the family. However, in Missouri and in New York, restrictions apply. In the famed Nancy Cruzan case, that of a young woman who had been in PVS for over 7 years following a severe head injury sustained in a motor vehicle crash, the Missouri Supreme Court denied withdrawal of nutrition and hydration. It also denied the removal of Nancy to another state on the basis of the state's responsibility to protect the individual's life. The case was taken to the

United States Supreme Court, which agreed that Missouri had the right to require continued feeding of a patient in PVS unless there was "clear and convincing evidence" that the individual would have wanted otherwise. Thus, in Missouri, individuals must give clear and convincing evidence of what they would want if they were to become permanently vegetative. This evidence can take the form of an advanced directive, discussions with friends and families, a written statement, or, as suggested by Nancy's father, Mr. Cruzan, a videotape expressing one's wishes.

Future ethical deliberations on the persistent vegetative state will not likely be affected by new ethical arguments in the foreseeable future. However, they may well be impacted by a better scientific understanding of PVS itself. It is possible that new imaging technologies or diagnostic techniques may more accurately predict if and when the PVS state becomes irreversible and thus assist families and physicians in decision making.

Brain Death

Most states have laws regarding the physician's duty in determining death by neurological criteria. These laws are based on the total and irreversible loss of brain and brainstem function. Published guidelines guide the physician in making the determination. Once brain death has been determined using these guidelines, the person has died and cardiopulmonary support is useless. Support is withdrawn, unless the family agrees to organ donation.

This "whole brain" definition of death has been effective, reproducible, and accepted by a majority of physicians and the public. Some ethicists, however, are critical of waiting for the loss of function of the whole brain prior determining the presence of brain death. They argue that, in patients who have widespread irreversible injury to the cortex even though they maintain brainstem function, the "higher brain," which houses cognition, reasoning, emotion, and those factors that make us human, is irretrievably gone, and, thus, the individual no longer exists. They also argue that, using a "higher brain" definition of brain death, more individuals would be defined as brain dead, and a larger number of organs would be accessible for transplantation—organs that would be life-saving for many individuals.

Arguments against the "higher brain" definition of brain death include the practical (How would organs be removed from a vegetative person who would likely move as the scalpel was used? Would anesthesia be required? If so, who is receiving the anesthesia?) and the "slippery slope" argument (Would patients with severe Alzheimer's or other cortically devastating neurologic dysfunction be declared brain dead?).

Future deliberations on brain death will likely not hinge on new ethical arguments, but on a deeper understanding brain function. Since the end of the 19th century, neurologists have correlated injury to the cerebellum with loss of coordination of the trunk or the extremities. Recent studies, however, suggest that the cerebellum may also be involved in many other brain functions, including cognition (12). While these studies are new and controversial, they nevertheless point to the possibility that our view of the cerebellum may change in the future and that at least a small part of the "individual" may reside in the posterior fossa, further solidifying the "whole brain" definition of death.

Euthanasia

Some seriously ill individuals who are competent and informed, claim a "right to die" with the assistance of their physician. Here the principles of nonmaleficence (to do no harm) and natural law theology (not to take a life) conflict with the duty to respect a patient's autonomy. This ethical dilemma is ongoing, and physicians should make their opinions known on this issue. It is likely that better management of terminal pain and suffering will result in less pressure to enact laws allowing euthanasia.

Human Gene Therapy

"Advances in biomedical science have placed humanity in the role of co-creator in the process of evolution. What has long been accepted as the 'natural' life and respected as the mysteries of life are becoming no longer natural or mysterious."

—William Atchley, President, International Bioethics Institute (Ethicus)

There are between 50,000 and 100,000 human genes, with the best current estimate given at approximately 80,000. There are two types of human gene therapy, and they differ significantly. The first is somatic-line alterations, which affect only the treated individual; the second is germ-line alterations, which will be transferred to future generations.

Neurological diseases that have been suggested as possibly responsive to gene therapy include Von Hipple-Lindau, neurofibromatosis, Parkinson's, Alzheimer's, Huntington's chorea, tuberous sclerosis, Down's syndrome, Duchenne muscular dystrophy, and rheumatoid arthritis. Thus, it is important for neurosurgeons to understand the ethical issues involved in these two types of therapy.

Somatic-Line Gene Therapy

In somatic-line gene therapy, a genetic disease is treated by adding genes to cells with missing genes or by substituting genes for malfunctioning ones. This type of therapy would prevent the disease from ever developing. Only the individual that would have developed the disease benefits, since somatic gene therapy affects only nonreproductive cells.

Ethically, somatic-line gene therapy is an extension of medical treatment as offered through the ages and is based on beneficence, while respecting nonmalefience and the individual's autonomy. Justice would advise us that these treatments should not be so expensive as to benefit only the well-to-do. The ethical challenge of somatic-line gene therapy will be ensuring fairness in patient selection.

In neurosurgery, the use of somatic-line gene therapy was pioneered by Edward H. Oldfield at the National Institutes of Health in the treatment of patients with malignant brain tumors.

Germ-Line Gene Therapy

Whereas somatic-line gene therapy is viewed an extension of current medical therapy, germ-line gene therapy is much more controversial. Indeed, some have asked whether this issue should be discussed at all (13).

Germ-line gene therapy treats diseases by adding new genes to germ cells with missing genes or substituting genes for malfunctioning ones. Supporters of germ-line gene therapy argue that it would be the best method of disease prevention. By correcting an error in the germ-cell line, not only is that individual protected from the disease, but so to are all future generations. The proposed uses of germ-line genetic therapy include the prevention of the transmission of genetic disease, such as cystic fibrosis, and as an alternative to selective abortion, as currently practiced by some families in the presence of genetic disease.

Several arguments have been put forward in support of germ-line gene therapy (13) and are listed below.

1. Germ-line gene therapy would be more effective than somatic-cell therapy, which must be repeated with each generation; it would treat the disease on one occasion, thus saving scarce resources.
2. Parents would avoid producing children who are carriers and thus spare their children from future genetic decisions.
3. Professionals have a "general obligation to seek out and offer the best possible therapeutic alternatives."
4. This type of therapy is in the "best accords with the health professions' healing role and with the concern to protect rather than penalize individuals who have disabilities."

While these arguments are be based on beneficence, justice, and autonomy, the arguments against germ-line gene therapy show that the potential of this technology is indeed challenging for humankind. The arguments against germ-line gene therapy are listed below (13).

1. Errors in the germ-line treatment could leave the individual more severely affected than before. This error could manifest itself in each subsequent generation. This would result in maleficence (harm) to the individual and to all subsequent generations unless procreation was restricted.
2. Germ-line therapy may be used for "genetic enhancement" of the embryo and, since it is likely to remain expensive, would be available only to the affluent.
3. Investigations in germ-line gene therapy would require testing in human embryos and, therefore, would raise issues regarding respect for the embryo.
4. Humans, or a small group of humans, would have "too much control over the evolution of the human race."
5. Malevolent use of the technology could occur. This century's experience with the Nazi racial cleansing program and the effort to create a "master race" point to the potential abuses of this technology.
6. The human rights argument is that "human beings have a moral right to receive from their parents a genetic patrimony that has not been subjected to artificial tampering."

Our principles of medical ethics, with their focus on the individual, provide limited guidance as to what to do with these new powers. Germ-line technologies result in effects not only for that individual, but for all the descendants hence. Only through open discussion by health-care professionals, researchers, and society can we hope to resolve these dilemmas.

Human Cloning

In February 1997, the Roslin Institute, located in a small village just south of Edinburgh, Scotland made an epochal announcement. A somatic nucleus removed from the udder of a 6-year-old ewe had been coaxed into expressing its full genetic potential. From this nucleus, a replica, or clone, of the sheep was made. The replica, named Dolly, is alive and well. Although 277 attempts were needed for this success, a line has been crossed. Indeed, the press viewed the event as on the order of the biblical story of the creation of Adam (14).

With the rapid pace of human genetic research at the end of this century, it appears likely that the line will also be crossed in humans within the next decade or two. Before humans are cloned, we must consider the ethical dilemmas posed. Will we view human cloning as a breakthrough or a cataclysm?

Consider the evolution of humankind as a series of links showing evolution from the first hominids 4 million years ago to the first tool makers 2.5 million years. Further evolution led to Homo sapiens 100 to 150 thousand years ago. Thus, for at least the 100,000 years in which Homo sapiens has existed, children have been created by the mixing of the male and female chromosomes. If human replication is possible, then a new method of creation of humankind is at hand. The nucleus of a somatic cell of child, woman, or man, could be coaxed to create a genetic copy.

One may ask why human cloning should be discussed in relation to health care, in particular to neurosurgical care? As reported by CNN (15), Dr. Ian Wilmut, the scientist that created Dolly, stated in his announcement that, "there are a number of genetic diseases for which there is no cure . . . and this will enable us to carry out research into the causes of those diseases and perhaps develop methods to treat them." This was soon followed by press speculation that insights may be gained into why spinal cords, heart muscle and brain tissue that won't regenerate after injury (14). Thus, it appears that neurosurgical disorders are a prime justification given by proponents of this technology. It is up to us to understand the issues and participate in the ongoing debate. The temporary ban on human cloning recommended by the National Bioethics Advisory allows some time for the profession to consider the issues involved (15). Some claim that discussion is futile, that the technique can be outlawed, but biology cannot be repealed, that even outlawing such a technique must fail because it is too simple, too replicable, and that no FDA or NIH regulation or even the FBI can stop it (14).

Scenarios for the use of cloning in medicine are being proposed. The child with an terminal environmental disease or disorder, such as meningococcal meningitis or traumatic brain injury, could have its nucleus harvested and a replica of the individual could be produced for the family. Other uses would be the cloning of portions of the genetic makeup, such as the instructions for the development of the spinal cord or brain, and then creating tissue from the clone to repair the effects of neurological trauma or stroke.

What are the implications of cloning within our ethical framework? For the sake of discussion, assume that 20 genetic copies of an individual were made. (The creation of 20 replicas, although unlikely, it is not beyond consideration, in view of humankind's recent dismal history with eugenics.)

1. Beneficence. The creation of replicas will not benefit the ill or injured original individual unless the replica is used to obtain organs or tissue. While the family may "benefit" by having a genetically identical individual to bring up, there would be no benefit to the ill or injured individual. Thus, human replication is not justifiable on the principle of beneficence to the "original" individual.

2. Nonmaleficence. It is difficult to imagine a scenario in which a copy of an individual reduces the likelihood of harm to that individual. Only if the copy had been created to treat or ameliorate a problem, a scenario that is not allowed by Kant's ethics of the categorical imperative (namely, to treat individuals as ends and not as means) would the replica reduce harm. If humans become a means to an end, we turn humanity into a product or service.

3. Autonomy. As we have seen, Kant's categorical imperative asks us to treat all individuals as autonomous beings worthy of respect. They should be treated as ends and not as means. If there are 20 genetically identical beings, we know from our understanding of twins that they would each be their own individual person. However, how would society view 20 identical individuals? Assume that the "individual of origin" develops a costly medical illness. Is society as likely to support the treatment of that individual if there are 20 other genetically identical individuals? Is it more likely that the resources will be withheld?

Thus, based on these ethical principles, human cloning is not justifiable. The only benefit that could be derived would come from treating the clone as a means, created and used for the specific purposes. Not only does this clash with Kant's ethics, but it also clashes with most humans sensibilities.

This is an enormously challenging issue. It is possible that humankind will not decide well. Nevertheless, we have marched down civilization making choices. We have chosen ideals, such as democracy and freedom, and defended them vigorously. More recently, we have championed human rights, women's rights, and rights for the disabled. In the issue of human genetic duplication, we are faced with a choice of what our ideals are—indeed, of what humankind is.

THE PHYSICIAN-SOCIETAL RELATIONSHIP

While managed care is considered by many to be the "driver" of the rapid change occurring in the delivery of health care, a closer look reveals that there may be an underlying ethical principle that drives our actions. For years, the contract for health care has been between the physician and the patient. Physicians agree to care for the patient as best they can. This contract is based on the ethical principles of beneficence and nonmaleficence, principles that have guided the medical profession for centuries. In modern times, they have guided physicians to strive for the highest quality of care possible, regardless of cost.

With the advent of managed care, physicians now make two contracts: the patient contract and the managed care contract. A look at a managed care contract reveals that physicians are not contracting to take care of the patient; they have contracted to maintain the health of "covered lives"or "plan members." Basically, the agreement is to maintain the health of a group of people, some of whom will get sick.

When considering the group, the ethical principle of justice must also be considered. As discussed above, justice leads to a consideration of fair opportunity. Since one of the goals is to maintain the health of the group, the theory of justice, with its emphasis on fairness, leads to a consideration of resources. If all are to be treated fairly, the available resources must be known. While beneficence and nonmaleficence direct physicians to strive for quality, justice directs them to take cost into account. Thus, the formula of quality/cost = value. By increasing the quality or decreasing the cost, the value of the care provided is raised. Thus, justice would dictate searching for the treatment that provides the best value. Once agreement is reached on the best treatment for the group, physicians are ethically bound to offer the same treatment to two patients in the same clinical situation.

Taking the principle of justice, together with the core principles of beneficence and nonmaleficence, the following ethical duties can be derived:

1. Physicians must work to maintain the health of the group. Prevention becomes an ethical duty, since it may allow more resources to be directed to those who are ill or injured.
2. Physicians must work to increase the resources available for medical care. Even in this era of limited budgets, it is their duty to strive for the resources necessary to care for the ill or injured, to provide high value care to all.
3. Physicians must continue to improve the quality of the care they provide. However, since there are limited resources, it is their duty to use treatments that have been shown to be effective. Thus, outcomes must be measured. Physicians must strive to determine which treatments have benefit, and discard those that do not.
4. Physicians have a duty to lower cost while maintaining or increasing the quality of care,

since this will increase the value of the services provided.

At times, ethical duties to the patient and to the group may be in conflict. Physicians are forced to decide between what is best for the individual and what is best for the group. Although the ethical priorities in this conflict will likely continue to be discussed for some time, the primary duty is to the patient. As the California Court of Appeals stated "The physician who complies without protest with limitations composed by a third-party payer, when his medical judgment dictates otherwise, cannot avoid his ultimate responsibility for his patient's care. He cannot point to the health-care payor as the liability scapegoat . . . " Thus, if a managed care plan denies care that in the best judgment of the physician would be beneficial for the patient, the physician has a duty to protest the decision.

ETHICS COMMITTEES

"(A) view of ethics . . . has been held by certain groups in certain periods of history, that only people with special skills or knowledge or training can know ethical truths . . . . It is a controversial position in modern society, however, one that many people have rejected in favor of a position acknowledging that all may have moral insight."

—*Childress*

Ethics committees, at their best, consist of representative members from a variety of sectors including medicine, nursing, law, clergy, social work, the lay public, and more. The committee provides a forum to stimulate and facilitate ethical discussions regarding the problem at hand. At their best, ethics committees should *facilitate* decision making; the committees do not make the decision.

The ethics committee at the University of Missouri Health Sciences Center in Columbia works as follows. Access to the committee is available to any party with an interest in the case, including physicians, nurses, family, students, or others with concerns about the care. A call system is published, with one member of the committee on first call and one back-up, 24 hours a day. The director of the call team takes the first call from the concerned party. A decision is made whether the case merits bringing the committee together (rarely are cases not heard). It is not uncommon that this phone call will result in an exchange that helps the health-care provider to resolve the ethical dilemma without calling a meeting. The committee meets within 24 hours during weekdays. In urgent cases, the on-call member works to locate as many members as possible who can convene on short notice. Whenever the committee plans to convene, the treating physician is notified.

The case is then presented by the treating physician or a resident physician. Case presentation is followed by a question and answer period that allows committee members, as well as other interested parties, to ask questions of the care givers. Without accurate clinical information, the ethical discussion may miss the mark. Clinical questions often focus on morbidity, mortality, life expectancy, degree of pain and suffering, and the burdensomeness of treatment. The committee may invite health-care specialists to participate in cases with complex or uncommon medical issues. Once the clinical situation seems to be well understood by the members and participants, open discussion is held regarding the ethical issues at hand. The issues raised vary greatly, depending on the case presented, but often center on autonomy, wishes of the individual (or the current understanding of those wishes), and benefits versus burdens of the treatment.

One of the more effective aspects of the deliberations is that the family members, physician, and care providers are more open about their respective feelings, concerns, and fears, and this alone often sets the stage for a just decision making process agreed to by the family and physician.

When the discussion has run its course, the parties that brought the case to the committee are asked if the committee can be of further help. At this point, the degree of satisfaction, or lack of satisfaction, is expressed. This process has been very effective in leading the parties to a resolution.

ORGANIZATIONAL ETHICS

There is a trend to expand the role of ethics within institutions beyond the traditional ethics committee (Hoffman, Renz, Schyve). Ethics committees focus on clinical ethics: the ethical issues involved in the direct delivery of clinical care to the patient. However, the changes occurring in health care resulting from managed care

and the consolidation of health facilities, have led to increased consideration of business ethics. As Schyve states "business decisions and practices in marketing, admissions, discharges, transfers, and reimbursement mechanisms can all affect patient care and, ultimately, patient health outcomes and patient satisfaction" (18). Hence, the trend toward combining clinical ethics and business ethics into *organizational* ethics, which will serve as the ethics infrastructure for the institution.

The characteristics of an ethics infrastructure have been defined by Renz (17) as follows: An ethics infrastructure has an "organizational systems orientation: a linked set of structures and processes," and not limited just to a committee. The "primary focus is on the entire range of ethical issues and decisions: individual, professional, and institutional." The organization is "responsive to the moral and ethical standards of all stakeholders to the institution, including the community and its diverse constituencies." The "time perspective is long term"and "all levels of organization are involved, including board members, health care professionals, patients and families, executives, and representatives of the broader community (via board or other)."

An ethics infrastructure encompasses all the activities of an institution, from individual patient care issues to the much broader issues of the responsibilities of the institution for the community. The recognition of the importance of the need for an ethics infrastructure was recently recognized, and is now required by Joint Commission on Accreditation of Health Care Organizations (18). This occurred in response to the public's concern "about abuses in which patients were admitted to hospitals unnecessarily and were discharged or transferred only after their insurance expired" (18).

In the 1996 edition of the *Accreditation Manual for Hospitals* of the JCAHO (18), the section on Patient Rights and Organization Ethics requires hospitals to "operate according to a code of ethical behavior" which "addresses marketing, admission, transfer and discharge, and billing practices." In addition, the code should address "the relationship of the (organization) and its staff to other health-care providers, educational institutions, and payers." Finally, it says that "An organization has an ethical responsibility to the patients and community it serves."

These changes impact the neurosurgeon in two ways. One, the neurosurgeon active in the ethical or administrative duties of the organization needs to become active in the development of the ethics infrastructure within the institution. The resulting structure may take many forms, but the process will develop through four stages: awareness of the issue, trial and experimentation, adoption, and institutionalization (17). The goal, according to Potter (19) is to "maintain a culture where ethical considerations are integrated into decision making at all levels."

The second impact is based on the view that organizational ethics is simply a reflection of the individual ethics of those who are part of the organization. Modern neurosurgery cannot be practiced outside of an organization. Thus, this organizational ethic applies to all neurosurgeons. Again, as stated by Potter (19), " individuals bear the responsibility for what organizations do . . . " and he says further: "In every organization, individuals must feel the ethical imperative to improve the ability of the system to do good, to anticipate unethical outcomes, and to correct an unethical action once it has occurred, e.g., to speak out when the salaries of CEOs become outrageous, when unnecessary technologies are used on patients who might better die with dignity, when the bottom line becomes more important than the mass of individuals for whom small increments in attention would pay big dividends on the human scale."

CONCLUSION

It is apparent from our reflections that medical ethics will need to continue to expand its scope. Most ethical principles, except for justice, focus on the individual. Is beneficence to one, or even many, enough, when others don't have the opportunity to receive care? Is there a social contract in addition to the physician/patient contract? Will a social contract be based on the theory of justice, or some other as yet unarticulated principle or theory? As perspective expands, a need arises to straddle the paradox. How can the focus on respect for the individual be safeguarded and yet encompass society as a whole? How can health care that impacts not only the individual, but all subsequent generations derived from that individual, be addressed?

Will the duty to uncover new knowledge gain increasing importance in the future? The development of the Salk vaccine has promoted more beneficence and nonmaleficence than most other treatments. It has allowed many, who may otherwise have been afflicted, greater ability to express autonomy, and it certainly has promoted justice by expunging a scourge that would drain enormous resources.

Thus, neurosurgeons have a duty to continue research on the prevention and treatment of neurological disorders, such as brain tumors, cerebrovascular disorders, and brain and spinal cord injury. The benefits in terms of beneficence, nonmaleficence, autonomy, and justice are clear.

What are the duties of the public with regard to health care? Some may argue that the public incurs no duty and that medical ethics apply only to the providers of health care. However, the public has significant control over many, often costly, disorders—such as those caused by alcohol abuse or by tobacco fume inhalation. The drain on scarce resources caused by these disorders limits the beneficence that can be shown to others with health-care needs. Autonomy becomes limited, by the limiting of health-care options available to others, and justice is constrained by the withdrawal of resources from other disorders to treat these.

If the concept of duty of the public seems foreign in health-care matters, consider the new societal contract previously discussed. Thus, in addition to the physician-patient relationship and its focus on the individual, there is developing a physician-societal relationship. It follows from this that not only the duties of the physician to society or the public, but the duties of society or the public to themselves in regard to health care, should be considered.

Bioethics is a living field of inquiry. It is slowly but continually evolving. New technologies and new issues pose new challenges. Neurosurgeons, by the nature of their work, bring a special perspective to ethical discussions. They should become involved in their hospital ethics committees to assist in advising fellow health-care practitioners in ethical decision making within their institutions.

REFERENCES

1. Munson R. Moral principles, ethical theories, and medical decisions: An introduction. In: Intervention and reflection: Basic issues in medical ethics. 3rd ed. Belmont, CA: Wadsworth Publishing Co, 1988, 347.
2. Beauchamp TL, Childress JF. Principles of biomedical

ethics. 2nd ed. New York: Oxford University Press, 1983.

3. Childress JF. The normative principles of medical ethics. In: Veatch RM, ed. Medical ethics. 2nd ed. Sudbury MA: John and Bartlett Pub, 1997: 2955.

4. Muehlbauer E. Judge rules on informed consent in MDL. NASS News 1996;10 (2):6.

5. Shumrick DA. The doctrine of informed consent—The issue of the 1990s. Ear Nose Throat J 1994;73(8): 508–510.

6. Murphy CJ. Maryland Court of Appeals: *Faya v. Almaraz.* U.S. Law Week 1993;61:2254.

7. Johnson. *Adler v. Kokemoor.* North Western Reporter 2nd series. 1996:495–510.

8. Reid D. Informed consent: An evolution from battery/medical negligence to potential invasion of physician privacy. Miss Med 1993;(6):275–278.

9. Smedira MG, Bradley HE, Grais LS, et al. Withholding and withdrawal of life support from the cirtically ill. N Engl J Med 1990;322(5):309–314.

10. Capron AM. In: Re Helga Wanglie. Hastings Center Rep 1991;26–28.

11. Callahan D. Medical futility, medical necessity. The-problem-without-a-name. Hastings Center Rep 1991; 30–35.

12. Raymond JL, Lisberger SG, Mauk MD. The cerebellum: A neuronal learning machine? Science 1996;272: 1126.

13. Palmer W. Ethics of human gene therapy. New York: Oxford University Press, 1997.

14. Krauthammer C. A special report on cloning. Time 1997;May 10:60–61

15. Clinton bars federal funds for human cloning research. Sci-Tech. March 4, 1997, CNN Interactive, http// www.cnn.com/TECH/9703/04/clinton.cloning/index. html.

16. Hofmann PB. Hospital mergers and acquisitions: A new catalyst for examining organizational ethics. Bioethics Forum 1996; summer: 45–48.

17. Renz DO, Eddy WB. Organizations, ethics, and health care: Building an ethics infrastructure for a new era. Bioethics Forum 1996: 29–38.

18. Schyve PM. Patient rights and organization ethics: The Joint Commission perspective. In: Accreditation manual for hospitals. Standards, Vol 1. Oakbrook Terrace IL: Joint Commission Accreditation of healthcare organizations, 1996: 44, 45.

19. Potter VR. Indivuals bear responsibilty. Bioethics Forum 1996;(summer):27–28.

CHAPTER 16

Medical-Legal Aspects of Managed Care

HAROLD D. PORTNOY, M.D., JAMES M. PIDGEON, ESQ.

INTRODUCTION

Neurosurgeons increasingly face new problems as managed care gradually sweeps across the country. They are finding themselves involved in a new paradigm of health care. No longer is their relationship with a patient simply an implied contract, paid either by the patient or the patient's insurer. Neurosurgeons now are immersed in an unfamiliar system, in which they are dealing not solely with the patient, but rather with a more involved system driven by managers and businessmen—the managed care organization (MCO). In contrast to the traditional medical insurance company, which accepted responsibility only for financing health care, the MCO also accepts responsibility for the delivery of that care to the population enrolled in its health plan. The legal responsibility of the neurosurgeon in this managed care environment depends on the type of MCO and the relationship the neurosurgeon has with the patient *and* the MCO. How MCOs are formed, as well as what federal and state regulations affect action, such as antitrust laws, must now be considered by the physician.

MANAGED CARE AND THE PHYSICIAN

The relationship between the physician and the MCO varies, and this relationship is important in determining the legal liability faced by the physician in a managed care arrangement. The MCO may be either closed panel or open panel. In a closed panel MCO, the health maintenance organization (HMO) contracts with a limited group of physicians. The panel may either be in the form of a staff model, in which the physicians are directly employed by the HMO as

are the supporting personnel, such as physician assistants and nurses; or it may be a group model, in which the HMO contracts exclusively with a physician group practice, prohibiting the physicians from contracting with any other HMO.

An open panel MCO contracts directly or indirectly with a broad and usually mixed panel of physicians, who provide the members of the HMO with medical care in the private physicians' offices. The physicians may organize an individual practice association (IPA), in which the physicians form an incorporated group that contracts with an MCO. The IPA contracts with the MCO to deliver its services, either on a non-risk fee-for-service claims basis, or on a capitated risk basis. If the IPA is capitated, it receives a single capitation payment for all physician services and, in turn, contracts with the physicians to provide the medical care either by a fee-for-service agreement or through individual or group subcapitation. In the network model, the MCO provides health care for its enrollees by contracting with more than one group of physicians, or even with other groups of providers, thus multiple groups of physicians and providers serve the needs of the MCO.

How closely the MCO controls the selection and direction of the physicians and physicians' groups can determine professional liability risk: whether a physician is sued alone by an unhappy patient or in conjunction with the MCO.

Credentialing

Managed care organizations try to minimize their liability by credentialing the physicians who take care of their enrollees. The credentialing process is usually similar for both closed

234

and open panel model MCOs. The credentialing process is similar to that which physicians undergo for admission to a hospital medical staff. Credentialing standards have been established by the National Committee for Quality Assurance (NCQA), an organization for MCOs similar to the Joint Commission on Accreditation of Healthcare Organizations (JCAHO) for accreditation of hospitals. In order for the NCQA to approve an MCO, the MCO must have established standards for credentialing its physicians (6). These standards include written policies and procedures for credentialing, recredentialing, recertification and reappointment of physicians; a governing body that reviews and approves the credentialing policies and procedures; a peer review panel for credentialing decisions; and recredentialing on a biannual basis with verification of license, staff privileges, Drug Enforcement Agency number, board certification, and malpractice insurance, along with the physician's liability history. As noted later, failure of an MCO to properly credential a physician can be used as a basis for legal action (6).

Liability

When a patient enrolled in a MCO feels improperly treated by a physician or hospital, the patient may resort to a law suit in order to gain compensation for the alleged complaints. Whether the MCO is sued along with the physician and/or hospital depends on the relationship of the MCO to the physician or hospital. In these days of utilization review with the hope of cost containment, the question arises as to whether a physician can be held responsible for decisions based on directives of the MCO.

The case referred to when there is a conflict between the physician and the cost containment efforts of managed care is *Wickline v. State of California* (32). In 1976, Mrs. Wickline was approved by Medi-Cal for admission to a hospital for the surgical treatment of obstruction of the terminal aorta (Leriche syndrome). The surgery was complicated by a blood clot in the graft, for which she underwent a second procedure. She then had considerable pain associated with spasm in the vessels of the leg. Several days later, she underwent a lumbar sympathectomy for relief of the pain. Her physician requested an 8-day extension of her hospital stay; however, only 4 days were approved, which *her physician failed to appeal*, even though such an appeal

only required a telephone call. Four days after discharge, she again developed leg pain with progressive discoloration of the leg. Nine days after discharge, Mrs. Wickline was readmitted as an emergency for an infection at the graft site, leading to a clot in the graft and subsequent below-the knee amputation of her right leg. Rather than suing her physicians, Mrs. Wickline sued the State of California and its utilization review organization. While the trial court awarded Mrs. Wickline $500,000, the appellate court reversed the trial court finding the State of California not negligent. The appellate court decision was final when the Supreme Court of California declined to review the case. Several opinions of the court, however, are important in understanding the relationship between a patient, MCO, and physician (22).

The door was opened for inclusion of an MCO as a defendant in a case of medical negligence when the court stated that a "patient who is harmed when care which should have been provided is not provided should recover from all responsible for deprivation of care, including, when appropriate, a health care payer." The court further stated that "Third party payers of health care services can be held legally accountable when medically inappropriate decisions result from defects in designs or implementation of cost containment mechanisms."

The physician was also held responsible. The court noted that a physician who complies with the decision of the utilization review process without protest "when his medical judgement dictates otherwise, cannot avoid his ultimate responsibility for his patient's care." The message is quite clear. A physician is responsible for the care provided or withheld from his patient and must assure that the patient's needs are fulfilled, when dealing with a third party payer. If a physician believes that the decision of the utilization review process is incorrect, it is the physician's responsibility to challenge the process by pursuing all avenues of appeal available to him.

Vicarious Liability

Vicarious liability, that is, the liability based on the relationship between an employer and employee, or master and servant, without regard for the participation of the master in tort or act causing the damage, arises out of the public policy that the one should be held to respond for the acts of the other (*Naddeau v. Melin*)(16).

There are various theories of liability under which an MCO may be held liable for the inappropriate care by a member physician. The theory of vicarious liability of an MCO is dependent on the model employed. Actual agency (doctrine of *respondeat superior*, let the master answer) is most persuasive when used against the staff model HMO. This doctrine states that an employer may be held vicariously responsible for the negligent acts of its employees that occur in the course and scope of employment (5). The primary test is that of control. When the principal is capable of controlling the servant, the principal may be held liable for the acts of the servant. In 1980, the Supreme Judicial Court of Massachusetts found, in *Gugino v. Harvard Community Health Plan* (9), that an HMO could be vicariously liable for injuries suffered by an enrolled patient as a result of the negligence of one of its physicians and a nurse. The plaintiff had a Dalkon shield inserted in 1972 and, after reading articles on the shield, sought the advice of the physician who assured her of the safety of the device. As a result of the shield, she later suffered injuries resulting in a hysterectomy.

In 1987, the appellate court in Indiana, in reversing a summary judgement for the HMO, found in *Sloan v. Metropolitan Health Council of Indianapolis, Inc.* (26), that Metropolitan, a staff model HMO, could be held liable for its staff physicians. This HMO advertised complete care for its members in return for prepaid payment. The member selects a staff physician who treats the member/patient, orders tests, and otherwise takes care of that member. The HMO argued that it was not liable, because it was not incorporated under the Professional Corporation Act. The court held that the HMO's medical director controlled the negligent staff physician and that an employer-employee relationship existed between the HMO and the physician. Specifically, the court stated that "It is, however, a *non sequitur* to conclude that because a hospital cannot practice medicine or psychiatry, it cannot be liable for the actions of its employed agents and servants who may be licensed (5, 6)."

Furthermore, the courts stretched vicarious liability to include the actions of an independent consulting physician in *Schleier v. Kaiser Foundation Health Plan* (23). A physician employed by Kaiser requested a consultation by an outside cardiologist. The court held that Kaiser could be liable for the actions of the cardiologist, because a master-servant relationship could have existed between the cardiologist and the Kaiser physician. The court noted five factors for review in determining whether *respondeat superior* theory could be applied in managed care: selection and engagement of the physician; payment of wages; power of discharge; power to control the behavior of the physician; and whether the work is part of the regular business of the MCO.

Ostensible agency arises when the appearance is created that one party is an agent of another party, and a third party reasonably relies on that representation (5, 19). Ordinarily, a hospital cannot be held liable for the independent acts of physicians practicing within its walls and merely using the hospital's facilities to treat the patient (*Grewe v. Mt. Clemens Hospital*)(7). In the context of managed care, to apply the theory of ostensible liability, the plaintiff must prove that the patient looked to the MCO rather than to the physician for care and that the MCO held out the physician as its employee, thus establishing a reasonable assumption by the member/patient that the physician was an agent of the MCO. The theory of ostensible agency is popular with plaintiffs, because an actual employer-employee relationship does not have to exist, thus offering the most flexibility for the assertion of negligence against an MCO.

In *Boyd v. Albert Einstein Medical Center* (1), the plaintiff/patient was enrolled in a Group IPA Model type of HMO, HMO of Pennsylvania. The case involved an alleged negligent breast biopsy leading to the death of the patient. The HMO had a gatekeeper system, in which a specialist had to be authorized by the patient's primary care physician, who prevented the patient from seeing a specialist, thus denying her care that possibly could have helped her. The plaintiff/patient alleged that because the HMO advertised that its physicians and care providers were competent and had been evaluated by the HMO, the HMO should be held liable under the theory of ostensible liability. The court indicated that, when an HMO represents itself to the public that its physicians are carefully selected for competence and the patient has a restricted choice, a finding of ostensible agency is likely if the patient is harmed.

Nondelegable Duty

This theory is usually applied to hospitals, in which the hospital owes an independent, nondelegable duty to patients to exercise reasonable care in selecting competent physicians. Furthermore, the hospital has a duty to maintain proper facilities and equipment, to supervise all individuals practicing in the hospital, and to have adequate rules and policies to assure quality care. Nondelegable duty is an established exception to the rule that an employer is not liable for the negligence of its independent contractors. The Supreme Court of Alaska in *Jackson v. Power* (13) noted that the importance to the community of a hospital's duty to provide emergency room physicians rivals the importance of the common carriers duty for the safety of passengers and stated, ''We simply cannot fathom why liability should depend upon the technical employment status of the emergency room physician who treats the patient. It is the hospital's duty to provide the physician, which it may do through any means at its disposal. The means employed, however, will not change the fact that the hospital will be responsible for the care rendered by physicians it has a duty to provide.''

The court premised its decision, in part, on the fact that the hospital where Mr. Jackson was treated was licensed as a ''general acute care hospital.'' As such, it was required to comply with state regulations designed to promote safe and adequate treatment of individuals admitted to hospitals in the interest of public health, safety and welfare. Those regulations provided, at the time of Mr. Jackson's accident, that an acute care hospital shall ''insure that a physician is available to respond to an emergency at all times.'' It also noted that the hospital was accredited by the JCAHO, and that JCAHO standards required that the emergency room be directed by a physician on the active medical staff, be integrated with other units and departments of the hospital, and have the quality of care rendered be continually reviewed, evaluated, and assured through the establishment of Quality Control mechanisms. Those requirements having been noted, the Court ruled that the hospital had a nondelegable duty to provide fit and proper medical care in its emergency room, which duty could not be delegated away by retaining an independent contractor (the emergency room physician) to fill the need.

Under such circumstances, where the hospital has a nondelegable duty to provide a particular type of physician, it cannot claim that the physician provided was not its agent and thereby escape liability for harm done by that physician.

Corporate Liability

Corporate liability is the theory of law that imposes liability on a hospital, MCO, or other entity for their own negligence. The negligence of the hospital arises from the breach of a duty to exercise reasonable care in selecting or credentialing physicians on staff at its hospital, whether those physicians are independent contractors or employees. To demonstrate breach of the duty owed to the public in the selection of physicians to work in the hospital, the plaintiff usually will attempt to demonstrate that the physician hired as an employee or extended a contract by the hospital as an independent contractor does not have the proper training or education necessary to fulfill the role he or she was hired to perform, has demonstrated a lack of competence in his or her chosen field by virtue of having numerous medical malpractice actions successfully brought against the physician, or has other instances of misfeasance that have been called to the attention of the hospital's credentialing board.

This theory was first applied to a hospital in *Darling v. Charleston Community Memorial Hospital* (3). The plaintiff broke his leg playing football. At the defendant hospital, he was placed in an improperly applied cast, after which he had severe pain and his toes became swollen and discolored. This subsequently led to amputation of the leg. The Illinois Supreme Court found the hospital liable for violating its duty to review the actions of its physicians.

In 1989, the Missouri Court of Appeals applied the theory of corporate negligence to an HMO in *Harrell v. Total Health Care, Inc.* (11). The plaintiff had consulted with the primary physician of this group IPA about a urological problem and was referred to a specialist approved by the HMO. The urologist negligently performed surgery. Physicians were solicited to become participating physicians in the HMO by mail and sent an application if they showed an interest. The plaintiff contended that the HMO failed to conduct any inquiry into the physician's competence and reputation. Had such an inquiry been made, the HMO would have discovered the record of multiple malpractice suits against the surgeon. Because of statutory immunity for a nonprofit organization, the Missouri Supreme Court subsequently affirmed a summary judgment in favor of the HMO. In the absence of the immunity, however, the court indicated that the plaintiff had established a cause of action against the HMO for negligent selection of the physician.

As noted earlier, the first case usually referred to regarding the cost containment efforts of managed care is *Wickline v. State of California*. However, the courts are reluctant to hold an MCO liable based solely on the basis of financial incentives. In *Pulvers v. Kaiser Health Plan* (5, 19, 20), the plaintiff claimed that the reason her husband's disease was not diagnosed was because the nonprofit HMO gave incentives to its physicians to withhold care. The court rejected this theory of a cause of action based on financial incentives, noting that the use of these incentives was recommended by professional organizations and specifically required by the federal HMO act. The court granted the defendant's nonsuit noting that there was no evidence that individual physicians in the HMO acted negligently or failed to obtain appropriate diagnostic procedures.

In deciding whether an MCO is liable under the theory of financial incentives, the courts consider the standard of care offered by the treating physician. The issue is whether the standard of care was met by the MCO physician, rather than whether the MCO violated any duty related to financial incentives (19).

Breach of Contract

The theory of breach of contract in regard to managed care is that the organization has breached its contract with the enrollee/patient by not providing a certain quality of care (19). A contract action has the advantage over a claim of negligence, in that the statue of limitations for filing a claim is usually longer.

In the *Depenbrok v. Kaiser Foundation Health Plan, Inc.* (4), the court ruled that a plaintiff could sue for breach of contract against an HMO for substandard care. The case involved a tubal ligation that failed and resulted in later pregnancy. While the claim was rejected in this case, the court stated that "if a plaintiff can prove to a properly instructed jury that a surgeon has clearly promised a particular result (as distinguished from a mere generalized statement that the result will be good), and the patient consented to an operation or other procedure in reliance on that promise, there can be recovery on the theory of warranty" (or, to give the theory its more accurate name: breach of contract).

The major drawback to this claim is that the plaintiff must prove that the MCO made a clear, unambiguous promise that a certain result would occur. This is distinct from exuberant advertising claims, since the courts are hesitant to hold these organizations to the letter of their advertising.

Arbitration

Some states allow an agreement between an MCO and its enrollees which requires that any negligence claim must be submitted to arbitration, a provision that may minimize the potential liability of the MCO. The Supreme Court of California, in *Madden v. Kaiser Foundation Hospitals* (17), upheld an arbitration provision in an enrollment agreement. The court ruled that the arbitration provision in the contract did not constitute an impermissible denial of the plaintiff's rights to trial by jury. The Maryland Court of Appeals, in *Group Health Association, Inc v. Blumenthal* (8), went further in ruling that mandatory arbitration provisions of Maryland's Health Care Malpractice Claims Act applied to an HMO on the grounds that the HMO was a health-care provider (19).

It is to the advantage of the MCO to have as part of the enrollment agreement an arbitration provision. Generally, courts will uphold such agreements, as long as these agreements are not unconscionable or contrary to public policy, since alternatives to litigation preserve judicial resources.

EMPLOYEE RETIREMENT INCOME SECURITY ACT

The Employee Retirement Income Security Act (ERISA) of 1974 was enacted by Congress for the purpose of assuring the equitable character of employee benefit plans and their financial soundness. Congress was concerned that a lack of uniform regulation governing employee benefit plans in the various states might result in financial instability of the plans, placing the pension and welfare plans of workers at risk. With ERISA, Congress created a comprehensive system to regulate employee welfare benefit plans through the purchase of insurance or other means of providing medical, hospital, or other care in the event of sickness, accident, disability, or death. Now, with the advent of managed care, many patients are insured by employee health plans offered by employers or unions that come under ERISA regulation. Claims of medical negligence against an MCO for the actions of its incompetent physicians or other providers may be dismissed because ERISA does not permit either federal or state remedy for these claims. Specifically , Congress included a preemption provision which provides that ERISA supersedes all state laws, insofar as they relate to any employee benefit plan. Therefore, the courts must decide whether a medical negligence claim is preempted by ERISA by determining whether the state malpractice statutes relate to the plaintiff's employment benefit plan in a way that necessitates preemption (5, 6, 18).

The United States Supreme Court in *Shaw v. Delta Air Lines, Inc.* (24) interpreted the ERISA preemption provision broadly, ruling that the phrase ''relates to any employee benefit plan'' meant having a ''connection with or reference to'' an employee benefit plan. In *Ricco v. Gooberman* (21), the plaintiff sued U.S. Healthcare for failing to advise her of an abnormal mammogram and other careless treatment. The court ruled that claims based on vicarious liability were preempted by ERISA and dismissed the claim against U.S. Healthcare. Thus, claims that allege that an HMO is negligent in employing or contracting with negligent physicians, failed to properly select or oversee a physician, or failed to establish quality assurance regulations will probably be preempted under ERISA.

The courts, on the other hand, have determined that claims based on the theory of ostensible liability are not preempted by ERISA. In *Independence HMO, Inc. v. Smith* (12), the court found that a medical negligence suit brought against an HMO under the theory of ostensible agency had nothing to do with any denial of the plaintiff's rights under the plan. ''Instead, she seeks redress for physical injuries in which the HMO's selection of an operating surgeon allegedly played a part.'' In *Haas v. Group Health Plan, Inc.* (10), the court ruled that ''when an HMO plan elects to directly provide medical services or leads the participant to reasonably believe that it has, rather than simply arranging and paying for treatment,'' a medical liability claim based on substandard treatment by an agent of the HMO was not preempted by ERISA.

ANTITRUST LAWS

The Sherman Antitrust Act (25) declares as being unlawful any contract, combination or conspiracy that restrains trade. In order, for a physician or physician group to be in violation, two or more independent physicians or groups must engage in *joint activity*, and the joint activity must *restrain competition* (30).

Joint activity does not occur when an individual physician takes an action, nor does it occur when a group of physicians participates in a fully integrated single practice in which the physicians share profits and losses and are not in competition. However, a joint activity may be as simple as two physicians agreeing not to sign a contract or two groups of physicians agreeing to set fees. An illegal agreement between physicians or groups of physicians need not be in writing; an implied agreement is equally illegal. Thus, a casual conversation between physicians that results in a loss to an MCO may be found to be illegal.

Joint activity is not illegal unless it restrains trade, that is, the effect of the activity decreases competition. This may take one of two forms. It may be illegal *per se*, such as price fixing, a group boycott, or the allocation of territories or patients. Price fixing is considered illegal regardless of the reasonableness of the prices, unless the activity places the members at substantial financial risk. Substantial risk is narrowly defined to include agreements to provide services under capitation or the creation of significant incentives for members to contain costs, such as basing compensation on meeting cost containment goals (2, 14, 30)

If the *per se* rule is not applicable, then the court applies the *rule of reason*. Under the rule of reason, the court balances the procompetitive and anticompetitive purposes and effects of an agreement and determines which of the two competitive situations outweighs the other. If the agreement is primarily procompetitive, then the agreement is considered legal; if not, it is illegal. As a general rule, an agreement that involves a pooling of assets that increases efficiency and benefits the consumer or involves the sharing of financial risk usually is sufficient proof to warrant a *rule of reason* review (2, 15).

The penalties for violating antitrust laws include the loss of a physician's license, imprisonment for up to 3 years, and/or fines of up to $350,000. Furthermore, the physician may be subject to actions by private parties, such as competing physicians, MCOs, or patients harmed by the anticompetitive activity who may bring civil suit for injunctive relief and recover treble damages as well as court costs and attorney fees.

In response to the recent changes in health care, in which MCOs of various sorts have become prominent, physicians and physician groups have tried to form their own MCOs, either alone or in combination with a hospital. These physicians, along with other health providers, have worried about their exposure to federal antitrust enforcement. In 1993 and 1994, the Department of Justice (DOJ) and the Federal Trade Commission (FTC) issued policy statements designed to provide guidance to parties planning to engage in activities that could possibly be construed as being anticompetitive (27, 28). The statements issued in 1994 included 'safety zones', or activities that would not be challenged under usual circumstances. Activities outside these safety zones may or may not be legal and would be subject to the rule of reason. Four of the nine safety zone guidelines relate to physician conduct.

Physicians may now collectively provide *non-fee-related* information to purchasers of health care, such as outcome data and practice parameters, in an attempt to affect a payer's decision on contract terms or other parameters. If, however, the same physicians imply a boycott or other similar action against the payer, then the *non-fee-related* activity would be unlawful. Physicians may also collectively provide *fee-related data* and *price and cost surveys* to purchasers with the following provisos:

- The fee or cost data is determined by a third party (payer, government agency, health-care consultant).
- Any information shared with physicians must be at least 3-months-old.
- The data must be gleaned from at least five physicians, of which no one physician can submit more than 25% of the data, and the data must be so commingled that no individual physician can be identified.

These rules ensure that competing physicians cannot join together to use the data to fix prices.

Finally, the guidelines allow *physician joint ventures*, such as independent physician associations (IPAs), preferred provider organizations (PPOs), or similar physician organizations. Separate safety zones are established for exclusive and nonexclusive joint ventures. The exclusive venture restricts physician members from affiliating with other networks or plans, while nonexclusive ventures do not restrict their members from participating in other ventures. The DOJ/FTC indicate that they will closely review the physicians that participate in a nonexclusive joint venture to be sure that they truly participate in other competing physician ventures. Generally, an exclusive joint venture that comprises 20% or less of physicians in each participating specialty in a given area and who share significant risk will not be challenged by the government. For nonexclusive ventures, a 30% limit is allowed. Joint ventures by physicians that do not fall within the safety zone guidelines may be lawful, but are subjected to *rule of reason* analysis. This analysis involves defining the scope of the consumers in the market and other suppliers of service in the area, evaluating the competitive effects of the joint venture as to whether the venture will raise prices or prevent the formation of other competitive ventures, evaluating the potential efficiency of procompetitive versus anticompetitive practices, and evaluating whether any collateral agreements included as part of the joint venture are reasonably necessary (15, 31).

The DOJ/FTC issued new guidelines on physician network joint ventures in 1996 (29) that indicate that these agencies will look favorably at a greater variety of collaborative efforts by physicians. As noted above, the DOJ/FTC had declared as being illegal *per se* those ventures that did not put its members at substantial risk. The new guidelines recognize that there are other ways that physicians can be placed at significant financial risk, beside capitation and incentives to contain costs, and the new guidelines end the practice of automatically designating as unlawful any physician network that does not place the members at risk. These agencies note that a physician network can also reduce costs by implementing an ongoing program to evaluate and modify practice patterns and thus develop interdependence and cooperation among the physicians to control costs and ensure quality. Furthermore, the network is more likely to select physicians that further these cost containment and quality goals. Though these guidelines are applicable to physician networks, they do not apply to networks comprised of physicians and hospitals. The new guidelines also do not protect physician networks from challenges by private parties or by state attorneys general (14).

COMMENTARY

Many of the instances cited above, demonstrating that a hospital may be held liable for the acts of a physician who is not its employee, should provide little solace to physicians who actually engage in their profession as independent contractors. Although some attorneys will not take the time to initiate suit against physicians who are uninsured (since there is little financial motivation to do so), if a hospital and HMO or another medical facility can be named along with a physician as a defendant in litigation, then the physician is going to find himself or herself involved, one way or the other, in the litigation brought by the injured party.

Although relatively rare, hospitals are more frequently entertaining the thought of initiating litigation against the physician whose alleged negligence has given rise to the litigation, seeking to have the physician indemnify them for the full amount of any judgment that may have been rendered against the facility. Such action may be taken by the health facility, whether or not the physician was originally named as a defendant in the litigation.

As a juror, it is much easier to return a verdict of a substantial amount against a pile of bricks and mortar, than it is to return a verdict against a live individual who has sat through the trial that the juror has witnessed. Theories against physicians and health-care facilities are continuously expanding, because, as Willie Sutton said, when asked why he robbed banks, ''That's where the money is.''

Although misery may welcome company, the possibility of health-care facilities being found to share liability with the neurosurgeon should not help physicians sleep any better at night.

REFERENCES

1. *Boyd v. Albert Einstein Medical Center*, 377 Pa.Super. 609, 547 A.2d 1229 (1988).
2. Clary BG. Physician collective bargaining. Antitrust prospects and pitfalls. Minn Med 1995;78:41-44.
3. *Darling v. Charleston Memorial Hospital*, 33 Ill.2d 326, 211 N.E.2d 253 (1965).
4. *Depenbrok v. Kaiser Foundation Health Plan, Inc.*, 79 Cal App. 3d 167 (1978).
5. DiCicco DC. Liability of the HMO for the medical negligence of its providers. Defense 1996;38:10–15.
6. Dorros TA, Stone TH. Implications of negligent selection and retention of physicians in the age of ERISA. Am J Law Med 1995;21:384–418.
7. *Grewe v. Mt. Clemens Hospital*, 404 Mich 240, NW2d (1978).
8. *Group Health Association, Inc. v. Blumenthal*, 453 A.2d 1198 (Md. 1983).
9. *Gugino v. Harvard Community Health Plan*, 380 Mass. 464. 403 N.E.2d 1166 (1980).
10. *Haas v. Group Health Plan, Inc.*, 875 F.Supp. 544, 548 (S.D.Ill. 1994).
11. *Harrell v. Total Health Care, Inc.* 781 S.W.2d 58 (Mo. 1989).
12. *Independence HMO, Inc. v. Smith*, 733 F.Supp. 983, 988 (E.D.Pa. 1990).
13. *Jackson v. Power*, 743 Pacific 2d 1376 (1987).
14. Landerbaugh RA. What surgeons should know about antitrust guidelines for joint ventures and networks. Bull Am Coll Surg 1996;81: 8–11.
15. Lawton SE, Leibenluft RF, Loeb LE. Antitrust implications of physicians' responses to managed care. Clin Infect Dis 1995;20:1354-1360.
16. *Naddeau v. Melin*, 260 Minn 369, 110 NW2d 29 (1961).
17. *Madden v. Kaiser Foundation Hospitals*, 131 Cal. Rptr. 882 (1976).
18. Mariner WK. Health law and ethics. Liability for managed care decisions: The Employment Retirement Income Retirement Income Security Act (ERISA) and the uneven playing field. Am J Public Health 1996; 86:863-869.
19. Mulholland DM III. Managing care and the risk for managing quality. Managing Care 1992;7:12 –22.
20. *Pulvers v. Kaiser Foundation Health Plan*, 99 Cal.App.3d 560, 160 Cal.Rptr. 392 (1979).
21. *Ricci v. Gooberman*, 840 F.Supp. 316 (D.N.J. 1993).
22. Sederer LI. Judicial and legislative responses to cost containment. Am J Psychiat 1992;149:1157–1161.
23. *Schleier v. Kaiser Foundation Health Plan*, 876 F.2d 174 (D.C. Cir. 1989).
24. *Shaw v. Delta Air Lines, Inc*, 463 US 85, 91 (1983).
25. Sherman Antitrust Act. 15 US Code §1.
26. *Sloan v. Metropolitan Council of Indianapolis, Inc*, 516 N.E.2d 1104 (Ind.App. 1987).
27. U.S. Department of Justice and the Federal Trade Commission, Statements of Antitrust Enforcement Policy in Health Care, Sept 15, 1993.
28. U.S. Department of Justice and the Federal Trade Commission, Statements of Antitrust Enforcement Policy in Health Care, Sept 27, 1994.
29. U.S. Department of Justice and the Federal Trade Commission, Statements of Antitrust Enforcement Policy in Health Care, Aug 28, 1996.
30. Weber RD. Antitrust law applicable to managed care contracting. Mich Med 1995;4:16–17.
31. Werner MJ. Physician-run health plans and antitrust. Ann Int Med 1996;125:59–65.
32. *Wickline v. State of California*, 228 Cal Rptr 661 (Cal App 2 Dist 1986), 239 Cal Rptr 805 (Cal 1987).

CHAPTER 17

Socioeconomic Issues in Neurotrauma

JOHN H. McVICKER, M.D.

INTRODUCTION

Neurotrauma has become the focal point for many of the primary issues facing neurosurgery. At the center of these issues are individual concerns over malpractice, Emergency Medical Transfer and Active Labor Act (EMTALA) mandates with the potential for federal liability, reimbursement issues that include trauma call stipends, managed care organization (MCO) contracts, indigent care, and sacrifices in personal life-style that reduce the perceived attractiveness of neurotrauma. The reported excess of the neurosurgical workforce stands in contrast to widespread difficulty in assuring neurosurgical emergency room coverage. Active neurosurgical involvement in the development of proliferating regional trauma systems is variable, and interaction with hospital systems and other specialties, most notably the American College of Surgeons Committee on Trauma (ACS-COT) and the American College of Emergency Physicians (ACEP), may occasionally assume an adversarial tone. Encroachment by other specialties into neurotrauma added to indifference among neurosurgeons may eventually result in neurosurgery abdicating its role in neurotrauma, further reducing its already contracting preeminence. If neurosurgery does not itself address these concerns, others may do so and impose opprobrious or burdensome sanctions on the specialty.

National standards of care may initially appear to be an admirable goal. In reality, large variations in regional demographics and the economics of trauma tend to render globally applied frameworks, such as the ACS-COT neurotrauma guidelines or Federal neurotrauma system templates, locally inflexible and potentially inapplicable. An appropriate approach will require a better understanding of the present state of affairs and attitudes over a representative demographic and regional cross section of the country, establishing the characteristics of systems that appear to be working, as well as where problems are perceived. Once defined, organized neurosurgery can proactively address problems by promoting awareness of the issues, informing, educating, and empowering neurosurgeons with tools to flexibly address regional neurotrauma problems. This information transfer will enable local neurosurgical participation in the development of trauma systems that meet local needs. The use of national standards to measure and improve quality across systems, and legislative action at all levels, can then take place in a cohesive, cogent fashion. Legislation in many states is already being used to address some of these problems; active participation of neurosurgery in this process should be encouraged. The goal should be to reinforce neurosurgery's preeminent role in the treatment of neurotrauma, maintain equity for neurosurgeons bearing the brunt of the neurotrauma burden, and maximize the quality of care received by neurotrauma patients. The purpose of this chapter is formulate a framework in which organized neurosurgery at all levels may begin to take action.

WORKFORCE

Current Trends

In the United States in 1996, there were approximately 4611 self-designated neurosurgeons (62). Approximately 3760 of these are qualified by the American Board of Neurological Surgery. Ten percent of these physicians are involved in aspects of neurosurgery, such as research, that make them unavailable to the pool providing neurotrauma care. The current overall ratio of neurosurgeons to population is 1 : 60,000–65,000 in the United States, with wide regional variation. There are, however, nearly 1000 more emergency facilities in the United States than there are practicing neurosurgeons.

Due to a perceived overproduction of neurosurgeons in the 1970s, training or "production" of neurosurgical trainees declined. The development of neurosurgical centers in smaller communities in the 1980s led to the establishment of new training programs with an increase in the number of first-year trainees from 100 to 140 per year by the mid 1990s. Currently, there are 96 neurosurgical training programs with 846 residents. There are 126 "approved" fellowship programs available. There may be up to 300 non-approved "fellowship" positions filled. A portion of these physicians provides neurosurgical trauma coverage in certain situations.

In spite of these numbers, the overall production of board certified or qualified neurosurgeons has remained remarkably constant over the last 10 years (83). In 1995 and 1996, 148 candidates took the oral certifying examination with a pass rate of 84%. Availability of advertised work positions has also been used in some studies to determine whether the work force is properly sized (67). In the CNS job exchange bulletin board at the end of 1996, there were 80 positions advertised and 130 applicants in the pool. The commercial "head hunters" advertised 45 to 50 positions.

The percentage of international medical graduates in residency programs has remained at less than 10% in recent years. The movement of Canadian neurosurgeons to the U.S. has also declined. This migration amounted to an additional 10% of United States output per year at its peak in the 1980s. The decline in Canadian immigration is mainly due to socioeconomic factors, both here and in Canada, as well as to the recent action of the American Board of Neurological Surgery not to accept Canadian-trained applicants for board examination.

Current variables that may lead to a reduction, or at least a leveling off, of the number of practicing neurosurgeons include:

- Decrease in funding for specialty training programs (52, 65)
- Consolidation of programs, especially in large urban centers on both coasts

- Additional years in training before starting practice, with resultant restriction of on call availability to a subspecialty
- Earlier retirement of actively practicing neurosurgeons (54)

Oversupply and Unmet Demand

Concern has been raised in a variety of forums over neurosurgical workforce. The Federal Trade Commission has disallowed direct inquiry into questions of workforce specifically as they relate to the control of numbers of neurosurgeons in training programs, unless quality (and not need) is the parameter for study or restriction (73). Broad surveys of multiple specialties have reported progressive excess in national neurosurgical workforce. The dilemma for neurosurgery is that while some statistical analyses suggest that there is an excess of neurosurgeons presently in practice in the United States, practical experience suggests that there are gaps in coverage for emergency care, particularly in trauma (23, 37). In economic terms, there appears to be both oversupply and unmet demand.

Two reasons for this apparent dilemma may be offered. First, the statistical analyses that suggest an overabundance of neurosurgeons examine only overall need for neurosurgical expertise in a community and do not specifically account for additional "on call" time or unscheduled emergency activities that may be additional to, or fall outside of, traditional work hours (63). Neurotrauma care requires the immediate availability of a neurosurgeon (such as is required at a Level One or Level Two trauma facility) or the ability to transfer a patient to a facility where a neurosurgeon is currently available (82). In either case, the neurosurgeon needs to be physically present and totally committed to the care of the patient. Since emergency trauma care cannot be predicted or scheduled and the need for the neurosurgeon is often urgent, either case precludes the neurosurgeon from pursuing other work commitments in the office or operating room while making the on-call commitment. This time is unproductive in terms of earning capacity while the neurosurgeon remains available to a trauma center, and it may also involve the need to cancel scheduled productive efforts (i.e., seeing patients in the office or doing elective surgery) to take care of emergency victims. Although these extra hours on call may interfere with electively referred patient coverage and customary office and operative room schedules, they have not been included in most analyses.

Second, workforce requirements for neurotrauma care have not been directly addressed. Trauma is often poorly reimbursed, due to the demographics of trauma populations, which frequently include uninsured or underinsured individuals; reimbursement is usually made by giving the on-call trauma neurosurgeon exclusive access to the general emergency room population, including nontrauma patients, or by providing direct reimbursement for on-call hours. The latter is more common at large urban trauma centers. Since both general neurosurgical emergency patients and neurotrauma patients are included in many analyses, it is difficult to separate trauma care from general emergency room on-call coverage in analyzing demand for neurotrauma care.

Additional factors affect neurosurgical manpower requirements to meet the demands of neurotrauma. Many neurosurgeons take emergency call as a requirement to maintain hospital privileges, often at several emergency trauma facilities at a time and as part of a cooperative effort with their colleagues to provide this service within their communities (50). In fact, 65% of neurosurgeons cover emergency facilities at more than one hospital when on call. That this obligation is disruptive to their personal life and scheduled work effort is no surprise. "On call for trauma" is probably the least-liked aspect of neurosurgical practice. Although 65% of surveyed neurosurgeons are required to take emergency call to maintain their hospital privileges, 95% of neurosurgeons would prefer not to take additional trauma time on call (36). Recognizing this, many, if not most, trauma hospitals make this coverage mandatory for the physician to maintain hospital privileges, and, in some instances, find they are forced to pay for what was a voluntary effort in the past.

Although it is difficult to obtain an accurate picture of neurosurgical workforce needs across the country, many of the concerns that have been raised stem from unrealistic expectations on the part of hospitals, lack of organized trauma systems that define the role of individual institutions within the system vis a vis neurotrauma, and failure of neurosurgeons who may be available for other neurosurgical consultations to willingly participate in trauma care. The problems associated with maldistribution of neurosurgeons, whether in rural areas or in urban areas without a well-organized trauma system, have been documented (44). Not every hospital that seeks emergency neurosurgical coverage is appropriate for such coverage within the context of an organized trauma system, either in terms of community necessity, or adequacy of facility and ancillary services, as revealed by ACS-COT surveys (55). Compounding this apparent overestimation of need, there remains a widespread perception that of all trauma-related specialties, neurosurgical emergency room coverage is the most difficult to assure. Some of the problem stems from defining what role specific hospitals should play within an organized trauma system, but the availability and attitude of many neurosurgeons involved in trauma care has at least something to do with this perception. Mitchell et al., have documented that the failure to obtain trauma center designation by the ACS-COT is most frequently associated with an inability to assure neurosurgical coverage in a timely fashion, even though all hospitals studied ostensibly had neurosurgeons nominally available (55, 56).

IMPROVING AVAILABILITY

Several options for improving neurosurgical trauma care availability have been proffered. The first is simply to increase the number of neurosurgeons available to emergency trauma centers by expanding training programs or encouraging immigration. At present, increasing the number of neurosurgeons has few proponents for a variety of reasons (73). The primary concern is that an overproduction of neurosurgeons would seriously compromise the current levels of neurosurgical quality and proficiency (15). In addition, the length of time needed to provide fully trained neurosurgeons to implement this process is 10 to 15 years, which constitutes an unacceptable delay (38). A variation of this option would be to train specialists specifically and uniquely for neurotrauma care. These individuals would be certified only in this limited area of neurosurgery. This degree of specialization appears to have few proponents and, for a variety of reasons, would likely be impractical.

Another option to improve neurotrauma availability would be the development of confluent regionalized trauma systems. This would theoretically allow optimization of resources for the delivery and availability of neurotrauma and emergency neurosurgical care, and, in essence, bring the trauma to the neurosurgeons most able and interested in this aspect of neurosurgery. Using present methods of patient transport, the risks of transferring a neurosurgical patient by paramedic helicopter for 15 minutes are considerably less than waiting 1 to 2 hours for a neurosurgeon to arrive at a rural hospital, which may then be ill-equipped to evaluate or treat that patient. While a favorite of trauma planners, it nevertheless does not enjoy broad-based support in the neurosurgical community. Without careful planning, it may not solve the problems of smaller communities or address the substantial economic impact such change invariably brings. A number of such trauma systems have been instituted but subsequently have failed to maintain economic viability or the support of member institutions. However, many smaller hospitals, rural hospital affiliations, or hospital chains already centralize their neurosurgical care for efficiency in utilizing available neurosurgeons, cost of the equipment involved, immediacy of care, and safety of patients.

These economic considerations lead to a third option, which has, in fact, been the most common and pragmatic solution to the mismatch of community neurosurgical requirements with availability. Market forces within and outside of neurosurgery have forced institutions and neurosurgeons providing neurotrauma care to work together to centralize that care. This often requires transfer of patients between competing institutions and cooperation among competing neurosurgeons. This trend has been jeopardized by recent EMTALA rules interpretations that, if adhered to, could prevent the appropriate transfer of suitable patients to a center of neurosurgical expertise (44). If this issue is successfully addressed, market forces themselves may be relied on to correct geographic imbalances or temporary local oversupply of neurosurgeons, since the overall production of neurosurgical trainees appears to be coming into balance with currently calculated requirements for the "average" practice of neurosurgery in the US. The necessity for multiple neurosurgeons to live and work in a rural community simply to meet the demands of an emergency or trauma call schedule would disappear, and the actual number of neurosurgeons in those communities would more closely approximate the "actual" workforce requirements.

For market forces to work, at least two changes in the current situation will be needed, either of which would require action at the federal or state level. The first, as noted above, would be a correction in the EMTALA rules to allow the continued best utilization of the available neurosurgical work force. The second will be to place neurotrauma care, including trauma call, on at least a nominally equal footing with other aspects of neurosurgery in terms of productive time. In this regard, a free market system of reimbursement serves as an incentive to neurosurgeons to offer emergency medical services in trauma centers that benefit the trauma patient, and it improves the likelihood of a neurosurgeon's commitment to a trauma program. This may require a significant change in current systems of reimbursement for trauma care and could be pursued in conjunction with other trauma specialists. Increased commitment at both the state and national level to trauma care will be required to fund these changes, not to mention underwriting the costs of trauma care in general. When confluent, regionalized trauma systems that mandate specific transfer requirements are instituted, they must address relevant social and economic aspects inherent to those transfers in order to maintain fiscal viability and to continue to serve their communities. The direction these issues are taking is addressed below.

REIMBURSEMENT

Professional Ethics, Business Environment

As a profession, neurosurgery is struggling with the reconciliation of business ethics that exploit supply-demand imbalances with professional ethics that eschew consideration of compensation in the delivery of needed care. Such often-derided business ethics have given rise to precisely the tactics that have allowed managed care to gain a formidable foothold in the healthcare delivery system. In addition, supply-demand imbalances do not always fall in favor of neurosurgery, as the Southern California experience, discussed below, demonstrates. Although many may consider a business orientation to be self-serving and distasteful, when economic considerations lead to the unavailability of emergency neurosurgical services for the critically injured patient, it is the patient who suffers the consequences.

Much has been written about the oversupply of neurosurgeons relative to the perceived need of society. Not surprisingly, this perspective has emerged in great part from managed care models whose interests lie in minimizing cost and maximizing profit. The estimates of workforce requirements generated in this way often have the additional effect of intimidating the specialty physician into accepting marginal contracts for depressed fee levels with little opportunity for negotiation. Before accepting the premise of neurosurgical oversupply in a service area, the physician must closely examine the demand side of the equation. There may be more neurosurgeons than are necessary to perform the elective procedures deemed appropriate by a gatekeeper whose function is to manage the services his patients are allowed to receive. However, there may not be an excess of neurosurgical manpower available to provide 24 hour emergency call coverage to one of the more than 5500 hospitals desiring such coverage, as evidenced by the apparent difficulty across the country in obtaining neurosurgical coverage for many such hospital emergency departments. This situation is exacerbated to the extent that many of the 3500 board-certified practicing neurosurgeons are concentrated among the 96 training programs, leaving less than one neurosurgeon for every two community hospitals. While a manifestation of this imbalance is to place a disproportionate call burden on many community neurosurgeons, it has also created a significant (although variable) demand for neurosurgical manpower. This opportunity is seldom fully exploited by neurosurgeons involved in contract negotiations with hospitals or payors.

MCO Responsibilities

Managed care plans represent a significant and increasing portion of the insurance coverage of trauma patients. Waldrep et al., have documented this trend and propose that national guidelines should be developed to guarantee quality and continuity of trauma care (79). It must be recognized that managed care organizations profit enormously from the economic safety net provided by a trauma system, yet take the position that they should have no responsibility in supporting it. Managed care organizations (MCOs) recognize that the cost of delivering a

unit of care electively is far less than making that same unit available to the health-care consumer 24 hours a day, 365 days a year, providing care whenever needed. In this regard, they have successfully exploited the economic dynamics of a situation that allows them to freely contract for the delivery of elective care at discounted prices, while relying on EMTALA (Emergency Medical Transfer and Active Labor Act) mandates to assure their insured's emergency needs are met. Under the EMTALA provisions, a physician on the call roster is mandated to provide emergency care to a patient presenting to the emergency department, even though the patient may be covered by a MCO that has previously elected not to contract with the same physician to provide elective services to their insured population. The MCO is even free to contract for provision of elective neurosurgical care completely outside a community in which local neurosurgeons are compelled to provide emergency care for the MCO's "covered lives." While the physician may be variably compensated for a specific patient, this mandate acts as a buffer for the MCO by freeing them from the necessity of having to negotiate with providers for emergency coverage that they have contractually obligated themselves to provide. If, in fact, the MCO had economic responsibility for emergency point of service care for their own insured, either by statute or through a contractual obligation with the health-care providers likely to be supplying the emergency care, this relative disadvantage to the physician would be greatly diminished. In addition, MCOs also profit from a functioning trauma system without supporting it, avoiding any of the substantial infrastructural costs of providing that emergency care.

A parallel circumstance may be seen in the physician who does not participate in Medicare, but is mandated by law to provide emergency services to Medicare patients at nonnegotiable rates whenever that physician participates in the emergency call roster. The fee to which the physician is held is, in many cases, less than it was 15 years ago; it is unilaterally fixed, and makes no provision for the emergency nature of the services rendered. This disparity will be amplified if the Health Care Financing Administration (HCFA) begins to require MCOs to enter competitive bids for service to the Medicare population, forcing reimbursement reductions for doctors with or without whom the MCO has previously contracted (19).

Reimbursement for Voluntary Trauma Participation

For a variety of reasons, many engaged in the practice of neurosurgery have not viewed trauma call as one of the more attractive areas of their practice. However, recognizing the emergency needs within the community, neurosurgeons have traditionally accepted the burden of participating in the emergency call roster. In the past, the flexibility and latitude available in adjusting elective fee schedules was such that, in aggregate, neurosurgeons felt adequately compensated for this burden. As a greater percentage of neurosurgical patients have become covered by Medicare, Medicaid, or tightly controlled managed care organizations, this has become progressively more difficult to do. The "cost shifting" in time and resources that permitted neurosurgeons to participate in this community service has been marginalized.

In a 1992 report from the Office of the Inspector General of the Department of Health and Human Services, the problem of call coverage for trauma was deemed most acute for neurosurgery (32). The reasons cited were based on direct surveys. Sixty-six percent of the specialty physicians surveyed stated that fear of increased malpractice liability had persuaded them not to participate in on-call activities. Forty-seven percent of the physicians considered that the COBRA laws were a serious drawback to participation in emergency care, and 44% stated that reimbursement for emergency services was inadequate. The OIG indicated that many specialists did not want to participate in trauma care because they were engaged in more reliably compensated activities, such as private practice with elective surgery only. Many physicians now opt out of taking emergency call, because they no longer perceive that the risk/reward benefit justifies participation, and they simply can not afford the loss of time and revenue this service entails (34).

Many, if not most, physicians view themselves as having a moral and social responsibility to provide coverage for hospital emergency departments (13). However, many difficult questions are necessarily raised by the premise of a moral or social obligation to provide call coverage. Does the societal responsibility of the neurosurgeon to the trauma patient supersede the contractual responsibility he has to the elective patient scheduled for surgery the next morning? Is the responsibility of the neurosurgeon to maintain her practice and personal life subordinate to her societal obligation to those who may be in need of emergency neurosurgical services? These questions, though rhetorical, raise a few of the issues to be considered if one is to accept the thesis of mandatory rather than volitional call participation.

In many communities, neurosurgeons are expected to take call as a gratis community service, while the hospital systems within which they work may be marketing, expanding, and in some cases profiting from their participation in trauma care delivery. As institutional participation in trauma care increases, the neurosurgeon's time available for elective activities, compensable at contractually agreed-on rates, diminishes. The availability of comparatively fewer neurosurgeons (relative to other high-demand trauma specialists) places a disproportionately higher burden on them as trauma workload increases. If a hospital or hospital system participates in the delivery of neurotrauma care, it is responsible for assuring the availability of such care without coercing physician participation. Neurosurgical participation in trauma call would be greatly facilitated by supporting the concept of voluntary contractual relationships between neurotrauma centers and trauma neurosurgeons, including reimbursement for guaranteed availability. Put another way, call stipends are a reasonable and appropriate way to assure adequate neurosurgical coverage by an institution that has made a commitment to trauma coverage.

Because hospitals are legally responsible under EMTALA for providing call coverage in emergency departments, if a hospital is unable to obtain adequate coverage, it may be forced to eliminate a particular service or, in extreme cases, close the emergency department altogether. Although neurosurgeons are not legally bound to be involved in arranging for the provision of call coverage, a lack of such involvement invariably leads to conflict with the hospital and medical staff. If the agreement to provide emergency neurosurgery services is the result of a voluntary contractual relationship, all parties have an obligation to work together to provide reliable call coverage. Comprehensive policies may be collaboratively and systematically developed that are appropriate to the facility, guided by the number and distribution of neurosurgeons available as well as the patient care demands of the hospital and the community, that incorporate reasonable expectations of the neurosurgeons who serve on the call panels. To avoid gaps in coverage and attendant risk of EMTALA violations, call activities should be date- and time-specific. It is important to remember that while serving on the call panel may be voluntary, once a neurosurgeon is designated as the person on call for a facility, there is nothing voluntary about responding to emergency room needs. The courts have held that it is the hospital that is principally at risk of a civil suit associated with violations of this statute (24, 45). Thus, the added burden imposed on the physician by these responsibilities addresses risk held largely by the hospital. This risk provides further impetus for an institution to negotiate reimbursement by the hospital to the physician for guaranteed neurosurgical availability.

Negotiating Market-Based Neurosurgical Reimbursement

When viewed within the above context, there is little doubt why neurosurgeons are presently so unwilling to accept additional call responsibility, which carries with it added malpractice risk, risks to their own health, and onerous lifestyle sacrifices for themselves and their families. The most pragmatic method of addressing the problem is to embrace a free-market approach that allows a neurosurgical group to negotiate appropriate reimbursement for the provision of neurotrauma services with an institution that is appropriate for the delivery of such care. Successful negotiation for trauma reimbursement requires an in-depth understanding of the economic realities of providing emergency care locally and regionally, set in the context of a diverse geographic and demographic spectrum nationally. A variety of concerns need to be addressed as neurosurgery and neurosurgeons negotiate reimbursement issues with hospitals, hospital systems, managed care organizations, and state and federal governmental agencies. Specific options or areas that need to be addressed include:

- Voluntary rather than mandated emergency call participation.
- Market-based reimbursement for on-call availability.
- MCO responsibility for emergency point of service care for their own insured populations.
- Tax credits for indigent emergency care.
- Trauma system funding.

- Tort protection for uncompensated emergency care.
- Reform and clarification of EMTALA regulations.

The problem of funding for neurotrauma, regarding both reimbursement for physicians and hospitals and the costs of developing and maintaining the trauma systems themselves, is an exceedingly vexing issue. The means of raising funds for an organized trauma system have been addressed with varying success and are highly dependent on regional demographics and public awareness. Particularly in regions with significant indigent populations, physician, hospital, and community participation are being encouraged through the use of tax credits or other economic incentives for the delivery of indigent health care (70, 72).

Many such plans attempt to shift the burden of emergency services away from government through individual responsibility, partially defraying the cost of expensive trauma networks by assessing monetary penalties on those convicted of illegal behavior that results in trauma, whose victims, by necessity, end up utilizing these facilities. Fines and monetary penalties for drunk or reckless driving, illegal use of firearms, spouse or child abuse, criminal negligence resulting in injury, among others, could help to sustain not only a trauma network but spinal cord and brain injury research. Model legislation exists or is being developed in California, Kentucky, Washington, and Oregon, among others. Not only would such a system help offset the cost of providing coverage, but might actually provide an incentive for behavior modification. These proposals, however, are subject to significant political influence. The efficacy of legislation intended to provide for trauma system development and support in California, for instance, has been significantly eroded as funds have been gradually diverted to meet other budgetary shortfalls. Some of these issues are more closely examined in the section on trauma system funding.

EMTALA
Rules and Regulations

The Emergency Medical Treatment and Active Labor Act (EMTALA), tagged on to the Consolidated Budget Reconciliation Act of 1985

(COBRA), and amended in 1989 and 1991, is a federal statute governing the transfer of patients between hospitals participating in the Medicare program. This federal legislation, supplemented by parallel legislation in many states, was designed to eliminate the practice of patient "dumping," which in essence is the transfer for economic reasons of potentially unstable patients, because they are uninsured or otherwise unable to pay for services. The unprecedented increase in patient transfers for economic reasons that occurred in the mid 1980s was primarily in direct response to major changes in Medicaid eligibility enacted in the early 1980s. This and other factors leading to enactment of this legislation have been recently reviewed elsewhere (17, 30). Although well intentioned, the law and subsequent rules and regulations that expand on it have had many unintended effects. It has been stated that "the country is now embarking on a permanent course in medical care delivery under a federal law that defines the standard of care according to law and not according to medical practice (33)."

Physicians and hospitals that violate EMTALA laws are subject to severe penalties, including fines, investigation, disciplinary action, increased liability exposure, and criminal prosecution. EMTALA has also created a private right of action in the federal courts for the alleged violation of the statutes, and, in addition, allows the individual to obtain "those damages available for personal injury under [state] law" and "such equitable relief as is appropriate." The rules apply to all hospitals that are enrolled in the Medicare program and to all patients who come to the emergency departments of these hospitals, not just to Medicare recipients (30). Further, in a result apparently not contemplated by Congress, EMTALA may be used by malpractice attorneys to pursue a federal cause of action along with, or instead of, traditional state law claims (51).

In response to the initial vacuum in interpretation of this statute, the United States Department of Health and Human Services, Health Care Financing Administration (HCFA) finally promulgated federal interim final regulations in June of 1994 (2). These regulations detail hospital responsibility for emergency care and the penalties for hospitals and physicians that violate the law, including termination of Medicare status and civil monetary penalties. The rules and accompanying regulations are a mixed blessing, clarifying some requirements, but greatly expanding certain other responsibilities. Any hospital that usually provides emergency services, whether or not they have a designated emergency department, must comply with the following requirements:

- *Obligation to screen:* Each person who presents at an emergency department must be provided with an "appropriate medical screening examination" by a physician for the purpose of determining whether that person has an "emergency medical condition" or is in "active labor." (1) The definition of "emergency medical condition" under federal law explicitly sets a legal definition for "emergency medical condition" that differs from most medical definitions, including definitions of emotional or psychological conditions (3).

- *Obligation to treat until stabilized:* Each person presenting at an emergency department who is determined to have an emergency medical condition must receive care, treatment, and/or surgery by a physician as necessary to relieve or eliminate the emergency medical condition. This includes the obligation to provide specialty consultation and treatment by any specialist routinely available to the hospital "when determined to be medically necessary jointly by the emergency and specialty physician." The emergency care and treatment must be provided before one asks about the patient ability to pay (4). Except under specific circumstances, discharge or transfer of the patient may not occur unless it will not contribute to a material deterioration in or jeopardy to the individual's medical condition or expected chances for recovery (4).

- *Restrictions on transfer:* Federal law does not restrict the transfer of stable patients, except in that it does require certain designated facilities to accept such transfers (4). With respect to unstable patients, federal law allows the transfer of these patients only if (*a*) a patient requests the transfer or (*b*) a physician certifies that the benefit expected from the transfer outweighs its risk. If a physician certifies that an unstable patient may be transferred, he must specifically summarize in writing the risks and benefits of the transfer and include his signature (6). The medical record must also include "the name and address of any on-call physician who has refused or failed to appear within a reasonable time to provide necessary stabilization treatment (5)."

• *Exceptions to transfer requirements:* There are two narrow exceptions to the transfer requirements for unstable patients. A transfer may take place for medical reasons if the patient makes a written request for a transfer after informed discussion about the benefits and risks. Otherwise, the physician must explicitly record that "the medical benefits reasonably expected from the provision of appropriate medical treatment at another medical facility outweigh the increased risks to the individual . . . . " of the transfer (8).

• *Hospital's obligations to accept transfers:* Hospitals participating in the Medicare program that have "specialized capabilities or facilities" (such as burn units, shock-trauma units, and neonatal intensive care units) or that are identified as federal regional referral centers must accept an appropriate transfer of an individual who requires such specialized capabilities or facilities, whether or not the patient has been stabilized (7). Even if a hospital is not officially designated as a trauma center but has a neurosurgeon on call, it could be considered to have specialized capabilities and therefore be expected to serve as a referral hospital for an emergency department without neurosurgical backup. If there is a neurosurgical unit at the referral hospital with facilities available, it can be in violation of EMTALA if it refuses to accept a neurotrauma patient. A neurosurgeon who refuses to accept the transfer is also at risk if the violation is reported. Hospitals have already been cited under this relative standard (30).

• *Obligations of physicians:* The duties to screen and treat patients presenting at the emergency department and certify patients for transfer rests with the emergency department physician. On-call neurosurgeons have duties under the law as well. The law does not require physicians to serve on call. It does require that a physician who agreed to be on call cannot refuse evaluation on the basis of a patient's race, ethnicity, religion, national origin, citizenship, age, sex, preexisting medical condition, physical or mental handicap, insurance status, economic status, ability to pay, or any other nonmedical reason. Federal law implicitly requires on-call physicians to come to the hospital when medically necessary within a "rea-

sonable period of time" and establishes a mandatory reporting obligation on the transferring hospitals when an on-call physician refuses or fails to appear within a reasonable time to provide necessary stabilizing treatment. The name and address of the physician who failed to respond must be submitted to the receiving hospital at the time of transfer, along with the patient's medical records (6).

• *Physician penalties:* Under federal law, all physicians, including those on call, face a potential fine up to $50,000 for each violation they have committed or for which they are responsible. Under certain circumstances, a physician may be excluded from the Medicare program (6).

• *Expanded liability:* Any person who is potentially harmed by a violation may bring an action against the responsible hospital or administrative or medical personnel to enjoin the violation. Court decisions have affirmed that the act does not directly allow a federal cause of action against physicians (24). However, actions against physicians can be joined with EMTALA suits against the hospital in federal court, with an adverse affect on physician liability. Hospitals may cross-claim for indemnity against those physicians. Such federal actions lie outside of state tort reform legislation, including defined settlement caps.

Ambiguities in Interpretation

Despite promulgation of interim final rules, many questions continue to plague physicians and hospitals in regard interpretation of the statute. There remains an urgent need for legislative amendments or interpretive regulations that address certain practical considerations. Specific ambiguities include the definition of "facility capability," what patient movement constitutes a transfer, the nature of an emergency medical condition, and the specific conditions required of the medical screening examination.

Federal law requires that treatment be provided as necessary to stabilize the patient "within the staff and facilities available at the hospital (4)." This is not defined in the law, but at least one federal appellate court has held that the provision of a medical screening examination within an emergency room's "capabilities" constitutes good-faith application of all the hospital's resources (22). In some states, the definition of "facility capability" is complicated by state law. If a hospital reports to the state that it routinely provides given services, those services must be available for emergency cases at all times (18).

The definition of "transfer" needs clarification. At present, EMTALA defines a transfer to include any movement involving the discharge of an individual outside a hospital's facilities. There are many reasons for a noneconomic transfer, including an error in diagnosis. In such an instance, the hospital may be inadvertently denying therapy to a patient and negligently failing to recognize the need for treatment. This suggests that EMTALA has transcended its antidumping origins and is taking a step closer to becoming a federal malpractice law (51). In addition, discharging a patient thought to be stable, or even transiently moving a patient to a nearby facility for further diagnosis, constitutes a transfer under present definitions.

The term, "emergency medical condition," gives rise to numerous questions in regard to what a court may consider "serious" and what "immediate" means in terms of minutes, hours, or days. "Emergency medical condition" is a broad concept that may include conditions that many physicians would not consider true emergencies. Therefore, physicians must be aware that the legal definition of an emergency medical condition for the purposes of compliance with the transfer laws is not necessarily the same as the clinical definition.

The statute requires that the scope of the required medical screening examination be based on the capability of the hospital's emergency department, which includes ancillary services routinely available to the emergency department. The preamble to the rule states that "Congress intended that the resources of the hospital and the staff generally available to patients at the hospital could be considered available for the examination and treatment of emergency department patients, regardless of whether staff physicians had heretofore been obligated by the hospital to provide services to those coming to the hospital's emergency department." Since many emergency departments have gaps in their neurosurgical coverage, the potential for such gaps to lead to an EMTALA violation with both civil penalties and private cause of action is significant.

Special questions arise with respect to physicians who have traditionally provided simul-

taneous on-call coverage to more than one facility. The law does not address this issue, so it is conceivable that state or federal authorities could attempt to impose liability. The issue is best addressed by developing a working arrangement among the facilities, neurosurgeons, and emergency medical service providers within a geographic area, with a neurosurgeon on call only at the facility designated as the neurotrauma center. Otherwise, multiple exposures to liability exist if neurotrauma patients are received simultaneously at two or three hospitals where the same neurosurgeon is on call.

Delay due to "legal concerns" in the appropriate transfer of neurosurgical emergencies requiring specialized facilities or care has the potential to become a significant problem, unless points of confusion within EMTALA regulations are clarified (39). Patient transfers should be based on type and acuteness of disease and the capabilities of the facilities involved, not on economic or legal criteria. As has been discussed elsewhere in this chapter, centralization of neurosurgical care is occurring due to workforce considerations, economic constraints on smaller hospitals, and the development of institutional centers of neurotrauma expertise within the context of organized trauma systems. Concern over the potential for violation of the statute may inhibit trauma system development, because the very structure of such a system may require a *de facto* violation based on a restrictive interpretation of presently unclear regulations. Appropriate and expected transfers of unstable patients that subsequently deteriorate during, but not necessarily as a result of, a transfer within a trauma system presently exposes the involved hospitals and physicians to litigation risk. Unless the issue is explicitly addressed by further HCFA rulings, EMTALA regulations may impede or delay appropriate and necessary transfers within the context of such organized systems of trauma care.

Many additional uncertainties in interpreting and implementing emergency transfer laws exist. Until these are clarified, specific policies defining institutional and physician roles in delivery of trauma care should be explicitly incorporated into medical staff bylaws, providing a degree of protection to the individual physician. On a national level, neurosurgery is lobbying for advisory involvement in further HCFA interpretation of EMTALA legislation. It is critical that neurosurgeons are part of the administrative process that defines and interprets EMTALA regarding hospital and emergency room capabilities and responsibilities, especially in the context of organized trauma systems. EMTALA rules and regulations that prohibit appropriate transfers for the ultimate benefit of the patient must be constructively challenged.

TRAUMA SYSTEMS
Trauma System Design

Maryland pioneered the development of a statewide trauma system in 1973. A 1979 study comparing preventable deaths in a trauma center with those in hospitals without trauma centers became a major impetus for the subsequent development of trauma systems throughout the United States (80). As of mid-1997, some form of mandated regional trauma system had been developed in 27 states and the District of Columbia (69). In 1991, a total of 457 operational state-designated or American College of Surgeons-verified trauma centers were identified in this country, and approximately 20 other hospitals were functioning as trauma centers even though they were not designated (25). The tendancy toward proliferation of trauma care systems has been aided by the enactment of the Federal Trauma Care Systems Planning and Development Act (PL101-590) in 1990. This act provides assistance to states for the planning, implementation, and monitoring of trauma systems.

Neurosurgeons have initiated and actively participated in trauma care planning in many communities. The principles for neurosurgical participation have been enunciated in several ways over the last several years (35, 59). The American Association of Neurological Surgeons (AANS) and the Congress of Neurological Surgeons (CNS) support the concept of organized neurosurgical trauma care consisting of the appropriate combination of prepared communities and institutions and adequate numbers of committed neurosurgeons (60).

Trauma care systems are designed to provide care to an injured patient from the time of injury through definitive therapy in an acute care hospital and subsequent rehabilitation. Ideally, the care is regionalized to match the seriousness of the injury with the available resources in a designated area. The system ideally provides a continuum of care and ensures means of measuring outcomes (28, 26). A variety of providers are needed in a comprehensive trauma system (10), and a series of steps must be taken to develop such a system (11). A step-by step process for the development, management, and analysis of a trauma care system has been described by West et al. (81), and an instructive document has been prepared by the National Highway Traffic Safety Administration for use at the state and county level (75).

Colorado provides an example of such a trauma system presently under development. The private Colorado Trauma Institute was initially responsible for the design of a voluntary system that was marred by disagreements between participating institutions. In 1995, the Colorado State Legislature passed a bill mandating the development of an inclusive statewide system of trauma care. The legislation called for the formation of a State Trauma Advisory Council (STAC) charged with developing prehospital triage guidelines and interfacility transfer criteria. Most significantly, it has the task of proposing a geographical template for Area Trauma Advisory Councils (ATACs) that will determine institutional membership and county alliances and shape trauma admission and transfer protocols. Proposed guidelines draw heavily on the published criteria of the ACS-COT (11). Every facility accepting emergency medical services patients must submit an application requesting a specific trauma level designation that meets designation criteria developed by the STAC. Each ATAC must choose a Level I or Level II Trauma Center as its key resource. Triage guidelines will mandate delivery of patients with physiological compromise to a Level I center only. Delivery of patients with "mechanism of injury" and stable vital signs to a Level II center will be allowed, if "available in less than 15 minutes of additional prehospital time." The time element is mandatory and will impact present referral patterns in the state significantly. It has already stimulated institutional efforts to upgrade their trauma programs to meet criteria for a higher level designation. Data collection by every facility in the state regardless of designation is required, and statewide quality improvement indicators will be measured systemwide.

Trauma System Dysfunction

The efficacy of trauma systems has been verified by multiple studies that show as much as a 50% reduction in preventable deaths subsequent to the organization of regional trauma systems (16, 21, 68, 74). Several studies indicate substantial improvement in trauma mortality, hospital length of stay, and hospital cost per injury after initiation of an organized regional trauma system (41, 53, 57). Paradoxically, as the ability to provide improved neurotrauma care has evolved, the entire trauma care system has been put at risk and in some areas is floundering or has never been established, due largely to failure to maintain economic viability or to interinstitutional disagreements. Despite evidence of efficacy, by 1991 less than 25% of the United States was served by such systems. Many states have not begun to develop trauma systems, and in a number of areas, systems that were started subsequently failed (20).

In a 1991 study, the General Accounting Office (GAO) reported that most trauma program closures occurred primarily because of financial losses sustained from treating uninsured patients and patients covered by Medicaid and other government-assisted programs (20). In a study of 25 trauma centers, Eastman and colleagues found that underfunding resulted from a combination of adverse factors, including above-average costs and a disproportionate number of indigent patients (29). These authors pointed out that the object of a trauma care system is to concentrate the most critically injured patients in a limited number of designated trauma centers and that this design is the primary cause of system failure. At least 60 trauma centers closed in the 5 years preceding the GAO report.

The development of neurotrauma care in rural areas is also a problem that must be dealt with as attempts are made to refine rural trauma systems in general. These areas face unique problems in providing neurotrauma care. They are generally large geographic areas with small numbers of people. This creates logistical problems, including prolonged travel times, difficult access, and small hospitals with limited financial and human resources. Mortality rates associated with motor vehicle accidents have been shown to be highest in counties with a low population density (14). This is partially related to inadequate access to trauma care in rural areas. There are significant patient transfer and antidumping issues that are of particular concern to smaller or isolated community hospitals with part-time or limited neurosurgical coverage that threaten to intensify unless federal antidumping regulations are amended or clarified.

The following description of trauma center failures in a major urban area, outlined recently by Kusske, highlights the problems that must be overcome (45). In 1984, the Los Angeles County Emergency Medical Services Agency (EMS) verified 23 trauma centers, including 10 Level I centers, 10 Level II centers, and 3 rural centers, utilizing criteria enunciated by the American College of Surgeons Committee on Trauma (ACS-COT). Two years later, seven hospitals had withdrawn from the system, including the third and fourth busiest hospitals, which provided 20% of the system's care. The loss left large areas of central and western Los Angeles, including the Los Angeles Airport, the intersections of the Santa Monica and Harbor freeways, and some of the most heavily traveled sections of the San Diego and Hollywood freeways, without an adjacent trauma center. Two major hospitals in the eastern portion of the county also withdrew, leaving large areas to the east of Los Angeles without a nearby facility, including the areas that had been the site of a severe earthquake several months earlier (61).

There were four reported reasons why these private hospitals that had been designated as trauma centers dropped out of the system. The first was the very high volume of uninsured patients. The second was the inability to transfer uninsured patients promptly to a county hospital because these hospitals were already operating at or beyond capacity. The third was the steadily growing numbers of trauma cases, which far exceeded the anticipated volume. The fourth was the fact that the volume of uninsured patients interfered with physicians' ability to manage their private practice patients for elective scheduled surgeries and the lack of space in the intensive care units.

A hospital that remained in the system was significantly affected by the closures of the other hospitals and saw its trauma caseload more than double, the number of uninsured patients climb from 25 to 55%, and the percentage of intensive care unit (ICU) resources devoted to trauma patients soar from 14 to 40%. The hospital had to initiate compensatory payments to its neurosurgeons, orthopedic surgeons, and cardiovascular surgeons because of the high volume of uninsured patients they had to treat. Eventually, the county had to redraw the hospitalís catchment area to reduce the volume of uninsured trauma patients in order to keep the center in the system.

By 1992, 10 of the 23 trauma centers in Los
Angeles County had left the system, and in
southern California, 14 of 32 centers had terminated their contracts with the various emergency
medical services (EMS) agencies (9). The result
of this is that many southern California communities no longer have reliable networks of EMS
hospitals, and many institutions have been
forced formally or informally to abandon full-
service emergency programs. Meanwhile, the
demand for emergency services, particularly
among the poor, continues to grow at a time
when capacity is shrinking (78). The Los Angeles experience may be reenacted in the future in
other large urban areas.

Trauma System Funding and Institutional Viability

At present, the establishment of trauma systems and the designation of trauma centers are
usually functions of the local emergency medical services (EMS) authority. The Trauma Care
Systems Planning and Development Act (Plan
101-590) of 1990 called for a Model Trauma
Care System Plan, subsequently written in 1992
(76). Recommendations in the model trauma
plan are compatible with the criteria established
by the American College of Surgeons (ACS) in
its most recent iteration of Resources for Optimal Care of the Injured Patient (27). However,
as experience has shown in major urban centers,
such as Los Angeles, unless adequate funding is
available, the well-intentioned plans of the ACS
will not necessarily lead to the establishment of
a viable system. Adequate funding of trauma
care is critical to the survival of the system.

Unfortunately, it is difficult to demonstrate
precisely what would constitute adequate funding for an entire system. Data demonstrating the
actual cost of trauma in general and neurotrauma
specifically is hard to come by. One such study
details the neuroregistry of the Orange County
Emergency Services Agency and covers a 6-year
period from 1985 to 1991 (46), in which a community of 2.3 million people was closely followed for total hospital charges and estimated
charges generated by neurosurgeons. For 1990,
1476 patients admitted through four receiving
centers and three trauma centers, undergoing
241 emergency procedures, generated costs of
$33,016,884. Another study detailing trauma ad-
missions in British Columbia found that problems of neurotrauma coverage were better ap-

preciated when intraregional differences in
neurosurgical volumes were known; it also
found that interhospital differences in cost and
median length of stay not explained by severity
criteria suggested that greater resource efficiencies could be realized (77). Little detailed information exists for many states, regions, demographic distributions, and economic
environments, and generalizing from this data
would be speculative. However, organizing
trauma systems by emphasizing centralization
of specialty expertise and utilizing cost containment and reimbursement strategies across all institutions could lead a failing trauma system into
solvency. A 1996 study by the National Public
Services Research Institute found trauma-related workers' compensation costs in 17 studied
states were 15.5% lower in those states with
mandated trauma systems; the study rather opti-
mistically concluded: "Extending trauma care
systems nationwide could lower annual medical
care payments by $3.2 billion. Including produc-
tivity losses due to premature death, the savings
could total $10.3 billion, 5.9 percent of national
injury costs (53)."

Inadequate, inaccurate, or nonspecific demographic and cost data specific to neurotrauma
(or, in some cases, trauma in general) hinders
attempts to finance institutional trauma programs. Examining collection rates or payer-class
mix without examining both costs and revenues
may lead to an erroneous conclusion about a
program's fiscal viability. Relatively small
changes in third-party coverage or income eligibility requirements can have a large impact on
the program's financial solvency and break-even
volumes (66). In addition, inaccurate records increase general overhead as charges in many
cases do not reflect all treatment actually rendered. By addressing these issues, substantial
improvements in cost recovery for institutional
trauma programs have been realized (42).

Medicare and Medicaid reimbursement that
does not fairly reflect the additional costs associated with trauma is a significant factor hindering
adequate trauma system funding. Although the
government mandates that all persons must receive emergency care without regard to their
ability to pay, governmental payment at both the
state and federal levels does not approach the
costs involved, and even those funds have been
decreasing as a result of federal and state attempts at cost containment. Unreimbursed

trauma care was estimated at $1 billion in 1988, representing approximately 10 to 12% of the $8.3 billion in unsponsored health care provided by United States acute care hospitals in that year (20). The use of Diagnostic Related Groups (DRGs) has been estimated in some states to adversely affect reimbursement in up to 9% of trauma patients (78). The conclusion of most authors is that a differentiation should be incorporated within the Medicare or Medicaid framework for trauma and emergency care, which recognizes patient acuteness, prolonged treatment times, and the resultant substantial increase in total cost of care. From a practical standpoint, however, recent budget reductions for both Medicare and Medicaid make it unlikely that there will be any adjustments for DRG differentials in trauma care in the foreseeable future.

Federal monies are unlikely to be available to aid in trauma system development or support. Under the Trauma Care Systems and Planning Development Act of 1990, Congress planned a budget of $60 million a year, 80% of which was to go to states to improve statewide trauma systems. By 1995, however, only $5 million was earmarked for the program, and Congress decided to eliminate the Division of Trauma and Emergency Medical Services in the Health Resources and Services Administration, the agency primarily responsible for the allotment of these funds (48).

Other opportunities may exist to establish equitable payment programs for hospitals and physicians who provide sophisticated neurotrauma care, but not without vigorous support and ongoing watchfulness. Options for supplemental support for neurotrauma care in the context of the trauma system funding have been outlined by Champion and Mabee (20).

1. Cigarette and alcohol tax
2. Surcharges on driver's license fees, traffic violation penalties, 911 telephone numbers, and motor vehicle registration fees
3. Trauma financing pool: a federal-state-private sector financing pool developed to reimburse qualified centers for documented uncompensated trauma care
4. Adjustment of DRG-based reimbursement
5. Increased reimbursement in return for regional trauma care

Unfortunately, experience with some of these options has not been encouraging. California Proposition 99 (1988), an additional tobacco tax, initially funded the California Healthcare for Indigents Program. The funds were routinely used by hospitals to cover bad debt resulting from EMS operations, and physicians were attracted to the call panels because of the funding provided by this measure. The tobacco tax was effective in stabilizing the EMS system in Southern California. However, the funds were subsequently diverted to other programs, with a 53.5% loss to the physician account and a 26% loss to the hospital account. Other California legislation, SB 612 (1988), gave counties the ability to establish an Emergency Medical Services Fund through an increased penalty assessment on traffic violations. Initially, these funds provided increased reimbursement for EMS providers, but the funds have also been partly directed to other uses by various local or county governments (9). In John Muir and Contra Costa Counties, however, these funds have been used to establish a viable neurosurgical call reimbursement system that continues to meet the needs of the community (47).

In the current era of managed care, neurotrauma must be provided in a cost-effective manner within the framework of organized trauma systems. Many of the managed care plans, including large staff model health maintenance organizations (HMOs), do not address the issue of trauma care at all. Most plans have out-of-network contingencies that provide payment for such services in emergency situations. The issue of managed care responsibility for a portion of the trauma system infrastructure is addressed elsewhere in this document. It is of utmost importance that neurosurgeons continue to support both local and federal legislative efforts to provide funding for trauma systems, as these issues can be and have been all too readily overlooked. For example, President Clinton's defunct healthcare reform proposal presented to Congress in early 1994 contained no provisions whatsoever that specifically related to funding for trauma systems in its entire 1342 pages (40).

Making Trauma Systems Work

The Office of the Inspector General (OIG) of the Department of Health and Human Services (HHS) has noted that the problem of specialty call coverage for emergency rooms throughout the United States was most acute for neurosurgery (32). Forty-nine percent of hospitals that offered neurosurgery in their emergency departments encountered difficulty ensuring coverage, for reasons that have been elucidated elsewhere in this report. Hospital administrators responding to the survey cited a shortage of specialty physicians as the leading factor in their inability to meet this demand. However, the OIG report did not consider the ancillary support needed to provide neurosurgical coverage. Many hospitals that do not have neurosurgical emergency coverage may not be suitable places to provide this service.

The regionalization of emergency neurotrauma care as suggested in the ACS plan is the most appropriate way to link available neurosurgeons with hospitals that have the logistical resources to provide efficient and safe care for these complex problems and achieve optimal patient outcomes. This concentration of care, however, also concentrates cost. Thus, the factor that contributes most to improved care becomes the single biggest factor in trauma system failure. A functional trauma system must be accompanied by a reliable means of funding or it is doomed to failure. Accuracy in trauma data collection, efficiency in billing and collections and in cost-containment, fairness in government-mandated reimbursement, trauma-related surcharges, fees and fines, and the combined responsibility of those using the system and those profiting by it have been able in some communities to provide for the resources needed to accomplish the task. The development of a trauma system requires a working arrangement among the emergency facilities, neurosurgeons, and local emergency medical services involved within a geographic area. There exists a spectrum of issues commensurate with each unique trauma system. The perspectives and requirements of each are regional and need to be addressed regionally. Marked community and demographic variability requires development of unique systems with neurosurgical input from the local community. Many of the answers depend on the willingness of the neurosurgical community to become more involved in the planning and operation of trauma systems. The active participation of neurosurgeons is paramount in assuring the smooth functioning of a neurotrauma system. Although neurosurgeons have been instrumental in the tremendous advances made in neurotrauma care, in certain communities they have also been identified as a weak link in the trauma-care chain.

The survival of the discipline of neurosurgery may, in part, depend on the willingness of neurosurgeons to identify themselves as being the responsible primary physicians for the care of central nervous system and spinal trauma.

NEUROSURGERY'S PLACE IN TRAUMA CARE

Relationship with Other Trauma Specialties

From a neurosurgical perspective, the relationship with the American College of Surgeons (ACS) and the American College of Emergency Physicians (ACEP) may at times be adversarial. There exists the perception that the American College of Surgeons Committee on Trauma (ACS-COT), in particular, has a prevailing attitude that is imperious and dictatorial. Neurosurgery, on the other hand, may be viewed by the ACS-COT as an aloof and unwilling partner in trauma care. This attitude is not without some substantiation. The ACS-COT trauma center verification system has documented widespread concerns regarding neurosurgical trauma coverage and availability (55, 56). Of failures to verify trauma programs (54 of 120 in the years preceding 1994), 35% failed in whole or in part secondary to ''inadequate neurosurgical response'' to neurotrauma responsibilities. Improvement on subsequent evaluation of the trauma center was least likely to occur with this deficiency. With these statistics in mind, how can neurosurgery maintain a significant leadership role and revitalize a partnership with the ACS in the treatment of neurotrauma?

One considerable problem remains a lack of open communication between different specialty organizations regarding issues of trauma care. There has been a neurosurgical representative on the ACS-COT for many years, and, although a very effective way of presenting a neurosurgical perspective to general surgery colleagues, this has been the only direct formal communication between trauma surgeons and organized neurosurgery. As trauma care becomes an increasingly important social and political concern, it makes sense that an attempt is made to integrate by reciprocal representation a variety of trauma specialty organizations, providing formalized conduits of communication between the organizations and encouraging cooperation. Specialty organizations that must stay in close communication include at least the AANS/CNS, ACEP, ACS-COT, and AAOS trauma subcommittee. It then becomes critical that the reasonable concerns of other specialties be communicated to rank-and-file membership through the Joint Council of State Neurosurgical Societies (JCSNS), the Joint Council on Neurotrauma and Critical Care Newsletter, Neurosurgery:\\On-Call, etc., and that their concerns in turn are heard by the leadership of other organizations. Increasing and maintaining communication within neurosurgical circles, especially between leadership and rank and file, is critically important to this process, and is being diligently addressed by the neurosurgical leadership (71).

On a state level, communication and cooperation between the different trauma specialists of the individual trauma specialty organizations could begin with already established state committees of the ACS-COT. It is not necessary for participants to be members of the ACS, but encouraging neurosurgeons to become Fellows of the American College of Surgery is a simple way for neurosurgery to increase representation in the organization which is the *de facto* leader in developing trauma care delivery systems and trauma policy. The ACS state committees can be a starting point for cooperation between trauma specialists and can form the nidus of a more organized system of trauma delivery within individual communities and throughout the state. Development of trauma systems is an intensely political task and requires broad-based support and galvanized public opinion. Whether the goal is to produce a tightly controlled, resource-based trauma system or a market-driven system with regional cooperation and collaboration, state trauma advisory boards can wield considerable influence and must have neurosurgical representation if the interests of neurosurgeons in the state and region are to be given their due.

Encroachment by Other Specialties

It must be neurosurgery's unwavering and objectively verifiable assertion that neurotrauma is best managed by neurosurgeons. As noted above, however, neurosurgery is at significant risk of losing its preeminence in neurotrauma care if it does not assiduously develop and maintain competence in delivering care to the neurologically injured. Neurosurgeons have come under criticism from other specialties in the treatment of neurotrauma, particularly regarding

availability (12). Proposals have been made to train trauma surgeons in operative neurotrauma care. Many intensivists have a better working knowledge of the principles of management of severe traumatic brain injury than do their neurosurgical counterparts, despite the availability to neurosurgeons of outstanding opportunities for continuing education in neurotrauma and critical care. Is enough being done to meet the criticisms and challenges raised by other specialties? If neurosurgery's role in the intensive care unit is abdicated to intensivists as a matter of convenience, neurosurgeons will risk losing their own competence in critical care medicine. How will this affect the community neurosurgeonís ability to manage head and spine trauma knowledgeably? How will this deferral to trauma surgeons and orthopedists improve neurosurgery's economic viability across the board? The very fact that there are almost twice as many community hospitals seeking to care for trauma patients as there are neurosurgeons to adequately staff them, as noted above, is both a collective benefit and risk. If neurosurgical availability becomes too difficult to assure, other specialties will, of necessity, obtain the training required to manage patients with neurotrauma. This is not a trend that has developed yet to any great degree, but the potential is high. Avoiding this scenario will only occur by increasing the community neurosurgeon's competence and enthusiasm in delivering neurotrauma care. This, in turn, will take place only as the neurosurgeon sees the opportunity for a tolerable and controllable lifestyle, fair compensation for both work and availability, reduced risk of liability, and the freedom to negotiate with hospitals and payors.

PROPOSAL FOR ACTION
Education

For many neurosurgical residents, trauma too often is viewed as a distasteful chore, rather than a critical component of neurosurgical education that requires an understanding of the central nervous system and the pathophysiology of brain and spinal cord injury in order to manage successfully. Is adequate time allotted to understanding the altered physiology of the injured central nervous system at all levels of training? Can organized neurosurgery do better at educating the practicing community neurosurgeon in appropriate neurotrauma methodologies? Very important strides have been made in this direction already through continuing education courses made available by the AANS and CNS. It must be made clear to the postgraduate neurosurgeon in the community that expertise in critical care and the management of head and spinal cord injury may necessarily become a significant portion of their practice, but is at risk of being lost to other disciplines (intensivists and trauma surgeons, among others), if special competence is not maintained.

In a socioeconomic context, neurotrauma education should include not only continuing education in neuroscience and clinical advances, but also information about the unique role neurosurgery plays in delivering neurotrauma care within a system of trauma care delivery, clearly addressing prevalent socioeconomic misconceptions. The means to interact effectively with those with whom neurosurgeons must negotiate in this environment is dependent on an understanding of neurosurgeryís value within a system of trauma care delivery. What is necessary is a clearer perception by community neurosurgeons of the role they play in the socioeconomics of trauma and trauma systems, the personal, legal, and economic risks involved, and how this may directly relate to the fiscal viability of their practice.

As an example, a prevalent perception among neurosurgeons is that trauma patients, particularly the indigent, are more likely to sue for malpractice than are other patients (31, 36). The available evidence suggests this is not true. An association of insurance companies has stated that participation in emergency services does not appear to affect the price or availability of malpractice insurance (32). In Maryland, it has been determined that claims filed by persons enrolled in Medicaid were lower than expected based on population statistics (58). The Government Accounting Office found that Medicare and Medicaid patients are less likely than are other patients to file malpractice claims (32). Another study revealed that indigent and uninsured patients are significantly less likely to initiate malpractice actions (49). The American College of Obstetricians and Gynecologists completed a review of Medicaid obstetric patients and found no statistically significant difference between the percentages of obstetrics-related malpractice suits filed by women whose care is funded by the Medicaid program and those filed by other

patients (43). The current informational void about malpractice risks for neurosurgical specialists in emergency departments clearly has to be corrected, and it could be addressed by a study directed specifically at claims arising from the emergency room activities of those specialists. However, the concern that this is a problem of significant magnitude is almost certainly misplaced.

Several approaches may be used to better inform rank-and-file neurosurgeons about these issues. Discussion of the socioeconomic aspects of neurotrauma in the AANS socioeconomic/managed care course, Joint Council of State Neurosurgical Societies (JCSNS) meetings, and state and regional meetings has been useful. Increased exposure to basic neuroscience, advances in neurotrauma management, and socioeconomic topics in neurotrauma could be featured at the national meetings. Special lectures on aspects of neurotrauma care would improve neurosurgical knowledge and clinical acumen with direct benefits that go beyond care of neurologic trauma only. A Socioeconomic Video Course segment dealing with EMTALA regulations and negotiations with hospitals for trauma coverage could be an additional step. This ''Socioeconomics of Neurotrauma'' course could include the role of neurosurgical participation in the development and administrative aspects of trauma systems. Key individuals with practical experience, able to teach the material, should be identified. Allowing neurosurgeons to use neurosurgical CME to satisfy local trauma CME requirements would encourage participation. A variety of educational vehicles to facilitate transfer of information and improve rank and file perceptions of neurotrauma are readily available.

Content must include neurosurgical demographics and manpower issues, an understanding of federal regulations regarding patient transfer, the impact of managed care on delivery of emergency services, and a review of trauma system design. The relationship of the neurosurgeon to his colleagues in other specialties, to the hospital or hospital system, and the trauma system as it may exist locally should be examined. The goal is to increase awareness of the issues that impact the neurosurgeon in the delivery of trauma care. Access to nationwide data and neurosurgeons with experience in these issues will be reassuring and provide the neurosurgeon with information needed to make a local impact on the delivery of neurotrauma care, and indeed, to help assure his own economic survival.

Within the context of statewide or urban trauma systems and given appropriate regional considerations, designation of centers of neurotrauma excellence would allow for the development of special expertise, interest, and educational opportunities in neurotrauma. A team approach, utilizing several neurosurgeons and other specialties and services as appropriate and necessary, would help to reduce fatigue and individual "burnout," allowing for diversion of neurotrauma to centers that are prepared and enthusiastic, and would address both lifestyle and quality issues. Encouraging programs such as the AANS Critical Care Workshop and expanding them as necessary to address new developments in the treatment of brain and spinal cord trauma would help foster greater interest in neurotrauma, better understanding of the significant advances being made in care of the neurologically injured, and greater confidence in treating these patients appropriately and aggressively.

Political Action

In planning an organized political response to the concerns outlined in this chapter, the core issues must be identified, regional and community differences must be acknowledged, and isolated or anecdotal information avoided. Substantive conclusions must be based on evidence in order to reach reasonable recommendations that represent a consensus of neurosurgical opinion before any action is taken on behalf of organized neurosurgery. Unfortunately, much of the most basic information regarding the attitudes and concerns of neurosurgeons have not been systematically defined, so gathering this data becomes a priority. A survey of neurological surgeons across regions and demographic characteristics, at all trauma center levels, will allow us to gauge attitudes for, and obstacles to, participating in trauma care, determine what neurosurgical stipends or reimbursement mechanisms exist for neurotrauma, and estimate the degree to which neurosurgeons are taking part in the development of trauma systems. In short, it would help determine what is working and what is wrong with neurotrauma across the country and provide useful data to individual neurosurgeons as they seek to influence the direction of trauma care in their own communities.

The proposed survey would target neurosurgeons in a wide range of demographic circumstances, but particularly those who are likely to have some opportunity or inclination to include trauma in their practices. It could utilize the AANS neurosurgical data bank and its data gathering expertise, and would certainly require the support of the AANS and CNS.

At the national level, an effort for legislative reform should be advocated to end the de facto unfunded mandate for coverage that EMTALA imposes. Neurosurgeons should lobby for direct involvement in HCFA interpretation of EMTALA legislation along with the ACEP, ACS, and others with vested interest, and seek to maintain active communication and, when appropriate, concerted action with those interests. It is critical that neurosurgery participates in the administrative process that defines and interprets EMTALA legislation regarding hospital and emergency room capabilities and responsibilities in the context of organized trauma systems. EMTALA rules and regulations that prohibit appropriate transfer of patients within the context of a trauma system and to the ultimate benefit of the patient must be constructively challenged. In addition, since managed care plans represent a significant and increasing proportion of the insurance coverage for trauma patients, national guidelines need to be developed to guarantee the quality and continuity of trauma care for their patients. MCOs must assume a fair share of the expense of maintaining trauma systems from which they directly benefit. Legislative action at either the state or federal level could then be developed around these guidelines. Trauma system legislation, perhaps as part of further federal or state health-care initiatives, must be closely scrutinized and appropriate neurosurgical positions formulated.

At the state and county levels, neurosurgeons must be active in the development and refinement of trauma systems to avoid unnecessary duplication of services, avoid financial disincentives for hospitals or physicians, foster centers of expertise and improve quality and timeliness of care. They should work to develop mechanisms for the funding of trauma systems in general and neurotrauma specifically, including funds for neurosurgical care, research, education, and prevention.

Finally, at the local level, neurosurgeons should be encouraged to negotiate reasonable stipends for trauma call with hospitals or hospital networks. They should be provided with nationally based, demographically defined data to assist them in such negotiations. Although neurosurgeons accepting emergency cases bear a responsibility to see patients without respect to individual patient reimbursement, they should not be forced to participate under threat of EMTALA sanction or loss of staff privileges in a neurotrauma system in which they had no developmental or ongoing input.

If organized neurosurgery once again assumes the mantle of leadership in the treatment of neurotrauma, its commitment to excellence and education will undoubtedly equip it to address the criticisms and challenges of other specialists, the medical community, and neurotrauma patients. Most importantly, neurosurgery will continue to provide a quality of care to neurotrauma patients that would be unattainable if it were to abdicate its appropriate and necessary obligation, and allow the mantle of service to those in critical need of neurosurgical expertise to fall to those less qualified.

REFERENCES

1. "Special responsibilities of Medicare hospitals in emergency cases," Title 42 Code of Federal Regulations, Part 489, §489.24(a), 1996 ed.
2. "Basic Commitments," Title 42 Code of Federal Regulations, Part 489, §489.20, 1996 ed.
3. "Special responsibilities of Medicare hospitals in emergency cases," Title 42 Code of Federal Regulations, Part 489, §489.24(b), 1996 ed.
4. "Examination and treatment for emergency medical conditions and women in labor," Title 42 U.S. Code, §§1395dd(b), 1994 ed.
5. "Examination and treatment for emergency medical conditions and women in labor," Title 42 U.S. Code, §§1395dd(c)(2)(C), 1994 ed.
6. "Examination and treatment for emergency medical conditions and women in labor," Title 42 U.S. Code, §§1395dd(d), 1994 ed.
7. "Examination and treatment for emergency medical conditions and women in labor," Title 42 U.S. Code, §§1395dd(g), 1994 ed.
8. "Examination and treatment for emergency medical conditions and women in labor," Title 42 U.S. Code, §§1395dd, 1994 ed.
9. Abbate A. Report to Governor Pete Wilson on trauma hospital reimbursement in Southern California. Los Angeles: Hospital Council of Southern California, May 1992.
10. American College of Emergency Physicians: Guidelines for trauma care systems. Ann Emerg Med 1987;16:459.
11. American College of Surgeons Committee on Trauma: Resources for the optimally injured patient. Chicago: American College of Surgeons, 1990.
12. Andrews BT, Narayan RK. Have neurosurgeons abdicated their leadership role in the management of head injury? Surg Neurol 1993;40:1–2.
13. Aprahamian C, Wallace JR, Bergstein JM, et al. Characteristics of trauma centers and trauma surgeons. J Trauma 1993 Oct"(4):562–567.
14. Baker SP, Whitfield MA, O'Neill B. Geographic variation in mortality from motor vehicle crashes. N Engl J Med 1987;316:1384.
15. Brook RH, Kamberg CJ, McGlynn EA. Health System reform and quality. JAMA 1996;276:476–480.
16. Calcs KH. Trauma mortality in Orange County: The effect of implementation on a regional trauma system. Ann Emerg Med 1984;13:1.
17. Emergency Services, Discriminating liability of facility or health care personnel. California Health and Safety Code 90 §§1317 et seq. 1973, amended 1987.
18. Emergency Services, Discriminating liability of facility or health care personnel. California Health and Safety Code 90 §§1317.1(h), 1973, amended 1987.
19. Carson P. HCFA demonstration DOA. Health Care Observer 1997;2(6).
20. Champion HR, Mabee MS. An American crisis in trauma care reimbursement. Washington. DC: Washington Hospital Surgical Critical Care Services, 1990.
21. Champion HR, Teter H. Trauma care systems: The federal role. J Trauma 1988;18:877.
22. *Cleland v. Bronson Health Care Group Inc.* 917 F.2c (6th Cir. 1990).
23. Cooper RA. Perspectives on the physician workforce to the Year 2020. JAMA 1995;274:1534–1543.
24. *Delancy v. Cade et al.* 986 F.2d 387 (10 Cir. 1993).
25. Eastern Association for the Surgery of Trauma: Preliminary survey of US Trauma Centers and state-by state analysis of trauma system development. Reston, VA: Timothy Bell and Co, 1991.
26. Eastman AB. Blood in our streets: The status and evolution of trauma care systems. Arch Surg 1992;127:677.
27. Eastman AB. Resources for optimal care of the injured patient, 1993. ACS Bull. 1994;78:22.
28. Eastman AB, Lewis FR, Champion HR, et al. Regional trauma care systems design: Critical concepts. Am J Surg 1987;154:79.
29. Eastman AB, Rice CL, Bishop GS. An analysis of the critical problem of trauma center reimbursement. J Trauma 1991;31:920.
30. Emergency Transfer Laws. California Physician's Legal Handbook. Sacramento: California Medical Association, 1994.
31. Esposito TJ, Kuby AM, Unfred C, et al. Perception of differences between trauma care and other surgical emergencies: Results from a national survey of surgeons. J Trauma 1994;37(6):996–1002.
32. Evaluation of Hospital Emergency Room Specialty Services. OIG Report No. OEI-01-91-00771. Subject: Specialty Coverage in Hospital Emergency Departments, August, 1992.
33. Frew SA. Patient transfers: How to comply with the law. Dallas: American College of Emergency Physicians, 1991.
34. Girotti MJ, Leslie KA, Inman KJ, et al. Attitudes toward trauma care of surgeons practising in Ontario. Can J Surg 1995;38(1):22–26.

35. Guidelines for establishment of trauma centers. J Neurosurg 1986;65:569.
36. Harrington TR. Joint Council State Neurosurgical Societies 1995 Survey Report. Chicago: AANS/CNS,1995.
37. Harrington TR. Neurosurgical manpower needs—Achieving a balance. Surg Neurol 1997; 47(4): 316–320.
38. Harrington TR. Report of Manpower Committee to JCSNS. Chicago: AANS/CNS,1994.
39. Harrington TR, Zabramski JM. Position paper: Neurosurgical availability for emergency coverage in hospital or freestanding emergency room facilities. Chicago: JCSNS, 1997.
40. Health Security, Medicare program revisions. (PL103–432, 31 Oct 1994) 105 US Statutes at Large.
41. Hedges JR, Mullins RJ, Zimmer-Gembeck M, et al. Oregon trauma system: Change in initial admission site and post-admission transfer of injured patients. Acad Emerg Med 1994;1(3):218–226 .
42. Helling TS, Watkins M, Robb CV. Improvement in cost recovery at an urban level I trauma center. J Trauma 1995;39(5):980–983.
43. Hospital survey on obstetric claim frequency by patient payor category. Baltimore: American College of Obstetrics and Gynecology, February 1988.
44. Kusske JA. EMTALA Rules 1996. Washington Committee Report to JCSNS, October 1996.
45. Kusske JA. Neurotrauma care—Problems and solutions. In: Wilberger JE Jr, Polvishock JT, Narayan RK, eds. Neurotrauma. New York: McGraw-Hill (Health Professions Division); 1996.
46. Kusske JA, Shaver TE, O'Rourke B, et al. Neurotrauma care: Orange County California. Poster Presentation. American Association of Neurological Surgeons, Boston, April 25, 1993.
47. Levy JM. Personal communication, JCSNS, 1996.
48. Macpherson, P. Trauma Drama. American Medical News, 1997;40(7):14.
49. McNulty M. Are poor patients likely to sue for malpractice? JAMA 262:1391, 1989.
50. McVicker J. Joint Council State Neurosurgery Societies Interim Report. Ad Hoc Committee on Neurotrauma. Chicago: AANS/CNS, 1997.
51. Metropoulos DG. Son of Cobra: The evolution of a federal malpractice law. Stanford Law Rev 1992;45:263.
52. Meyer GS, Blumenthal D. TennCare and academic medical centers: The lessons from Tennessee. JAMA 1996;276(9):672–676.
53. Miller TR, Levy DT. The effect of regional trauma care systems on cost. Arch Surg 1995;130(2):188–193.
54. Miscall BG, Tompkins RK, Greenfield LJ. ACS survey explores retirement and the surgeon. Bull ACS 1996; 81:19–23.
55. Mitchell FL, Thal ER, Wolferth CC. American College of Surgeons Verification/Consultation Program: Analysis of Unsuccessful Verification Reviews. J Trauma 1994;37(4):557–564.
56. Mitchell FL, Thal ER, Wolferth CC. Analysis of American College of Surgeons Trauma Consultation Program. 1995;Arch Surg 130(6):578–584.
57. Mullins RJ, Veum-Stone J, Hedges JR, et al. Influence of a state-wide trauma system on location of hospitalization and outcome of injured patients. J Trauma 1996;40(4):536– 545.
58. Musman MG. Medical malpractice claims filed by Medicaid and Non-Medicaid recipients in Maryland. JAMA 1991;265:2992.
59. Narayan RK, Saul TG, Eisenberg HMI, et al. Neurotrauma Care. In: Resources for the Optimal Care of the Injured Patient. Chicago: American College of Surgeons Committee on Trauma, 1993;41–46.
60. Neurotrauma care and the neurosurgeon: A statement from The Joint Section on Trauma of the AANS and CNS. J Neurosurg 1987;67:783–785.
61. Oversight hearing on the financial problems of trauma centers in Los Angeles County. California Legislative Special Committee on Medi-Cal Oversight. Los Angeles, October 22, 1987.
62. Pevehouse BC. 1995 Comprehensive neurosurgical practice survey. Park Ridge IL: American Association Neurological Surgeons, 1996.
63. Popp AJ, Toselli R. Work force requirements for neurosurgery. Surg Neurol 1996;46:181–185 .
64. Preliminary Report on Neurotrauma Emergency Coverage. Joint Council State Neurosurgical Societies. Park Ridge, IL: American Association of Neurological Surgeons, 1996.
65. Salsberg ES, Wing P, Dionne MG, et al. Graduate medical education and physician supply: New York State. JAMA 1996;276(9):683–688.
66. Saywell RM, Cordell WH, Nyhuis AW, et al. The use of a break-even analysis: Financial analysis of a fast-track program. Acad Emerg Med 1995;2(8):671–672,739–45.
67. Seifer SD. Changes in marketplace demand for physicians. JAMA 1996;276(9):695– 699.
68. Shacksford SR, Hollingsworth-Fridlund P, Cooper GF, et al. The effect of regionalization upon quality of trauma care as assessed before and after the institution of a trauma system: A preliminary report. J Trauma 1986;26:812.
69. Somerson MD. States tout benefits of mandatory systems. Columbus Dispatch, 1997 Feb 2;5B.
70. Tanner L. Funding emergency: Task force deems $40 million trauma facility crucial to emergency-care plan. But who will pay? Dallas Business Journal 1993 Mar 26;16(30), Sect 1:1.
71. Tator C. Letter from the Chairman. Joint Council on Neurotrauma and Critical Care Newsletter 1997; Spring.
72. Turner J. Legislature 1997: Trauma bill advances, with new fuel. News Tribune 1997; Local/State: Apr 8: B1.
73. Tyson GW. Competition in neurosurgery. Part II. Surg Neurol 1996;46:599–601.
74. U.S. Dept. of Transportation, National Highway Traffic Safety Administration. Medical services program and its relationship to highway safety.Technical Report DOT HS 806832. Washington, DC: Office of Enforcement and Emergency Medical Services, 1985.
75. U.S. Dept. of Transportation, National Highway Traffic Safety Administration. Development of trauma systems: A state and community guide. Washington, DC: Office of Enforcement and Emergency Medicine, 1991.
76. U.S. Public Health Service. Model trauma care system plan, September 30, 1992. Rockville, MD: U.S. Department of Health and Human Services, United

States Public Health Service, Health Resources and Services Administration, 1992.

77. Vestrup JA, Phang PT, Vertesi L, et al. The utility of a multicenter regional trauma registry. J Trauma 37(3): 375–378,1994.

78. View of the Future. Los Angeles: Hospital Council of Southern California, 1992.

79. Waldrep DJ, Hiatt JR, Cohen M, et al. Future shock: Trauma in the managed care era. Am Surg 1994; 60(11):892–894.

80. West JG, Trunkey DO, Lim RC. Systems of trauma care: A study of two counties. Arch Surg 1979;114:455.

81. West JG, Williams MJ, Trunkey DO, et al. Trauma systems current status: Future challenges. JAMA 1988; 259:3597.

82. Wilberger J. Trauma care guidelines: Update 1996 neurotrauma. Chicago: American College Surgeons, 1996.

83. Wilkins RH. American Board of Neurological Surgery, Specialty Board Reports. Bull ACS 1996;81:48.

CHAPTER 18

Views of Neurosurgery Around The World: Why We Are Losing the Battle

JAMES I. AUSMAN, M.D., PH.D.

INTRODUCTION

In order for neurosurgeons to develop a strategy for dealing with the health-care changes in the future, it is helpful to understand the experience of others around the world. The purpose of this chapter is to review the experience of neurosurgeons in selected countries around the world, to develop a view of the world in the next 25 years, and to understand how this perspective impacts neurosurgery. It is important for us to know where neurosurgeons stand as a worldwide neurosurgery corporation and as neurosurgeon negotiators so that we can develop strategies not only in the United States, but in other areas of the world based on this background information.

WHAT IS HAPPENING IN NEUROSURGERY IN COUNTRIES AROUND THE WORLD? (1)

Solo Neurosurgical Practice—The Early Period

In the **Philippines**, there are 46 neurosurgeons for 60 million people, a ratio of 1 to a million. Thirty-six of the neurosurgeons are located in Manila leaving only 10 to serve the rest of the 55 million people in the Philippines outside the Manila metropolitan area. Parts of the country are without neurosurgery service whatsoever. The Filipino neurosurgeons are not well organized. The health-care system is governmentally financed, although there is some private insurance.

In **Peru** and **Venezuela,** most neurosurgeons are in solo practice. The national societies are not well organized. Each neurosurgeon is very individualistic, leaving neurosurgery without much concentrated power. In these three countries, the development of neurosurgery is similar to that in the United States or Japan in its early period.

The Early Growth Period of Neurosurgery—Too Much to Do for Too Few

In **China**, which has a growing economy, neurosurgery is more developed. There are 6000 neurosurgeons, either in practice or training. Three thousand are fully trained and 3000 are in residency. China has a population of 1.2 billion people. When all Chinese residents are fully trained, there will be 1 neurosurgeon for every 200,000 people. Neurosurgeons in China, particularly at the Beijing Neurosurgical Institute, do little spine surgery until the problems reach the level of the neck. Because Chinese neurosurgeons are so busy, orthopedists do virtually all of the spine surgery up to the cervical region. The neurosurgeons perform some of the interventional neuroradiological procedures, but this effort is in its early stage.

The major problem in China is the lack of sufficient neurosurgeons to serve the population. Because the neurosurgeons are overwhelmed with work, they allow other specialties to work in areas that neurosurgeons are fighting to regain or retain in other parts of the world. The economy in China is socialized, and there is government control of health care. Hospitals are on strict budgets. A Chinese hospital director indicated that doctors were looking for new equipment, but there was not enough money to support these requests. Eventually, the physicians were able to obtain the needed equipment, so that, presently, there are 800 MR scanners, 2000 to 3000 CT scanners and 14 gamma knives in China. The Chinese are developing their own version of the gamma knife at half the price of the competitor's product. The Chinese are very capable neurosurgeons and see large volumes of patients. Their expertise is in clinical neurosurgery, not in research, although some of their research is on the leading edge, particularly in genetics and brain tumors. In many respects, neurosurgery in China is similar to that in the United States in the 1950s and 1960s.

THE MIDDLE PERIOD—THE GOLDEN AGE OF NEUROSURGERY—FINANCIAL REWARD

In **Thailand,** there are 150 neurosurgeons serving 60 million people, for a ratio of 1 neurosurgeon for every 200,000 people. As the country's economy has boomed with a growth rate of between 8 to 10% per year, neurosurgical incomes have quadrupled. Neurosurgeons work in multiple hospitals and urge the acquisition of more advanced equipment by these hospitals. This scenario seems to mimic that of the growth of medicine in the United States in its ''golden age'' in the 1950s, 1960s and 1970s.

What will happen to Thailand as more and more resources are acquired and neurosurgeon incomes increase? Will health-care expenditures ultimately accelerate to a point where some restraint must be introduced? What will happen as more medical students aspire to neurosurgery and the specialty becomes overpopulated?

Recently, Thailand's economic growth rate fell because the country was financially overextended. There was too much construction and too little demand, and other countries have emerged as having more favorable business climates.

THE LATER PERIOD—TOO MANY NEUROSURGEONS

The results of an oversupply of neurosurgeons can be seen in **Spain** and **Italy** where there are too many neurosurgeons.

In **Russia**, as in other countries around the world, one of the common answers to the question to young neurosurgeons, What is the major problem you see for your future in neurosurgery? was Will I have a job? The facilities in Russia are behind those of Western countries.

In **Greece**, there are 160 neurosurgeons for a population of 10 million (2). This means there is approximately 1 neurosurgeon for every 50,000 people. According to prediction, the numbers of neurosurgeons will double, and, thus, the neurosurgeon to population ratio will decline to roughly 1 to 25,000 people. At the present time, each neurosurgeon performs only 21 neurosurgical procedures per year on average. When the neurosurgical program directors discussed the issue of oversupply on neurosurgeons in Greece, it was decided to limit the number of trainees. However, when the question became important enough to initiate this process, no one wished to reduce the number of neurosurgeons they were training. This scenario occurs in many countries around the world. Is this a strategy that is compatible with survival of neurosurgery? Does this position represent an unwillingness to view and accept the future?

In **South Korea**, there are 1000 neurosurgeons for a population of 40 million. This represents 1 neurosurgeon for every 40,000 people. Neurosurgery is practiced in academic centers or the major hospitals. Neurosurgeons in private practice are not able to do neurosurgical procedures. The neurosurgical professional society in Korea tried to limit the number of neurosurgeons being trained. However, one of the neurosurgeons contested this proposed restriction and won in the courts. Ultimately, the only hope South Korean neurosurgeons have is for their number to be reduced to equal about 1 per 100,000 population. At this point, there is little they can do to control the situation.

In **Argentina**, there are 280 certified neurosurgeons and 500 who are not certified and who have not had a quality training experience. For a population of 30 million, these 800 neurosurgeons produce a ratio of 1 neurosurgeon for every 37,500 people. Many of the neurosurgeons are in larger cities. The Argentinean neurosurgeons are very individualistic and independent, and they openly state that they are unable to work together. Thus, in the market place, insurance companies force neurosurgeons to compete against each other. Quality is of no concern, only price. If the price is not right, the insurance companies seek a cheaper alternative. Aneurysms are treated by interventional approaches and arteriovenous malformations by radiosurgery, as these approaches are believed to be cheaper alternatives. Yet, in Argentina, the anesthesiologists have united as a group and are even regarded as a "Mafia." By being united, the anesthesiologists were able to stop services and force the payers to acknowledge their position, thus preventing the reduction of payments to them. Because the neurosurgeons in Argentina are so disunited, and since there is an oversupply, there is little the neurosurgeons can do to correct their problem. Neurosurgeons in Argentina are perhaps in the worst political and socioeconomic situation of any developed country, outside Belgium and Russia.

THE LATE PERIOD—GOVERNMENT CONTROL

In **Belgium**, neurosurgeons face depressing circumstances. There is an excess of neurosurgeons. Belgian politicians would like to have even more neurosurgeons—to have a neurosurgeon at each hospital in each community. Thus, politicians gain political capital by demonstrating to the public that they are providing specialty health care in their constituents' locale. Because there are too many neurosurgeons, the number of procedures per neurosurgeon has declined, and the quality of health care has diminished. Neurosurgeons' incomes are falling, because they are powerless to reduce the number of trainees. The situation is one over which they exercise no influence or control, and the situation is extremely distressing to them. Is this what happens when the political system prevails?

As health-care costs spiral, the government intervenes. In **Canada** there is central governmental control of health care. In each province, health care represents 33% of the budget. The provinces are reducing their health-care expenditures by 10 to 15%. These budgetary cuts have resulted in layoffs of hospital employees and hospital closures. In the fall of 1996, physicians were being taxed if they billed more than a predetermined amount of money for the care of their patients. As their billing exceeded a specified level, the tax rate on the amount the doctors earned over the predetermined level rose to 75%. This disincentive to do additional work stimulated the orthopedists, gynecologists, and other

specialists to go on strike, refusing to provide any new medical consultations. The government immediately capitulated and came to the bargaining table.

In **France**, there are 260 neurosurgeons for 60 million people giving a ratio of 1 for every 200,000 people. The health-care system is strictly government controlled. All hospitals are given tight budgets to which they must adhere. As neurosurgeons and physicians are asked to do more, given the restricted budgets, this financial constraint produces tremendous financial pressures on the physicians and their disbursement of medical care. The only way to obtain new equipment is successfully to compete in the budget allocation process. Expensive equipment is unlikely to be purchased. Costly or advanced procedures are unlikely to be done, because they will not fit within the health-care budget. Generally, a high quality of health care traditionally has been dispensed in the French system; however, with these serious financial constraints, this quality is believed to be in jeopardy. The only additional ways to get money would be to raise the revenue from private resources. Is this the ultimate endpoint of government-controlled health care and budgeting?

In **England,** government health care exists for everyone. However, health care is dispensed without choice of physician. Patients must visit specified government hospitals and endure waiting lists, or "queues," for their illnesses to be diagnosed and treated. There is rising interest in private insurance that allows the patient freedom of choice among physicians and hospitals. Thirty-one percent of the public now has private insurance. A form of managed care has been introduced to the English health system. Is this the future for the United States and other countries as they rebound from government medicine?

THE ENTRENCHMENT OF LEADERS IN NEUROSURGERY—A WORLD-WIDE PROBLEM

In many neurosurgical societies around the world, there are older leaders of neurosurgery who have been entrenched for years and who are out of touch younger neurosurgeons' needs and desires. This generation gap only serves to cripple neurosurgery and prevent it from planning for the future. Are we repeating this history in the United States?

SOLUTIONS FOR THE PRESENT AND FUTURE—EXAMPLES FROM TWO COUNTRIES

Two countries should be recognized for of their ability to deal with health-care problems and provide solutions that may be of value to others.

Japan has 4000 neurosurgeons for 125 million people, for a ratio of 1 neurosurgeon for every 30,000 people. The fact that there are the same numbers of neurosurgeons in Japan as in the United States serving half the population means that neurosurgeons in Japan inevitably will operate on fewer cases. For this reason, Japanese neurosurgeons publish numerous case reports, since they are not able to accumulate large individual series of cases. Because their experience is more limited in neurosurgery, anatomy courses have been rising in popularity as a way for neurosurgeons to learn more surgical anatomy. Although some neurosurgeons believe there are too many neurosurgeons in Japan, others believe that this is not an issue.

For many years Japanese neurosurgeons have been dominant in the clinical neuroscience field. Almost 80% of cerebral angiography is performed by the neurosurgeons and in 50 of the 80 academic centers, neurosurgeons are doing the interventional work. Neurosurgeons are also involved in physical medicine and other specialty areas. Since the Japanese do not have as many procedures to perform as neurosurgeons in the United States, the doctors have more time for research. The research in neurosurgery in Japan is superb and highly competitive with that in the United States and other advanced countries.. It is possible that, in some areas, the Japanese have eclipsed other nations in neurosurgical research. Thus, in Japan, the neurosurgeons have dominance in all fields dealing with the nervous system, and they continue to exercise it. They are incorporating new advances, such as the endovascular approaches to aneurysms, under the umbrella of neurosurgery.

In **Brazil**, as recently as 5 or 6 years ago, neurosurgery was organizationally in a shambles (3). Through the efforts of a number of prominent neurosurgeons, who are also leaders in Brazilian society, neurosurgery has become united

and strong over the past 4 to 5 years. One physician, Carlos De Sousa, spent 6 months or more traveling around the country, speaking with neurosurgeons, their local societies, and local groups to assess the concerns of neurosurgeons and to develop a unified point of view. Brazilian neurosurgeons had their first national meeting in Belo Horizonte in 1995, a meeting that generated large sums of money for the new organization. This collective funding allowed the central neurosurgical organization to flourish and to begin to invest in resident training standards and projects of common interest to all neurosurgeons. In a 4-year period, the neurosurgical society has developed a computer network that tracks the performance of every neurosurgical resident in the country. Exams are held once every year, and training standards are being adopted nationally by all neurosurgeons.

Because of Brazilian neurosurgery's successful efforts at unifying, the neurosurgical leaders recently approached the government with an offer to reduce the length of stay of patients undergoing neurosurgical procedures. In exchange for this pledge, the government agreed to raise reimbursement for neurosurgeons, which had been a fifth of that paid to cardiac surgeons. As a next step, the Brazilian neurosurgical society is asking manufacturers of shunts to offer large volume purchase prices so that this equipment may be purchased at a reduced rate for all the neurosurgeons in Brazil. *Thus, the neurosurgeons in Brazil have shown that by unifying, they can develop power and then can deal with other large organizations to their benefit and to the benefit of their patients.*

THE SIGNIFICANCE OF THIS HISTORY TO NEUROSURGERY TODAY AND TOMORROW

What is the importance of these experiences in other countries to neurosurgery in the United States? From the above discussion, one can see that there is a transition from the solo practitioner stage in countries like Peru and Venezuela and the Philippines to a more organized state as seen in China, where, (as was true in the United States in the mid-20th century) with insufficient neurosurgeons to meet demand, neurosurgeons are giving away neuroradiology, some spine surgery, peripheral nerve surgery, and cerebrovascular work to other specialties as the Chinese have already done. The transition occurring now in China, and which occurred in neurosurgery in the United States 15 to 30 years ago, will lead to similar problems as the neurosurgical numbers increase, as they have in Italy, Spain and Greece, where neurosurgeons find themselves with few procedures to do individually.

Thailand reflects the next stage of the evolution in American medicine, with growth in the economy and in the incomes of neurosurgeons associated with large expenditures for equipment and hospitals undertaken to satisfy the needs of a growing population. Ultimately this growth in Thailand will lead to a problem with costs, costs that the government will eventually be unable to pay for because it is unable to sustain a high economic growth rate. There will be an oversupply of both equipment and hospitals for which, in an increasingly competitive environment, industry will not be able to pay. Such a scenario is occurring in the United States today. Where governments are involved in the distribution of health care, as in England, France, and Canada, accelerating health-care costs are brought under control by government intervention. With this central control come government restrictions in payments to hospitals, closures of hospitals (as in Canada), and limitations on the neurosurgeon's income. This perhaps is the next step toward which the United States is headed.

IS THERE A SOLUTION?

Should steps not be taken to prevent governmental control and the socialization of medicine from occurring? Neurosurgeons must be alert to this possibility and undertake steps to stem the spiral of costs, which they can control by developing unified positions. Ultimately, the situation can lead to despair, as evidenced in Belgium and Korea, where the excess number of neurosurgeons is promoted by government policy and is associated with a diminishing quality of health care and income.

One lesson learned from the Brazilian and Canadian neurosurgeons and the Argentinean anesthesiologists is that there is power in numbers. *Neurosurgeons need to unite around common interests to create a powerful organization representing the interests of significant numbers of neurosurgeons. The greater the number of neurosurgeons represented, the better the negotiating position. Only by developing the power of numbers will neurosurgeons have a chance of effecting change in any country in the world.* Without power, as in Argentina, Greece, Canada, Belgium, and many other countries, the political interests of neurosurgeons will be lost.

Another solution is to allow the individual citizen different options in obtaining health insurance. For example, under a plan termed Medical Savings Accounts in the United States. each person would be able to purchase the health insurance that would be personally affordable and desirable. This money could be provided as it is now by employers, but would be at the sole disposal of the employee to use as desired. Money left over in such employee health-care accounts provided by the employer could be taken as income by the employee or could be saved for future health-care costs. While this system might not cover all people, particularly in the developing countries, it is certainly worth consideration. It has been shown to reduce health-care expenditures in companies where it has been used. A second variation on this system is to allow the public to buy a high-deductible insurance policy with money set aside for benefits at their place of employment and then to permit the public to use additional money of their own to purchase the health-care policy with the options desired. The company would offer a series of benefit options, but totaling only a fixed amount that the company could afford to spend. The employee could choose the benefits desired from these options, which would total the amount allowed by the company. An employee could choose, perhaps, to spend all the benefit money on health insurance and not take a holiday option. Such a solution would solve several problems, relieving the company of the criticism of limiting the health-care options of the employee, making the individual responsible for his/her own health, and promoting a free market system for health-care services, which would allow fair competition for the health-care customer.

THE WORLD IN 2025 (4, 5)
Population Growth

In the next 28 years, significant changes will occur in the world, which will affect health care and neurosurgery. The population of the world will double from its present size (4.5 to 5 billion) to between 8 and 11 billion people. This growth will occur primarily in the developing parts of the world in Asia, Africa, and Latin America. The population in China and India will be controlled and will be a little over 1 billion each, while those in Europe and North America will grow at a much slower rate. This Third World population growth means that within the next 25 years there will be an explosion of young people and a tremendous worldwide need for pediatric neurosurgeons.

Urbanization of the Population

Most people (over 50%) in 2025 will live in cities. At present, in countries all over the world, cities are becoming the center of industrialized economies and are attracting people from agrarian communities searching for higher paying jobs and more income. However, many rural migrants have found only unemployment in the cities, and, thus, live in abject poverty, placing tremendous pressure on the social, economic, and environmental services of each community.

Social Effect of Population Growth

These social, economic, and environmental pressures in urban centers will become even larger problems in the future. When the Minister of Health in Peru, who is a cardiac surgeon, was asked what he would do if the World Bank gave him 1 billion dollars to be used only on health care, his response was that he would use it for the improvement of sanitation. In many countries, as in Peru, neurosurgery is regarded as a luxury. When asked what neurosurgery could do to help him with the problem of health care, Peru's Health Minister was surprised and shocked at the question, thinking that there was little neurosurgeons could contribute to solve the immense health problems of his country. When the suggestion was made that neurosurgeons could save the government millions of dollars in health-care costs by educating the community about prevention of head and spinal cord trauma, he was extremely interested in this prospect. *Thus, neurosurgery, as it looks at the changing economy in the community, can offer to develop community health education programs on important medical conditions, such as trauma, stroke, and nervous system infections, which could save millions of dollars for the country. Perhaps, then, organized neurosurgery would be in a position to ask for some of these saved resources.*

Political Effect of New Generations

As the young become more and more prominent in political affairs, intergovernmental relationships will be conducted by people who have no remembrance of World War II, the Korean War, or even the Viet Nam War. Thus, they will feel no obligation or debt to the United States or any other country that helped them during those periods. Each country will come to the table on an equal basis and bargain to their best advantage.

In addition, the developed world will have an increasingly older society, which will consume resources generated by the young and rely on tax support financed by the young. The aged will become a greater economic burden on younger generations, creating more resistance to supporting older citizens as a result. What will happen in this conflict between the older and the younger generation is yet to be determined.

IMPACT ON MEDICINE AND NEUROSURGERY OF THESE SOCIAL CHANGES IN THE NEXT QUARTER CENTURY

What will be the impact of all these changes in the next quarter century on medicine and neurosurgery? With the growth of populations around the world and the desire to serve the needs of these populations, corporations are becoming international in scope and are developing and manufacturing in parts of the world where the costs of labor can be reduced. While some economists in the United States believe that a low economic growth rate will contain inflation, others believe that a high growth rate is necessary to generate the revenues necessary to pay for social programs. Competition will lower the costs of goods and services. In order for corporations to remain successful, they must compete in larger markets. This means that as corporations compete for a larger share of the world market, they will be committed to containing their health-care costs as a part of their corporate expenses. *There will be no place for uncontrolled, spiraling health-care costs in the corporate budget. These unlimited and passively absorbed heath care costs were part of the policy of the past. This corporate change does not necessarily mean that the business community is not interested in quality, but at the present time, concern for cost is predominates over concern for quality. Neurosurgeons need to understand this concept as the business world is evolving.* This limited budgetary allowance for health care will be a matter of course in corporations and a fact of life in society. Gone are the days of uncontrolled health-care charges.

The significance of all these changes in the world in the next 28 years is that as the population of the world doubles and a large proportion of this population growth is in the pediatric age group, there will be a growing need for pediatric neurosurgeons. *The United States can help by allowing neurosurgeons to train in fellowships in pediatric neurosurgery in the United States and by supporting the pediatric neurosurgeons who have developed worldwide education courses and programs to meet this future demand.* The growth of cities will put pressure on the social and economic resources of communities and governments that have restricted financial budgets. In a world economy, local governments will be reluctant to raise taxes because of a concern about losing local businesses and industries to other competing areas. *Thus, neurosurgeons must cooperate to find ways to reduce expenses to the community.* This would be particularly relevant in public health programs for the prevention of head and spinal cord injury and stroke, two of the leading causes of death and disability in the United States.

The major significance of these changes in the world in the next 28 years will be the globalization of national economies and of industries. Industries will no longer be able to feel safe competing within their national borders; instead they will have competition from companies in countries all over the world. Labor costs for the production of goods will be lower in the developing world and corporations will seek to have their goods manufactured in those in overseas labor markets. *In an effort to compete worldwide, companies will want to control their health-care costs, which means that—unless there is an excess of money from high growth economies, as in Thailand—medicine will have to find ways to provide quality health care under controlled costs. This pressure to economize in health care will be inevitable as the globalization of the world economy occurs.*

THE WORLDWIDE NEUROSURGERY CORPORATION AND ITS STATUS (6)

Assume that you have been appointed president of an international corporation, which is the Neurosurgery Corporation. This corporation has a sales force of 23,000 worldwide, many of whom are located in the same city, selling the same products, to the same customers. In effect, they are competing with each other. In addition, other corporations have now entered these same markets and are selling similar products but have a better marketing strategy. As president of the corporation, what would you do to rescue a business that is losing revenue to its competition? There are three choices. One is to reduce the number of sales people, which is exactly what your competition would like, since they will then enlarge their markets into your areas. The second is to develop special training courses so that your sales people can become specialized in various areas of neurosurgery, and, thus, compete effectively in the marketplace. Because the knowledge base is expanding, these neurosurgeons would be specialists, devoting their time to a limited area, which would allow them to encompass all the relevant literature well. The third alternative is to unite with some of your competitors to form a combined group. This third alternative would reduce the time necessary to develop these specialty interests and, looking to the future, might be the most economical solution. Obviously, the latter two choices are preferable to the first.

A LOOK AT NEUROSURGEONS AND THE WORLD THEY LIVE IN
The Neurosurgical Personality

Neurosurgeons, like neurologists, cardiologists, and internists, have specific personality traits. These traits may influence how neurosurgeons, as a group, deal with changes in the health-care market.

The neurosurgeon is a product of a school environment that rewards the student for excellent performance and for achieving high grades in classes. To accomplish these goals, the neurosurgeon must be organized, thoughtful, and willing to sacrifice some immediate personal desires for a distant planned goal or goals. This success requires an obsessive-compulsive nature. The neurosurgeon has self-confidence, intelligence, and self-dependence. In the operating room, a neurosurgeon learns to give orders and to be authoritarian. This type of person does not easily to listen to another's advice. Yet a neurosurgeon by training is not a "risk taker." Patients do not come to neurosurgeons to take risks with their lives. A neurosurgeon learns by training that there is little room for error. The results of a neurosurgeon's work are immediately apparent in the patient's neurological function. This is not true of other specialties, except perhaps plastic surgeons or ophthalmologists.

The Neurosurgical Personality Versus the New World Order

The neurosurgeon is now thrust into a new world and faced with business people who are encouraged and rewarded for taking risks. These are the business people who run insurance companies and the businesses that are behind the cost containment policies of health care; people who specialize in business organization, finance, contract negotiation, and marketing.

The neurosurgeon brings to this confrontation an obsessive compulsive temperament, an authoritarian nature not used to compromise, and a risk-averse personality coupled with a fierce individuality, which is based on self dependence. How will the neurosurgeon survive in this new world of business and finance? Will some changes in behavior be necessary for the neurosurgeon in order to succeed in this modern business-driven world of health care? The answer is unequivocally, YES!

In today's market, in which there is a corporatism of virtually every enterprise, business people are required to surrender their individuality to work for group goals and take risks in competition—personality traits that are the antithesis of what neurosurgeons embody. *Thus, neurosurgeons are ill prepared by virtue of their profession, training, and personality to deal with the demands of the marketplace, which require a different personality structure.*

THE HEALTH-CARE INDUSTRY AS AN OPPORTUNITY

The Trillion Dollar Opportunity

In the United States, the health-care business consumes one trillion dollars annually. This is more money than has ever been spent on health care in the history of our country. The real challenge confronting neurosurgeons and physicians is, Can they compete in a creative and innovative way to demand a share of that very large health-care marketplace, or will they surrender this opportunity to others? Presently, this opportunity

is being surrendered to others who are winning the competition for this financial bonanza.

The Changing Method of Delivering Health Care: A Specialists' Opportunity

Leo Henikoff, M.D., the CEO of the Rush Medical Systems in Chicago, has thoughtfully analyzed the direction of health care in the United States. He contends that the public is interested in costs, freedom of choice, process, quality, and customer satisfaction with service and outcome. The public wants the security of knowing that their health insurance will continue and that they will have access to health care. According to Dr. Henikoff's analysis, comparing fee for service, managed care, and the Canadian system using these parameters, both fee for service and the Canadian system are preferable to managed care in the public's view. He feels further that the reason the fee-for-service system would succeed over the Canadian system is that the Americans do not want government-controlled health care or that they would not find a Canadian-style socialized medicine acceptable. Thus, he asks, is there another form of health care which will emerge in the future? The answer most probably is, Yes.

There is evidence in the United States that the gatekeeper approach to medicine utilized in managed care plans is highly inefficient, with the costs of the management of disease by a primary care physician being three times that of a specialist. *Insurance companies are becoming more convinced that Americans are interested in specialists and specialty care and, for that reason, the insurance industry will capitate specialists and allow the patients to go to them directly.* This change would favor the emergence of specialty networks. Perhaps these specialty networks are the alternative health-care system that would fit into Dr. Henikoff's equation. The problem at the present time is that insurers, doctors, and hospitals are locked in a pitched battle to prevent each other from gaining ascendancy in the health-care market. In some markets, this battle has already been fought and won—usually by nonphysicians. Yet, in other areas, the battle is still raging, and the outcome is yet in doubt.

WHY WE NEED TO PROVIDE VALUE
Economic Realities in Each Country

In economies around the world, the challenge to medicine and to neurosurgeons is to provide the best quality health care at the lowest possible cost. Although at this time corporate America and the corporate world are interested primarily in the lowest cost for health services and interested very little in their quality, inferior quality will not be accepted by the customer. Neurosurgeons and physicians should not abandon the quest for quality, because the public will not, in the long term, accept mediocrity.

In the present and in the future, there is not an unlimited amount of money for health-care spending. *The economies in each country have limitations. Thus, medicine and neurosurgery must work within that economic reality.* In the booming economies of countries in Asia, however, a golden age of medicine, as seen three decades ago in America, is a phase which some are experiencing now. How long they will be able to sustain this spectacular growth in health-care expenditures into the future is uncertain, but they likely will reach the same point experienced by other economically successful countries around the world. Planning must be done in order to manage this eventuality. For example, in Thailand, as neurosurgeons' incomes have quadrupled in an economy that is growing at 8 to 10% annually, more equipment is being purchased, hospitals are being built, and operating funds are being allocated to health care. This increasing spiral of expenditures can only be sustained by continuously expanding economies, a situation that has not occurred in other countries around the world.

So, the challenge for neurosurgeons is to learn to provide quality health care at the lowest price and to accommodate to inevitable resource limitation.

Growth in Knowledge as a Basis for Superspecialization

There will be continued exponential growth in knowledge. At the present time, it is difficult for any neurosurgeon to be an expert in all areas of neurosurgery. In fact, this is an impossibility. *As knowledge and research expand in each unique area, this information explosion will require that individuals become specialized in these areas of study and research. It is inevitable that specialization and superspecialization will occur. Not only can this specialization provide better knowledge and higher quality health care, but it can provide better service and probably lower cost.*

Centralization of Resources

It will become mandatory that, in a limited economy, continued steep growth in expenditures for health-care resources will not be possible, and these expenditures will have to be allocated in a business-like manner. This allocation will require a centralization of resources and equipment, which would be utilized by all of the physicians or neurosurgeons in a community.

The Inevitable Change in the Practice of Neurosurgery

Neurosurgeons are provincial about their specialty. Many believe, in countries around the world, that neurosurgery will be the same in 25 years as it is now. But the following is an example of a likely change. Interventional radiology and the use of coils for the treatment of intracranial aneurysms has been introduced as treatment. It is the opinion of this author, speaking as a vascular neurosurgeon, that, in properly selected cases, this approach will be valuable in the treatment of selected aneurysms. Yet, neurosurgeons around the world are reluctant to accept this change. Already, patients have been treated successfully without a craniotomy and discharged from the hospital after a brief stay at a lower cost. Ultimately, it can be expected that decisions about selection of care will be made not by physicians, but by health-care executives, who will examine the cost for standard neurosurgery versus that of endovascular surgery. The selection will be made based on equivalent outcomes for the lower cost procedure.

Gerard Debrun (an interventional neuroradiologist) estimates, as I do, that at least 50% of the aneurysms will be treated by coils in the future; others believe the figure will be 80%. Are neurosurgeons prepared to change their approach in aneurysm surgery or are they in a period of denial, criticizing the technique and assuming that this new approach will not prevail? I believe not only that the technique will prevail, but that newer modifications in the technique will advance the approach even further technologically. Is neurosurgery prepared for this change? The choices are to abandon vascular surgery, to teach neurosurgeons to become interventional or endovascular surgeons, or to incorporate interventional radiologists in neurosurgical practice. The first choice is unacceptable and will lead to ultimate failure in neurosurgery. The other two choices are the most viable for practice success and providing value in a changing health-care market.

THE CORPORATE EQUATION—RETURN ON INVESTMENT

In corporate terms, investors are interested in a return on their investment. Profitability can only occur when revenues exceed expenses. An example can be taken from automobile manufacture. In the 1980s in Detroit, as the automobile manufacturers began losing revenue because their products were not competitive, their response was to cut expenses by reducing the number of employees and factories. They regained profitability, but their share of the automobile market plunged from 52% to 35%. This result cannot be viewed as success, because the companies ultimately lost 40% of their market share, even though the return on investment for each shareholder increased (6, 7).

In the last decade, a prominent, worldwide corporate strategy to increase return on investment has been to cut expenses. This reduction has been done by restructuring and reengineering, two catch words that amount to cutting the workforce and trying to provide more customer-friendly services. These changes alone are not enough to propel a corporation into the future. *To increase revenues, one must generate new ideas that will generate new business* (7). In neurosurgery terms, one may ask how many neurosurgeons are interested in pain medicine as a means of generating new revenue sources? In the United States, this is not a specialty area commonly practiced by neurosurgeons. However, in Turkey, this is not only a successful area of neurosurgery but one that is very popular among young trainees and residents because of the leadership of Dr. Yucel Kanpolat. How many neurosurgeons are interested in radiosurgery, peripheral nerve, vascular surgery, or the management of stroke? There are five times more intracranial metastases than there are primary brain tumors. How many neurosurgeons are interested in this area? How many are interested in stereotactic and functional neurosurgery? These are areas for new business and the generation of growth in neurosurgery rather than the generalist neurosurgical position, which has been adopted by neurosurgeons in countries around the world. This position will not be competitive in a future

with the tremendous explosion of knowledge and the need for specialization (6).

"DONE BEATS PERFECT"

Recently a health-care consultant mentioned the principle that, in corporate America, "done beats perfect." This principle is the antithesis of that by which neurosurgeons have been trained, because, for neurosurgeons, "perfect beats done." This dilemma illustrates the major conflict between the neurosurgical mentality and the business mentality of the world in which they are being forced to compete. The neurosurgeon who fails to understand the mentality of "done beats perfect" will fail to survive in competition in that marketplace.

SOME IDEAS TO WIN IN THE MARKET PLACE AND FOR THE FUTURE OF NEUROSURGERY

Group Practice

Given the increasing corporatism of health care, the only choice available to medicine is to abandon the "mom and pop store" of the solo practice, in which 50% of the neurosurgeons are involved in the United States and even a larger percentage in other countries around the world, and to merge to form larger groups with more bargaining power (5). This means neurosurgeons must subordinate their very individualistic, independent, and ego centered tendencies and instead work in groups for the opportunity of a greater reward—rather than pursuing a solo strategy, which is bound to die in a globalized economy. Efficiencies and value, as discussed, will be the key, and these can be provided better in groups than they can be in solo practices. Thus, larger group practices of neurosurgeons or neuroscientists will need to emerge to provide service to the community.

Superspecialization

Because of the explosion in knowledge, superspecialization is inevitable. The neurosurgical societies in North America and around the world will have to accommodate to the fact that superspecialization is inevitable and must be accepted and supported if fragmentation of the specialty is to be prevented and which will certainly occur if this approach is denied (6). One of my associates is interested in critical care; unless neurosurgery offers this opportunity to him, he will be forced to obtain certification from another specialty. Neurosurgery does not need this attrition in its membership. Such a near-sighted approach only strengthens the position of other specialties. Pediatric neurosurgery has done an incredibly successful job of uniting and providing educational courses around the world. Organized pediatric neurosurgery has been severely criticized by organized neurosurgery for establishing their own independent pediatric neurosurgical board and training program accreditation in pursuit of superspecialization. This superspecialized approach, as demonstrated by the pediatric neurosurgeons, is inevitable.

As a member of the board of directors of a corporation, I and others recently sought help from a law firm in Washington to deal with the Food and Drug Administration (FDA). We went to a firm with 425 lawyers. In that firm, 25 lawyers specialized only in FDA litigation and of those 25 lawyers, each had further superspecialized. One lawyer also had a Ph.D. in biochemistry, one a Ph.D. in statistics, another in engineering, and so forth. With this level of superspecialization, our success in dealing with the FDA was clearly enhanced, because of the highly focused, specialized knowledge these individuals possessed. We discharged a firm we had previously hired, because they did not have the superspecialized skills and could not deal as effectively with the FDA as the new firm. The superspecialization of the second firm made it easier for us to accomplish our goals. *Thus, as in other professional areas, neurosurgery needs to understand that superspecialization is the wave of the future.* (Note: The reason the word superspecialization is chosen over subspecialization is that it impacts on how one markets one's abilities. The perception of a subspecialist is less positive than that of a superspecialist. Thus, neurosurgery also must understand how to market its products.)

Academic—Private Practice Linkages

It is essential that academia and practicing neurosurgeons work in concert. Although there is a prevalent belief that all training can be done in academic centers, this approach is neither practical nor sustainable in the future, as more and more general neurosurgical procedures are done in the community by excellently trained former residents. Academic centers will progressively become repositories for patients requiring complex care. Under these circumstances, it is imperative that residents rotate in the community with nonacademic neurosurgeons to gain experience with general neurosurgical cases in addition to those cases attracted to academia.

Academia must understand that it needs to provide help to neurosurgeons in the community by finding solutions to problems, rather than producing a "town-gown" confrontation. This confrontation provides no value to the customer and is an ineffective long-term strategy for success. Many academic centers believe that after the residents are trained they will go into the community and just take care of patients with head injury and send the rest of their patients to the academic center. This is neither a realistic or cost-effective view, nor does it acknowledge the high level of training being given in academic centers to residents who eventually practice in the community.

Consortia of Neurosurgeons

In Chicago, a consortium of neurosurgeons is being developed, linking academic neurosurgeons with practicing neurosurgeons in multiple communities and different states. This amalgamation is being done to provide a product for the marketplace, integrating neurosurgeons from a wide geographic area and all levels of complexity of care. It is called Midwest Neurocare. It is a consortium of over 40 neurosurgeons and interventional neuroradiologists, mostly from the practice community. Two academic centers are included. The group provides quality neurosurgical services from a wide geographical base, while covering neurosurgical problems from simple to complex with experienced neurosurgeons providing the services. Perhaps this type of arrangement also can be utilized to include neurologists, other neuroscientists, and physical therapists.

Specialty consortiums are also being developed in orthopedics, oncology, cardiology and eventually will come to the neurosciences. These can be disease oriented, such as treating back pain, stroke, dizziness and a variety of other problems in a multi-disciplinary fashion.

Power

As stated previously, neurosurgeons will only be able to achieve their goals for their patients and themselves by having the power to be heard. A solo neurosurgical voice is inaudible. It represents nothing of importance to the players in the health-care market, who represent large power bases. To be an effective bargainer at the table, neurosurgeons must have a negotiator who represents a large number of neurosurgeons, preferably all neurosurgeons. Thus united, neurosurgery would speak with a single voice and negotiate (or refuse to negotiate, which itself is power) from a position of power. Who else can provide what neurosurgery can do? No one.

A business friend has said that he does not understand how doctors have allowed themselves to be reduced to the defenseless position they are in, allowing anyone to dictate term to them. He stated that there is no one else who can produce the product that doctors do. Thus, at any moment, doctors can shut down the health-care system, and there is no alternative. This is power, but physicians and neurosurgeons by personality, temperament, and lack of political training are unwilling to use it. Yet, the world is a huge arena, and there is power in numbers in the arena.

Politics

The political reality of "you do something for me and I'll do something for you," must be understood by neurosurgeons. Neurosurgeons can no longer simply ask to have resources allocated to them in a world in which resource allocation is becoming severely compromised. In order to achieve this goal, they must be able to show that they can reduce the costs of health care in other areas, so that the health-care planners will be willing to devote resources to neurosurgery.

CONCLUSION

As neurosurgeons look at the world of the future, many changes will have occurred in population size and growth of cities by the year 2025; these changes will produce social changes which, in turn, will have an impact on the practice of neurosurgery in countries around the world. In order to compete in this new world, neurosurgeons will have to recognize the limitations their training has structured into their personalities, limiting their ability to deal with these changes and business structures. They will have to understand the economic realities of an expanding population with limited resources and find ways to meet the challenges the new world offers. Group practice, superspecialization, centralization of resources, and integration of physicians in the community to provide quality health care widely available to the public will be strategies certain to succeed in the new world. Will neurosurgeons be able to make these changes? I believe that they will.

REFERENCES

1. Ausman JI. What is happening in neurosurgery around the world. Surg Neurol 1997;47:205–208.
2. Stranjalis G. The overproduction of neurosurgeons jeopardizes future neurosurgical care. Surg Neurol 1996; 45:304–319.
3. Ausman, JI. Neurosurgery notes. Surg Neruol 1995; 44:91.
4. Kennedy P. Preparing for the twenty-first century. New York: Random House, 1993.
5. Ausman JI. The future of neurosurgery: A perspective on the next 30 years. Surg Neurol 1995;43:408–412.
6. Ausman JI. A strategy for your future. Surg Neurol 1996; 46:304–307.
7. Hamel G, Prahalad CK. Competing for the future. Boston: Harvard Business School Press, 1994.

Index